Manual of
PRACTICAL MICROBIOLOGY
and
PARASITOLOGY

Manual of PRACTICAL MICROBIOLOGY *and* PARASITOLOGY

P Chakraborty MD (Path & Bact)

Ex-Prof. and Head, Dept of Microbiology
Medical College, Kolkata, India
Author of
Textbook of Microbiology, Textbook of Medical Parasitology
Practical Pathology

Nishith Kumar Pal MD (Microbiology), DCP

Prof. and Head, Dept of Microbiology
Institute of Postgraduate Medical Education and Research (IPGME&R)
Kolkata, India

New Central Book Agency (P) Ltd

LONDON
HYDERABAD ERNAKULAM BHUBANESWAR
NEW DELHI KOLKATA PUNE GUWAHATI

NCBA

OVERSEAS

NCBA (UK) Ltd, 149 Park Avenue North, Northampton, NN3 2HY, UK
email: ncbauk@yahoo.com

REGD OFFICE

8/1 Chintamoni Das Lane, Kolkata 700 009, India
email: ncbapvtltd@eth.net

EXPORT

NCBA Exports Pvt. Ltd, 212 Shahpur Jat, New Delhi 110 049
email: ncbaexports@ncbapvtltd.com

BRANCHES

212 Shahpur Jat
New Delhi 110 049
email: ncbadel@ncbapvtltd.com

House No. 3-1-315, 1st Floor
Nimboliadda, Kachiguda, **Hyderabad** 500 027
email: ncbahydb@ncbapvtltd.com

Shop Nos. 3 & 4, Vinayak Towers
681/B Budhwar Peth, Appa Balwant Chowk
Pune 411 002
email: ncbapune@ncbapvtltd.com

GSS Shopping Complex, 1st Floor
Opposite College Post Office, Convent Road
Ernakulam 682 035
0484-4021054/53

Shop No. 15, Bharati Towers, Ground Floor
Forest Park, **Bhubaneswar** 751 001
email: ncbabub@ncbapvtltd.com

Radhamayee Complex (Second Floor)
Opp. SBI, Panbazar, Jaswanta Road
Guwahati 781 001
email: ncbaguwahati@ncbapvtltd.com

MANUAL OF PRACTICAL MICROBIOLOGY AND PARASITOLOGY • P Chakraborty, Nishith Kumar Pal

First Published: January 2008
Reprinted: July 2008
Thoroughly Revised and Updated Second Edition: 2011
Reprinted: 2012, 2014, 2018

7283_19318

PUBLISHER AND TYPESETTER
New Central Book Agency (P) Ltd
8/1 Chintamoni Das Lane, Kolkata 700 009

PRINTER
New Central Book Agency (P) Ltd
Web-Offset Division, Dhulagarh, Sankrail, Howrah

COVER DESIGNER
Soumen Paul

TECHNICAL EDITOR
Dr Mita Sen, MBBS

PROJECT COORDINATOR
Nochiel Radhakrishnan

PROJECT TEAM
Dr Atreyee Chakraborty, Dr Tamal Das

ISBN 978 81 7381 926 1

Price ₹ 350.00

यः स्वधर्मेण मां नित्यं निराशीः श्रद्धयान्वितः।
भजते शनकैस्तस्य मनो राजन् प्रसीदति ॥ ९ ॥

yah svadharmena mam nityam
nirashi shraddhayanvitah
bhajate shanakaistasya
mano rajan prasidati

The Supreme Personality of Godhead, Lord Vishnu, continued : My dear King Prthu, when one situated in his occupational duty engages in My loving service without motive for material gain, he gradually becomes very satisfied within.

Shrimad Bhagavatam, Part IV, Ch. 20, Shloka 9

Dedicated

to the most pleasant memories of

Dr. Maitrayee Chakraborty, MBBS, DNB (I), WBHS

daughter of senior author

and student of

both senior and junior authors.

She served the ailing patients

till the last moment of her life

Preface to the second edition

The authors are overwhelmed by the response to the first edition of this book from the students of Microbiology of MBBS, DMLT, and B.Sc (Microbiology) courses. Communications were received from many students and teachers suggesting improvement of the publication. Keeping in mind their suggestions and criticisms many changes have been incorporated in most of the chapters.

The sole objective of the first edition was to present the students a handbook for their preparation of practical class and examination. The format of the first edition has been preserved in the second edition but major changes and additions have been incorporated to help the students develop skill and analysis in day-to-day clinical sample processing.

A new chapter is added on antimicrobial susceptibility test. The chapter includes the test methods commonly adopted in a clinical microbiology laboratory, in addition to tests adopted for research purposes. The tests like detection of MRSA, ESBL, AmpC-β-lactamase and Metallo-β-lactamase are described in such a manner that common labs without automation can include these tests in their daily practice.

We have also included (newly) a zone size interpretative chart (*according to CLSI-2007*) based on results obtained using Mueller Hinton Agar for the benefit of our various readers.

We acknowledge the help and support of Dr. R.K. Singh, Dr. Atreyee Chakraborty, Dr. Mita Sen, Mr. Nochiel Radhakrishnan, Mr. Sudarshan Chakraborty, Mr. Prasenjit Halder.

We also wish to thank Mr. Amitabha Sen, Director, New Central Book Book Agency (P) Ltd., for the generous support given throughout and also for his sincere effort to bring out the book within the stipulated time.

We admit that every chapter could have been enriched further with more information. Constructive suggestions from users will be our guide in our future efforts.

May 17, 2011
Buddha Purnima

EC 63, Salt Lake
Kolkata 700 064

PRANABESWAR CHAKRABORTY
NISHITH KUMAR PAL

Preface to the first edition

With the continuing expansion of the practice of microbiology, the biggest challenge in the preparation of Manual of Practical Microbiology and Parasitology has been to provide a concise volume with all uptodate technology.

The book contains more than 200 colour plates and 50 illustrations that set out the basic facts and principles clearly and briefly which are essentially visual in impact.

Chapters 2 to 10—dealing with staining procedure; identification of bacterial cultures from specimens and culture plates; stool examination; immunoassays and identification of spots — are aimed for students pursuing undergraduate studies in medical and dental sciences based on the course of studies of Asian and African universities. It will also prove useful for other groups such as Veterinary Science students, medical laboratory scientists specialising in microbiology, and to postgraduate students of Microbiology.

Chapter 11 deals with management of hospital waste; Chapters 12-16 deal with laboratory diagnosis of bacterial, viral, fungal, parasitic and sexually transmitted diseases, respectively; and Chapter 17 deals with bacteriology of water, milk and air. These chapters are also very useful. A chapter on laboratory animals (Chapter 18) dealing with care of the animals, animal disease and experimental procedures is included for the benefit of postgraduate students in microbiology and for clinical microbiologists. In Chapter 19, methods of preparation of media are described. Appendices contain current question papers in Microbiology of MBBS and MD examinations for information of the students.

At the end of each chapter, a question-answer format has been included in order to acquaint the students with the type of oral questions that she/he has to face in the examination.

We are deeply indebted to the authors of many texts and reference books which we have frequently consulted but their references have not been cited. We welcome suggestions and comments from all quarters to make the book better in subsequent editions. Please mail your suggestions and new ideas on our e-mail : ncbapvtltd@eth.net.

Our special thanks to Dr. (Mrs.) Mita Sen for editing the manuscript. Our sincere thanks to Shri Soumen Paul for colour processing and designing the cover of the book, Smt. S. Dutta and Shri Subas Maitra for proof-checking, and Shri Nochiel Radhakrishnan for composing, computer graphics and supervising the book. We also extend our special thanks to Shri Amitabha Sen, Shri Jogendranath Sen and all the staff of New Central Book Agency for their constant help and sincere endeavour in publishing the book.

4th January 2008
Sufaliekadashi
EC 63, Salt Lake
Kolkata 700 064

Pranabeswar Chakraborty
Nishith Kumar Pal

Preface to the first edition

Contents

Contents

Introduction

1

STRUCTURE OF BACTERIA

Bacteria (*sing.* **bacterium**) are unicellular prokaryotic microorganisms which divide by binary fission. They do not possess nuclear membrane and the nucleus consists of a single chromosome of circular double-stranded DNA helix (Fig. 1.1).

Flagella

These are long filamentous, cytoplasmic appendages, 12-30 μm in length, protruding through the cell wall and contain contractile protein flagellin. These are organs of locomotion.

Fimbriae or pili

These are thin, short filaments (0.1-1.5 μm × 4 to 8 nm) extruding from the cytoplasmic membrane, also called pili. They are made of protein (pilin).

Capsule

It is an outer covering of thin jelly-like material (0.2 μm in width) that surrounds the cell wall. Only some bacterial species possess capsule. Capsule is usually made of polysaccharide (e.g. pneumococcus), occasionally polypeptide (e.g. anthrax bacilli) and hyaluronic acid (e.g. streptococcus).

Cell wall

It is a tough and rigid structure of peptidoglycan with accessory specific materials (e.g. LPS, teichoic acid etc.) surrounding the bacterium like a shell and lies external to the cytoplasmic membrane. It is 10-25 nm in thickness. It gives shape to the cell.

Nucleus

The single circular double-stranded chromosome is the bacterial genome.

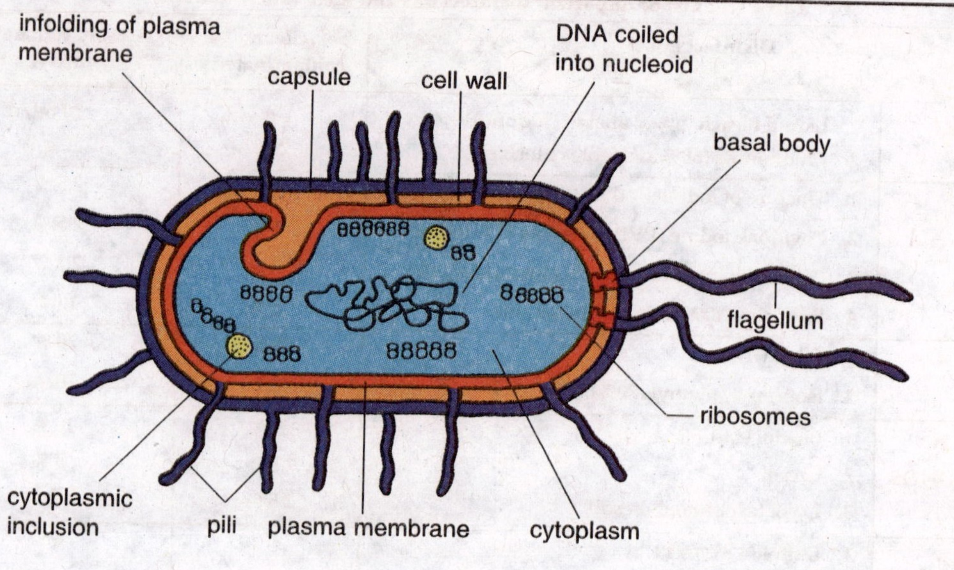

Fig. 1.1 : Section of a bacterial cell

Other structures include cytoplasmic membrane, mesosomes, ribosomes and cytoplasmic inclusions. Unlike eukaryotes cytoplasm does not contain ribosome, golgi, cytoskeleton.

COMMON APPARATUS AND EQUIPMENTS

Commonly used apparatus and equipments include:

1. **Platinum or nichrome wire (Bacteriological)** loop mounted on a glass or **metal rod**.
2. **Gas burner**.
3. **Incubator** to maintain a constant temperature at 37°C, sterilised.
4. **Petri dishes**.
5. **Test tubes, Flasks** and other containers for collecting materials for culture.
6. **Sterile swabs stick** (cotton wool swabs in test tubes plugged with cotton wool).
7. **Faeces container (tube/bottle), MacIntosh and Fildes' jar for anaerobic culture.**
8. **Test tube racks.**
9. **Bijou bottles, MacCartney bottles,** etc.

PERSONAL CARE

1. Use of **gown or aprons**.

2. **Gloves** : Gloves should be worn for touching blood, body fluids, mucous membranes, non-intact skin of all patients, and for handling items or surfaces soiled with blood or body fluids. Gloves should be changed after contact with each patient.

3. **Masks** and protective eyewear or face-shields should be used during procedures that are likely to generate droplets of blood or body fluids to protect the mouth, nose and eyes.

4. **Precautions** should be taken to prevent injuries caused by needles, scalpels, etc.

5. **Health-care** workers with exudative lesions of skin should refrain from direct contact with patients.

6. **Pregnant** health-workers should take extra precaution to avoid perinatal infection (e.g. HIV) resulting from transmission.

7. **Disposables**, e.g. syringe, needles are preferred.

8. Use of properly **sterilised** and **disinfected** equipments.

Safe disposal of specimens

Decontamination of contaminated materials is most effectively done by autoclaving (sterilisation). In Table 1.1, a list of important disinfectants and the concentrations in which they are to be used in clean contaminated and grossly contaminated conditions are given.

Table 1.1 : List of important disinfectants and their concentrations

Disinfectants		Clean contaminated	Grossly contaminated (dirty)
CHLORINE	1. Liquid bleach (5% available chlorine)	2 ml/dl	20 ml/dl
	2. Chloramine (60% available chlorine)	2 g %	20 g %
IODINE	1. Tincture of iodine (Iodine 0.5% + alcohol 70%)	2.5 %	2.5 %
	2. Povidone iodine (PVI), Betadine (1% iodine)	2.5 %	2.5 %
	3. Glutaraldehyde (*Cidex* : 2% glutaraldehyde)	2.5 %	2.5 %
	4. Formalin (40% soln. formaldehyde)	5 %	10 %
ALCOHOL	1. Ethyl (70%)	70 %	70 %
	2. Isopropyl/methyl (70%)	70 %	70 %
PHENOLIC COMPOUNDS	1. Phenol (carbolic acid)	5 %	10 %
	2. Cresol	2.5 %	5 %
	3. Lysol (saponified cresol)	2.5 %	2.5 %
CHLORO-XYLENOLS	1. Dettol (4.8% v/v)	4 %	6 %
	2. Dettol + 1% EDTA	3 %	6 %
DIGUANIDE	1. Chlorhexidine (1.5% v/v, e.g. Hibitane)	5 %	10 %
	2. Chlorhexidine + cetrimide (Savlon)	5 %	10 %

Methods of Morphological Study of Bacteria

2

Low or high-power objectives of light microscopy is usually adequate for the study of fungi and protozoa, whereas oil-immersion microscopy is necessary for identification of bacteria.

I. UNSTAINED WET MOUNT

Drops of liquid specimens of 3-6 hours growth in fluid media at room temperature (22°C) are examined mainly for study of bacterial motility. The method is also used for demonstration of spirochaetes from clinical materials by D.G.I.

Hanging drop preparation (Figs. 2.1-2.4)

Procedure :

(a) Four beads of plasticin or vaseline is placed over the middle part of a clean glass slide (Fig. 2.1).

(b) With the help of sterile bacteriological loop place a large drop of young broth culture at the centre of a clean cover glass (Fig. 2.2).

(c) Glass slide with adherent plasticin/vaseline beads is inverted gently on the cover glass with culture drop. This will make the cover glass adherent to the slide.

(d) Then the glass slide with adherent cover glass is reverted making the culture drop hanging from cover glass (Fig. 2.3).

(e) The hanging drop is then examined, first under low power (x 10) to focus the periphery of the drop, and then under high power (x 10) to note the motility (Figs. 2.4 and 2.5).

[**Caution** : Elevation of beads should not be too high to interfere focusing and too little allowing drop to touch the slides. A dry drop is unsuitable for examination].

Observation :

(a) Non-motile bacteria are either static or show

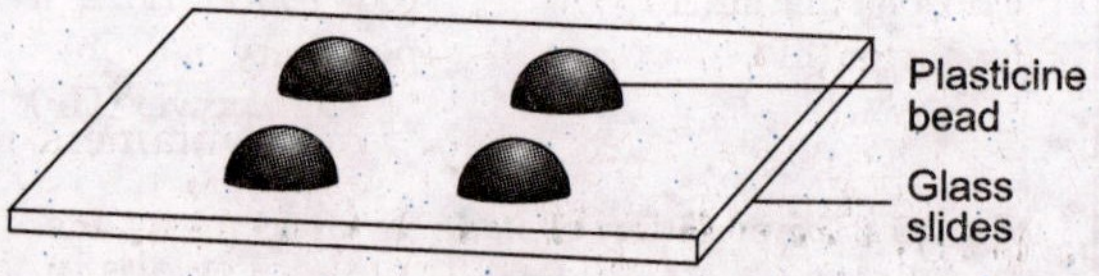

Fig. 2.1 : Glass slides with plasticine beads

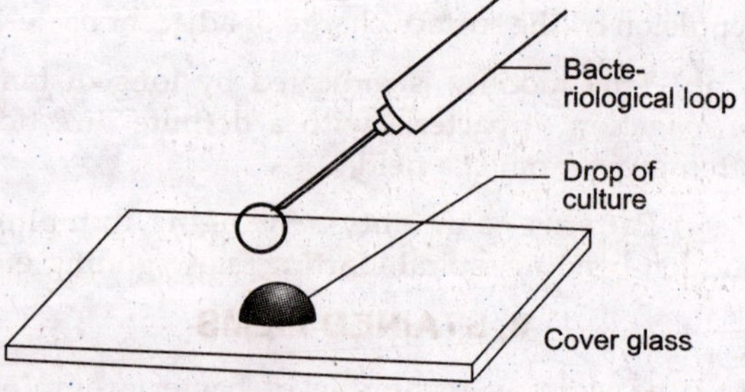

Fig. 2.2 : A large drop of culture in liquid medium placed on cover glass using a loop

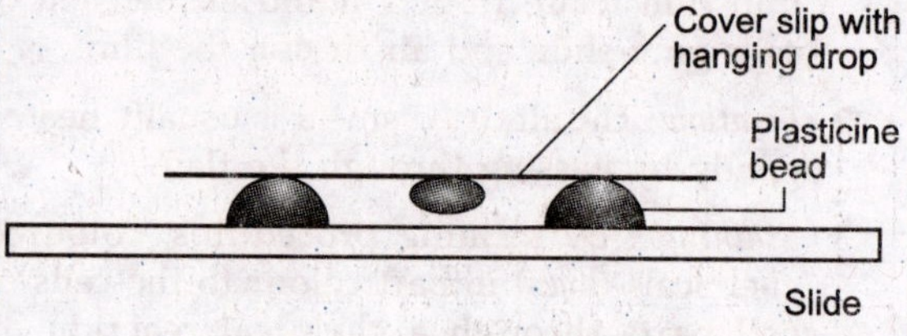

Fig. 2.3 : Glass slide with plasticine is first inverted on the cover glass, then reverted to make the drop hanging

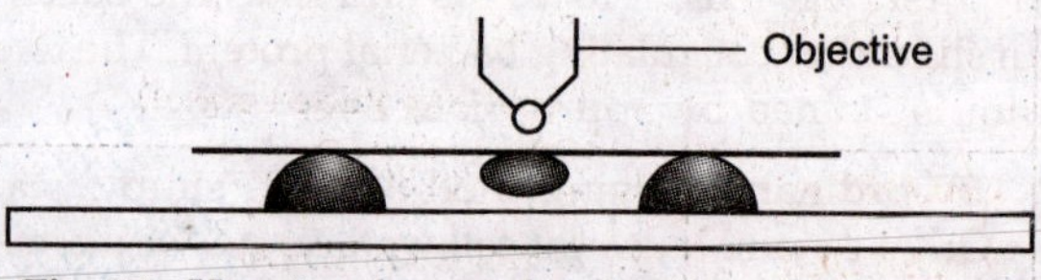

Fig. 2.4 : Hanging drop under objective of microscope

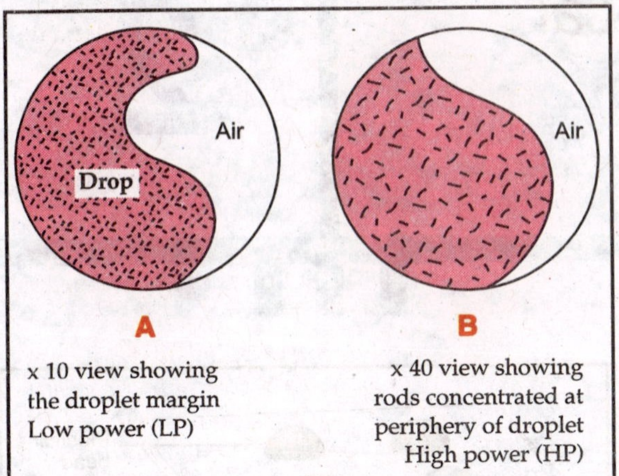

Fig. 2.5 : Examination of hanging drop under the microscope

brownian movement, i.e., in different directions without any definite propagative movement, due to repulsion by the surface charge of adjacent bacteria.

(b) True motility is indicated by long distance propagation of bacteria with a definite direction, often away from the field.

(c) Patterns of motility : Swinging, tumbling, sudden bending, spiral, darting, slow gliding etc.

II. STAINED FILMS

Routine staining technique of bacteria employs smear preparation, drying, fixation and staining of smears :

1. *Smear* : The technique consists of spreading a thin film made from a liquid suspension of cells on a slide and air drying the film.
2. *Fixation* : The air dried smear is usually heated gently by passing through the flame.
3. *Staining* : By staining procedures, coloured chemicals (*dyes*) impart colour to the cells or cell parts through a chemical reaction by affixing to them.

Smear made from bacterial cultures or specimens are first heat-fixed. Heat kills and fixes the bacteria on slide after coagulating bacterial protein. The fixed film is stained by appropriate dyes.

By ordinary staining method (e.g. simple stain or Gram's stain) bacterial cell wall cannot be stained. The coloured body seen under light microscope represents cell protoplasm only. In the chain of bacteria, the coloured bacterial bodies are separated by gaps which represent unstained connecting cell walls.

Common staining techniques

1. *Simple stains* : Watery solution of a single basic dye such as methylene blue or basic fuchsins are used as simple stain.
2. *Negative staining* : Bacteria are mixed with dyes (India ink or nigrosin). The background gets stained leaving the bacteria contrastingly colourless. The technique is useful in demonstration of bacterial capsule.
3. *Impregnation methods* : Bacterial cells and appendages that are too thin and delicate cannot be seen under ordinary microscope. These delicate structures are thickened by impregnation of silver (*special stains*) on the surface to make them visible under light microscope, e.g. demonstration of spirochaetes and bacterial flagella.
4. *Differential stains* : They impart different colours to different bacteria or their structures.

In a stained film, bacterial shape, arrangement and presence of other cells (pus cells) are noted. The two commonly used differential stains are **Gram's stain and Acid-Fast stain.**

GRAM'S STAIN

It is the most widely used stain in medical bacteriology. The stain was originally devised by Christian Gram (1884) as a technique of staining bacteria in tissues. There are four steps in the technique.

Bacterial culture in plate or tube is provided to students.

Preparation of smear

(a) Using a sterile bacteriological loop, a drop of sterile normal saline is placed on a clean grease free slide.

(b) Pick the tip of a bacterial colony on solid medium with loop or straight wire, and make a small emulsion with saline. Next spread it into a thin smear.

(c) Air dry the smear.

Fixation of smear

Dried smear is fixed by passing it several times over a flame. Gentle heating kills the bacteria and coagulation of protein fixes it on slide. Care is to be taken not to overheat to char the bacteria.

Staining Method

1. Primary staining of heat fixed smear of specimen or bacterial culture is made with a pararosaniline dye, e.g. crystal violet, gentian violet or methyl violet solution for one minute. Usually the smear is fully covered with crystal violet solution.
2. Pour off crystal violet and add dilute solution of iodine, such as Gram's iodine—keep for one minute.
3. Wash with water.
4. Decolourisation with an organic solvent (alcohol or acetone or iodine-acetone 1 : 1 mixture) — 10 to 30 seconds till faint blue colour persists.
5. Wash with water quickly to avoid over-decolourisation.
6. Counterstain with a dye of contrasting colour 1 : 20 dilute carbol fuchsin, safranin or neutral red for 1/2 to 1 minute. Safranin is commonly used as counterstain.
7. The smear is washed with water and then air or blot dried.
8. The smear is examined under oil-immersion objective (×100) with condenser up.

Observation (Fig. 2.7)

Gram-positive bacteria resist decolourisation and stain violet. Gram-negative and other cells (pus cells) are decolourised and stain pink with counterstain. The Gram-positive bacteria may sometimes appear Gram-negative under certain situations, such as in ageing cultures and when the cell wall is damaged.

On the basis of Gram's staining, bacteria are divided into two categories :

1. *Gram-positive bacteria* : All cocci except *Neisseria, Moraxella* and *Branhamella* are gram-positive.
2. *Gram-negative bacteria* : All bacilli are Gram-negative except *Corynebacterium, Mycobacterium, Bacillus, Clostridium, Actinomyces, Listeria, Lactobacillus, Propionibacterium* and *Erysipelothrix* which are Gram-positive.

Reagents

A. *Crystal violet solution*

Crystal violet	...	0.5 gm
Distilled water to make	...	100 ml

First make a thick solution of crystal violet in absolute alcohol, then make up the volume to 100 ml with distilled water.

B. *Gram's iodine*

Iodine	...	1 gm
Potassium iodide	...	2 gm
Distilled water to make	...	100 ml

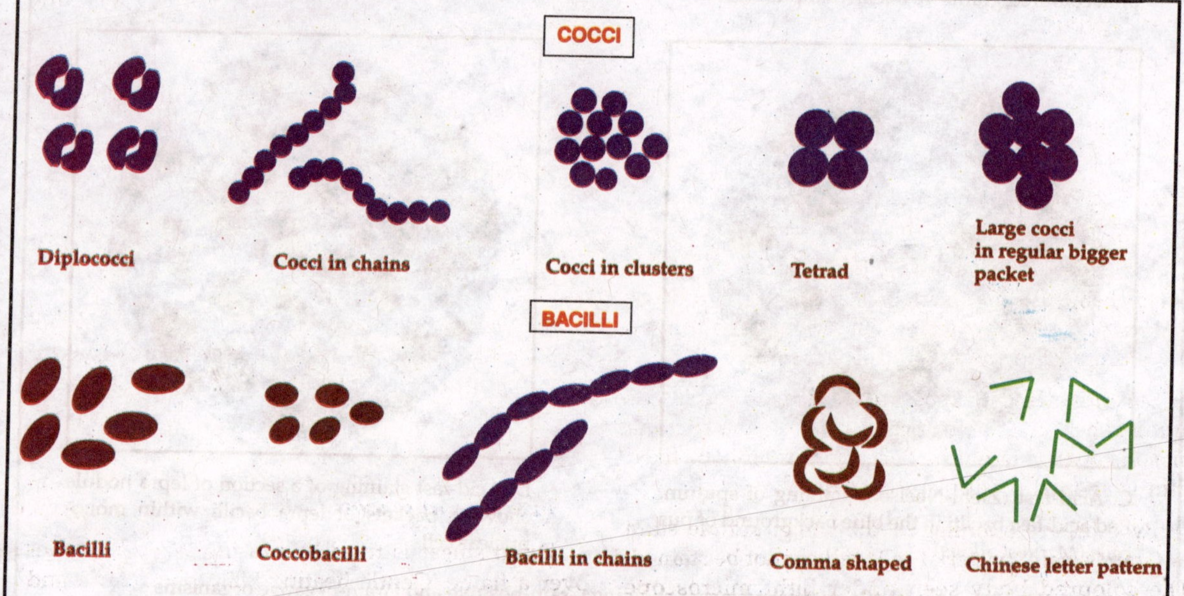

Fig. 2.6 : Morphology of bacteria

At first dissolve pot. iodide in 50 ml water. Then add iodine and dissolve in it. Add more water to make the volume 100 ml.

C. *Acetone or alcohol*

D. *Safranin*

Sufranin	...	0.5 gm
Distilled water to make	...	100 ml

Mechanisms of Gram's stain

The exact mechanism is not understood. There are two major theories in this respect :

1. *Protoplasmic pH* :The hydrogen ion concentration of the protoplasm of Gram-positive bacteria (pH 2-3) is higher than that of Gram-negative bacteria (pH 4-5). The iodine treatment makes the cytoplasm further more acidic and serves as a mordant, i.e. iodine combines with the dye and then fixes the dye in bacterial cell.

2. *Cell wall permeability* : The Gram-reaction probably depends more on the permeability of bacterial cell wall and cytoplasmic membrane. A dye-iodine complex or *lake* is formed within the cell after staining with crystal/methyl violet and

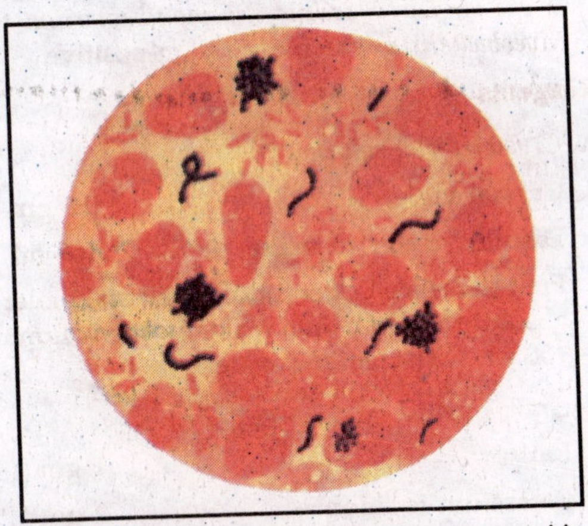

A. Gram staining (pus): Violet gram +ve cocci in clusters (staphylococci), in chain (streptococci); pink coloured gram –ve bacilli and pus cells

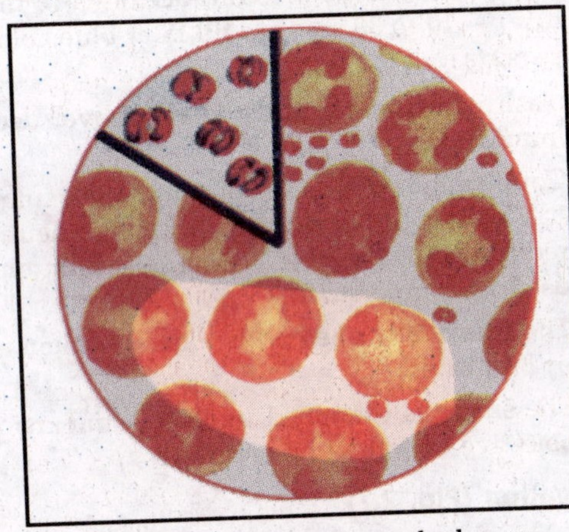

B. Gram –ve diplococci in urethral smear

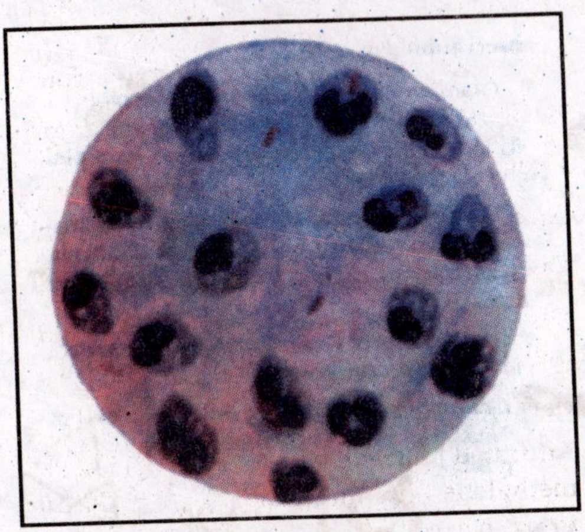

C. Acid-fast (Ziehl-Neelsen) staining of sputum. Red acid-fast bacilli in the blue background of pus cells (*M. tuberculosis*)

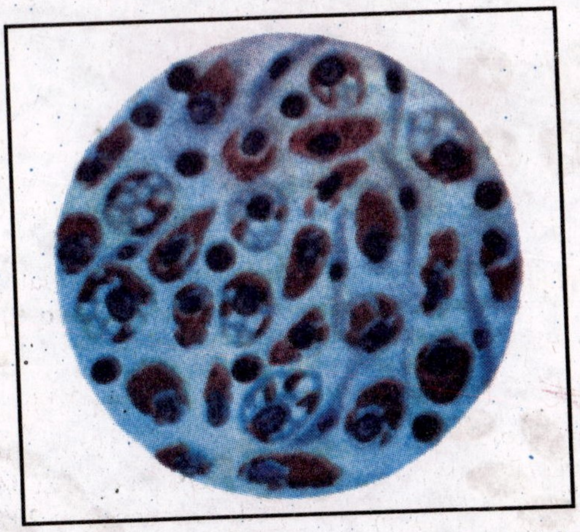

D. Acid-fast staining of a section of lepra nodule showing packets of lepra bacilli within mononuclear cells

Fig. 2.7 : *(A + B)* : Gram-stained smear showing Gram-positive and Gram-negative organisms. *(C + D)* : Acid-fast organisms treatment with iodine. This dye-iodine complex is insoluble in water but moderately soluble and dissociable in alcohol or acetone used as the decolourising agent. Under the action of the decolouriser, the dye and iodine complex diffuse freely out of the Gram-negative cell, but not from the Gram-positive cell, presumably because the cell wall of the latter is less permeable. Gram-positive bacteria become Gram-negative when their cell wall is ruptured or damaged or deficient (L-form).

ACID-FAST STAIN

It is extremely difficult to stain mycobacteria with ordinary stain like Gram's stain. Staining of *Mycobacterium* (tubercle and lepra bacilli) can be done by Acid-fast stain (Ziehl-Neelsen technique) or by auramine-rhodamine stain. The latter is more sensitive than the acid-fast stain but requires fluorescence microscopy.

The acid-fast stain was discovered by Ehrlich and subsequently modified by Ziehl and Neelsen.

Procedure

Smear preparation

(a) With the help of a sterile swab stick a portion of sputum is picked up and smeared on a clean slides. From culture smear is prepared in normal saline. In cases of *M. leprae*, scrapping of tissue from slit skin of lesions, using a scalpel blade, is smeared directly on slide. Air dry the smear.

(b) Smear is fixed by gently heating by passing the slide over a flame several times. Care is taken not to overheat.

Staining method

(a) Hot and steaming carbol fuchsin solution in a test tube is poured over the smear to cover it. It may need intermittent heating of the reverse side of the slide using a spirit flame. Wait for 5-10 minutes. Be careful not to dry the stain. If required add more stain.

(b) Pour off the stain and wash in tap water.

(c) Decolourise the smear with 20% H_2SO_4 till very faint pink colour persists. In case of *M. leprae* 4-5%. H_2SO_4 is used. Alternative to 20% H_2SO_4, 3% acid-alcohol (3 ml conc. HCl in 97 ml of absolute alcohol) may be used in special circumstances, e.g. demonstration of *Cryptosporidium* oocyst in stool, or to differentiate *M. tuberculosis* complex (both acid and alcohol fast) from some M.O.T.T. bacillus.

(d) Next counterstain using 2% alkaline methylene blue or malachite green (same as Albert I) solution for 1-2 minutes.

(e) Gently wash with tap water and air or blot dry.

Examination : Scan the slide thoroughly, at least 200 fields, under oil immersion objective with condenser up.

Observation (Fig. 2.7C&D)

Acid-fast bacilli appear red in blue background of pus cells and epithelial cells in smear of sputum.

Acid-fast organisms

1. *Mycobacterium*–Tubercle and lepra bacilli.
2. *Others*–Bacterial spores, ascospores of some yeasts, *Actinomyces* clubs (in animal tissue), some *Nocardia* species and *Cryptosporidium* oocysts. The bacterial spores are weakly acid-fast where the decolourising agent used is 0.5% H_2SO_4.

Principle of acid-fast staining

Acid-fastness has been attributed to the high content of lipids, fatty acids and higher alcohols, which constitute almost 40% of the dry weight of tubercle bacilli. Mycolic acid (a wax), acid-fast in the free state, is found in all acid-fast bacteria. The integrity of the cell wall is also important for acid-fastness of bacteria.

Reagents

1. Ziehl–Neelsen's Carbol fuchsin solution

Basic fuchsin	....	1 gm
Phenol (crystalline)	....	5 gm
Alcohol (95% or absolute)	....	10 ml
Distilled water to make	....	100 ml

Dissolve the dye in the alcohol and add the the same to 90 ml 5% phenol solution.

2. Methylene blue (2%)

Saturated solution of methylene blue in alcohol	....	30 ml
KOH, 0.01% in water	....	100 ml

ALBERT'S STAINING

Albert stain is done to differentially stain the metachromatic granules and cytoplasm of *Corynebacterium diphtheriae* and diphtheroid bacillus.

Procedure :

(a) Fixation of smear is done by gentle heating over a flame avoiding overheating to char.

(b) Cover the smear with Albert-I staining solution. Keep it for 5 minutes.

(c) Pour off the stain. Do not wash.

(d) Next stain the smear for 2 minutes with Albert-II staining solution (iodine solution).

(e) Pour off the Albert-II solution from slide. Do not wash.

(f) Blot to dry the smear.

(g) Examine the smear under oil immersion lens (× 100) with condenser up.

[**Note** : Like other methods of bacterial staining, in Albert method, washing is avoided as malachite green is highly soluble in water and stain quality fades].

Staining reagents

A. Albert I or Albert stain

1. Toluidine blue	....	0.15 gm
2. Malachite green	....	0.20 gm
3. Glacial acetic acid	....	1 ml
4. Alcohol (95% ethanol)	....	2 ml
5. Distilled water to make	....	100 ml

Dissolve the dyes in alcohol and add to the water and acetic acid, allow the stain to stand for one day and then filter.

B. Albert II or Albert's iodine solution

1. Iodine	....	2 gm
2. Potassium iodide	....	3 gm
3. Distilled water to make	....	300 ml

Dissolve KI in water and then add Iodine and dissolve in pot. iodide.

Observation : Body of the bacilli appear green and metachromatic granules blue-black (Fig. 3.1).

Internal quality control of staining :

Quality of staining reagents and procedure is checked every time when new staining solution is prepared (or procured) and at the time of staining, identification of unknown bacteria in culture and clinical material.

Bacterial smears with known staining character are subjected for staining. If the results are in expected line, the reagent and the procedural quality is validated.

Example :

(a) *Gram stain* :

Positive control	....	Staphylococcus
Negative control	....	E. coli

(b) *Acid Fast stain* :

Positive control	....	Mycobacterium tuberculosis
Negative control	....	E. coli

(c) *Albert stain* :

Positive control	....	Corynebacterium diphtheriae
Negative control	....	None

Some points to note :

- Morphology by staining is best studied in stationary phase of growth of bacteria.
- Gram stain cannot stain bacterial spores, which appear as clear 'halo' inside the cell cytoplasm.
- Spores may be stained by cold carbol-fuchsin, followed by decolourisation with 0.5% H_2SO_4.
- Albert I staining solution imparts green stains to the cytoplasm of all gram +ve and –ve bacteria.
- An old gram +ve bacterial culture may appear gram –ve or gram variable.
- Spirochaetes needs D.G.I and metal-shadowed preparations for study of morphology.

Staining of Supplied Smears

3

INTRODUCTION

In microbiology practical examination of MBBS course, students are supplied with 2 smears and asked to stain and examine one by *Albert's* method and another one by *Ziehl-Neelsen* method.

I. ALBERT'S STAIN

Usually examinee is provided with a fixed smear prepared from *C. diphtheriae* grown usually on Loeffler's serum slope or occasionally from blood tellurite agar medium (Fig. 4.1C). If it is an unfixed smear, fix it by heating gently by passing it over a flame several times. Then proceed it for staining.

Method

1. Refer to chapter 2 for technique in details.
2. Microscopic examination of stained smear is done using × 100 lens (oil immersion objective) with condenser up.
3. Show the examiner, a well stained area focused under the microscope. Importance is given on quality of stain.

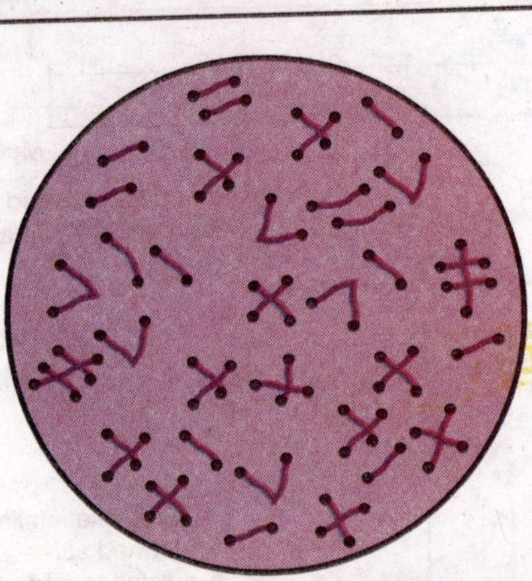

Fig. 3.1 : *Corynebacterium diphtheriae* on Albert's staining : Green bacilli with metachromatic granules (*Diagrammatic representation*)

Observations

Bacillary body and metachromatic granules of *Corynebacterium diphtheriae*, take green and bluish black colours respectively. Arrangement shows angular patterns of V, X, Y, H etc, often described as *cuneiform* or *chinese letter*. Draw a faithful diagram of focused field and label it (see Fig. 3.1).

CORYNEBACTERIUM

Corynebacteria are pleomorphic, Gram-positive, non-acid-fast, non-sporing, non-motile bacilli measuring about 3 µm × 0.3 µm. They often show club-shaped swellings (*Koryne* — club).

Classification

A. Pathogenic

(a) *C. diphtheriae*, classic model of bacteria, is the causative agent of diphtheria.

(b) Other pathogenic corynebacteria : These are primarily animal pathogens. *C. ulcerans* causing acute pharyngitis, *C. pseudotuberculosis* causes chronic lymphadenitis in axilla and *C. jeikeium* is an opportunistic pathogen in man.

B. Non-pathogenic

C. Xerosis—a commensal of conjunctival sac and *C. hofmannii* (*C. pseudodiphtheriticum*), a commensal of oral mucosa.

CORYNEBACTERIUM DIPHTHERIAE

There are three subspecies of *C. diphtheriae* :

1. *C. diphtheriae gravis* with 13 serotypes.
2. *C. diphtheriae intermedius* with 4 serotypes.
3. *C. diphtheriae mitis* with 40 serotypes.

Gravis type is associated with severe form, intermedius type with intermediate form, and mitis type with mild form of diphtheria. Infection due to *C. diphtheriae mitis* is common in India.

Diphtheria toxin

The production of exotoxin depends on the presence of a *tox* gene in chromosome of lysogenic *C. diphtheriae*. The toxin is a heat-labile polypeptide (MW 62,000) and consists of two fragments — A and B — linked by a disulphide bridge. Both fragments are essential for cytotoxicity. The aminoterminal portion of the toxin, fragment A (21 KDa), contains the enzymatically active site of the toxin. Fragment B (37 KDa) binds the toxin to eukaryotic cell. The toxin is thought to inhibit protein synthesis of host cell acting at the ribosomal level by splitting the molecule of NAD (nicotinic adenine dinucleotide) — an essential co-factor for the transferase involved in peptide bond formation by ribosomes.

The toxin can be rendered non-toxic but still antigenic by treatment with formaldehyde and application of heat. Toxoid thus formed is used in prophylactic immunisation.

Pathogenesis

1. ***Local effect*** : The bacteria remain localised at the site of entry (usually upper respiratory tract) and multiply on the mucous membranes and produce exotoxin. The toxin causes necrosis of the mucosal cells along with superficial inflammatory reaction. The necrosed epithelium together with fibrinous exudate, leucocytes, red cells and bacteria form a grey, adherent pseudomembrane.

2. ***General effect*** : After absorption into blood stream, the toxin acts systematically on the cells of the myocardium, nervous system (only motor nerves) kidney and adrenals.

Laboratory diagnosis

Patient suspected of having diphtheria is treated immediately with antitoxin without waiting for laboratory report as the toxin is powerful and rapidly fatal.

Specimens : Swabs from throat, nose or larynx depending on the site of lesion. Membrane may be found in skin ulcer or inside vagina.

Microscopy

Albert-stained smears show long, thin and curved greenish rods arranged in Chinese letter patterns, often beaded due to presence of dark staining volutin granules in the rods. Nonpathogenic *C. xerosis* also contains sparse number of volutin granules. The volutin granules are best demonstrated by Albert's staining method in film preparations from luxuriant media (e.g. Loeffler's serum medium). The morphological similarity of *C. diphtheriae* and *C. xerosis* demands that they should be differentiated by further tests.

Culture

The material is inoculated in (1) Loeffler's inspissated serum medium and (2) Tellurite blood agar medium and incubated at 37°C for 12 hours and 24 hours, respectively. (3) When the specimen is inoculated in blood agar colonies appear after 24-48 hours incubation. Albert's staining of smear made from colony is examined to see the bacterial morphology.

Biochemical reaction

Isolated organism is inoculated in Hiss's serum medium containing sugar (glucose, maltose, sucrose, mannitol). The toxigenic strains usually produce acid in glucose and maltose, whereas the diphtheroids ferment sucrose and mannitol.

Toxigenicity test

1. ***Guinea pig inoculation*** : Suspension of isolated strain of *C. diphtheriae* (0.3 ml) is injected subcutaneously into thigh of two guinea pigs, one protected intramuscularly with 500 units of diphtheria antitoxin 18-24 hours before the test.

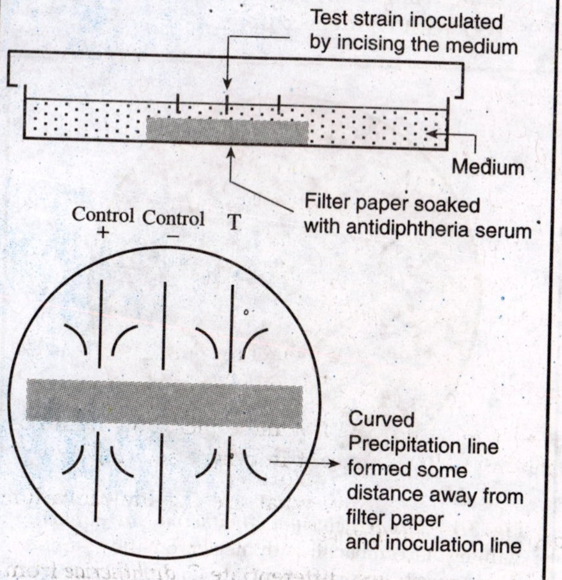

Fig. 3.2 : Elek's agar-gel precipitation test

Observation : The unprotected animal dies within 2-3 days with evidence of haemorrhage in the adrenal glands.

2. ***Gel-precipitation (Elek) test***: A rectangular strip of filter paper previously incorporated in diphtheria antitoxin (1,000 units/ml) is incorporated into serum agar plate before it has set. The testing strain is then streaked across the plate at right angles to the filter paper strip and incubated at 37°C for 24-48 hours.

Observation: The lines of precipitation radiate a little distance away from the intersection of the strip and bacterial growth.

Typing

The isolated strain of *C. diphtheriae* is further subdivided by serotyping by agglutination tests, phage typing and bacteriocin typing for epidemiological studies.

Test your knowledge on *C. diphtheriae*

QUESTIONS

1. What is Kleb-Löeffler's bacillus?

2. What is the gram stained property of *Corynebacterium*?

3. Why Albert staining is done for corynebacterium?

4. Why the bacillary body of any bacteria is stained green by Albert stain?

5. What is the Albert stained property of *C. diphtheriae*?

6. Why metachromatic granules are stained bluish-black?

7. What is the position of metachromatic granule on bacillary body?

8. What is the importance of microscopy in diagnosis of *C. diphtheriae?*

9. Is the presence of metachromatic granule is the property of *C. diphtheriae* only?

10. Can you name few more inclusion bodies or volutin granules present in other bacteria?

11. In microscopy, what are the identification points of *C. diphtheriae*?

12. How can you differentiate *C. diphtheriae* from *diphtheroids* by morphology, biochemical and other studies?

13. What factor is responsible for the characteristic arrangement of *C. diphtheriae* or diptheroids in smear?

14. Is it possible to demonstrate metachromatic granules in gram or methylene blue stained smear?

15. What are the sites of formation of diphtheritic patch?

16. Is it possible to develop complication of diphtheria in a properly immunised individual?

17. Are all isolates of *C. diphtheriae* toxigenic?

18. How a nontoxigenic *C. diphtheriae* strain becomes toxigenic?

19. Name some commensal, pathogenic and opportunistic pathogenic diphtheroids and the diseases they cause.

20. What are the biotypes of *C. diphtheriae?*

21. What is the most prevalent biotype in India?

22. How the biotypes are differentiated?

23. Name the traditional selective medium for isolation of *C. diphtheriae*?

24. Comment on the usefulness of the medium as regards effective selective medium and colonial morphology of biotypes of *C. diphtheriae*.

25. Name the medium and composition for best demonstration of microscopic morphology of *C. diphtheriae*.

26. What are the biochemical tests done for confirmation of identity of *C. diphtheriae*?

27. What is the base of the biochemical test medium for a fastidious bacteria like *C. diphtheriae*?

28. How to test *in vitro* and *in vivo* the toxigenicity of an isolate of *C. diphtheriae*?

29. Name the standard toxigenic strain of *C. diphtheriae* for demonstration of toxin production?

30. How *C. diphtheriae* exotoxin acts?

31. Which test is most important for lab diagnosis of diphtheria? (a) Culture, (b) Toxigenicity test, (c) Direct smear examination by Albert stain, (d) Culture followed by biochemical and toxigenicity test.

32. Which medium is used for early growth of *C. diphtheriae*? (a) Potassium tellurite blood agar, (b) Dorset Egg, (c) Löeffler serum slope, (d) Blood agar.

33. Which corynebacterium shows haemolysis on blood agar medium?

(a) *C. diphtheria* biotype *mitis*, (b) *C. xerosis*

(c) *C. erythrasma* (d) *C. haemolyticum*.

34. How can you assess the susceptibility of a person to diphtheria? Describe in detail.

35. Who first demonstrated presence of antitoxin to *C. diphtheriae* toxin in human serum?

36. What is pseudomembrane of diphtheria? What other infections may cause similar membranes on fauces?

ANSWERS

1. *Corynebacterium diphtheriae* is often called as Kleb-Löeffler's bacillus after the names of discoverers Kleb and Löefflers of the bacteria.

2. Gram +ve rod.

3. Metachromatic granules, an important identification point of *C. diphtheriae* is better and differentially stained by Albert's method.

4. Albert-I staining solution contains malachite green dye, which stains cytoplasm of all bacteria green.

5. Bacillary body stains green and metachromatic granules stain bluish black.

6. Chemically metachromatic granules are polymetaphosphate which is stained metachromatically by Albert stain.

7. Metachromatic granules may be present in any part of the body, but bacillary ends are common locations.

8. Diphtheria can be diagnosed quickly and efficiently by microscopy, which is highly sensitive. So for presumptive diagnosis this simple test is always advocated. However, microscopical diagnosis is to be confirmed by culture and toxigenecity test.

9. Some diphtheroid bacilli may contain metachromatic granules.

10. Other inclusion granules : Polymerised β-hydroxybutyric acid, glycogen and starch granules.

11. Long slender (0.3 μm × 3 μm) rods. Shape and size vary. There are bulging usually at the ends, but may be present anywhere of the bacillary body due to presence of metachromatic granules, stained bluish black or violet. Arrangement of bacilli tend to be in angular pattern of V, X, Y etc., resembling chinese letters.

12. See Box – 1 below :

BOX – 1	*C. diphtheriae*	*Diphtheroid*
Gram stain	Less gram + ve	Intensely gram +ve
Pleomorphism	More prominent	Less prominent
Metachromatic granules	Usually present	Usually absent
Shape	Long slender bacilli, with tappered ends.	Short, plump may be curved and may show swelling due to metachromatic granules.
Arrangements	Angular pattern	Parallel or in pallisades
Glucose	Ferments	Ferments
Sucrose	Nonfermenter	Ferments
Diphtheria toxin	May elaborate toxin	Usually non-toxigenic

13. *C. diphtheriae* multiplies by longitudinal fission and the daughter cells lag separation, leading to angular arrangement.

14. All aniline dyes, including primary stain of gram method, stain metachromatic granules metachromatically.

15. Sites of diphtheritic patch : (i) fauces and adjoining regions, (ii) anterior nares, (iii) conjunctiva, (iv) skin and (v) vagina.

16. An immunised person may develop diphtheritic patch, but he is immune to the toxin of diphtheria, so no toxigenic complication develops.

17. Only a clone of *C. diphtheriae* lysogenised with a bacteriophage (β-phage) carrying toxigene produce toxin. Otherwise an isolate is a nontoxigenic one.

18. See answer to question 17.

19. Most of the diphtheroids are commensals of skin and throat. Some are pathogenic and opportunistic pathogens (Box–2) :

BOX – 2	Name	Disease
(a) Pathogenic	*C. ulcerans*	Diphtheria like feature, when toxigenic
(b) Opportunistic pathogens	*C. pseudotuberculosis*	Respiratory tract infection
	C. auris	Middle ear infection in children
	C. urealyticum	Acute and chronic encrusted U.T.I.

contd. next page

BOX 2 contd. from previous page	Name	Disease
	C. jeikeium	Bacteraemia in immunocompromised persons.
	C. minutissimum	Erythrasma
	C. xerosis	Variety of infection
	C. striatum	Variety of infection

20. Biotypes : gravis, intermedius and mitis.

21. Most prevalent biotype in India is mitis.

22. Differentiating properties of biotypes of *C. diphtheriae* are shown in Box – 3.

BOX – 3			
Character	**Gravis**	**Intermedius**	**Mitis**
(a) Colony on Tellurite blood agar	Daisy head	Frog's egg	poached egg
(b) Consistency	Brittle	Intermediate between two	Soft
(c) Glycogen	Acid	Negative	Negative
(d) Virulence	Severe	Moderate	Mild
(For details see text book, page 275)			

23. Potassium tellurite blood agar.

24. Not a good selective medium. *Neisseria* and *Staphylococcus* may grow over it. Traditional teaching says colonial morphology of 3 biotypes are better demonstrated in this medium.

25. In Löeffler's serum slope, *C. diphtheriae* grows rapidly and by 6-8 hours shows best morphological features. Composition : Sterile OX, Sheep or Horse serum – 75 ml, Nutrient broth base – 25 ml, Glucose 0.25G.

26. Ferments glucose, produce acid in glycogen, urease–negative and sucrose-non fermenter.

27. Hiss's serum sugar broth or serum sugar slope.

28. In vitro test — Elek test and toxigenicity test in tissue culture.

In vivo test — Animal inoculation test — (a) subcutaneously and (b) intracutaneously

(For details see text book page 277).

29. *'Park-Williams–8'* strain of *C. diphtheriae*.

30. See Text Book – page 10.

31. Ans. (c). 32. Ans. (c). 33. Ans. (d).

34. By performing Shick test, adequate amount of neutralising antibody against diphtheria could be assessed. For details — see Textbook.

35. Von-Behring.

36. Pseudomembrane constituted of necrotic tissue debris of underlying squamous epithelial cells with few WBCs and bacteria. Diseases producing pseudomembranes or like features :

(i) Diphtheria, (ii) Acute streptococcal tonsillitis, (iii) Vincent's angina, (iv) Infectious mononucleosis and (v) Candida albicans.

II. ZIEHL-NEELSEN (ZN) OR ACID-FAST STAINING

Generally, a fixed smear is supplied in examination as stress is made mostly on the staining procedure. If, the smear is unfixed, fix it by gently heating the smear on flame.

Method : ZN staining already described in Chapter 2. Examine the stained smear under oil-immersion objective (× 100) of microscope.

Observations :

1. *Mycobacterium tuberculosis* are seen as bright red bacilli (AFB). See Fig. 3.3.
2. Draw a labelled diagram of your findings and focus under microscope.

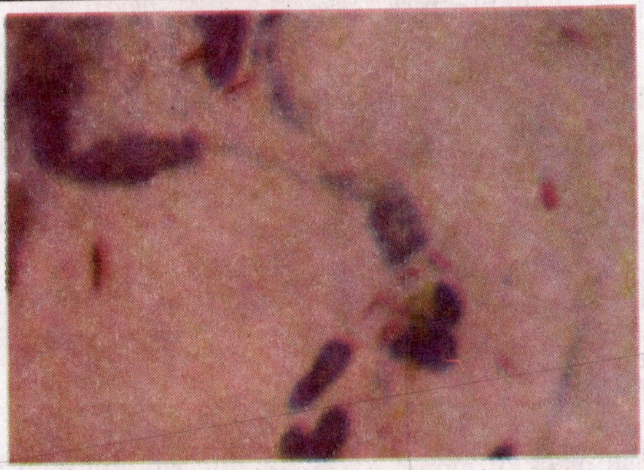

Fig. 3.3 : *Mycobacterium tuberculosis* on *Ziehl-Neelsen (ZN) staining* : Acid-fast bacilli (AFB). Diagrammatic representation when seen under X 100 magnification.

MYCOBACTERIUM

Mycobacteria are non-motile, non-sporing, non-capsulate, slender acid-fast bacilli and sometimes exhibit filamentous forms resembling fungal mycelium (Greek *Myces* meaning fungus) and, hence, they are so named. Hansen (1868) discovered the first member (Lepra bacillus), Robert Koch (1888) isolated mammalian tubercle bacillus, and Johne (1895) described *M. paratuberculosis* (Johne's bacillus).

Mycobacterium species

The genus *Mycobacterium* contains over 50 well-defined species. In developing countries, the major pathogenic species are *M. tuberculosis*, *M. bovis* and *M. leprae*. A tentative classification of those species capable of producing human disease are listed in Box 4.

BOX – 4

MYCOBACTERIA

Cultivable — **Non-cultivable**

M. leprae – leprosy in man

A. Strict pathogens

1. Human type – *M. tuberculosis* — Generalised tuberculosis in man
2. Bovine type – *M. bovis*
3. Human type – *M. africanum* — Causes tuberculosis in man

B. Atypical / MOTT mycobacteria

Group I – *Photochromogens* (e.g. *M. kansasii*)
Group II – *Scotochromogens* (e.g. *M. scrofulaceum*)
Group III – *Nonchromogens* (e.g. *M. avium*)
Group IV – *Rapid growers* (e.g. *M. fortuitum*)

C. Saprophytic mycobacteria (non-pathogenic)

1. *M. smegmatis* – Present in smegma (grows at 52°C)
2. *M. phlei* – Present in grass
3. *M. stercoris* – Present in dung
4. *M. thermoresistible*
5. *M. butyricum* – Present in putrefied butter

D. Animal pathogens

1. *M. microti* – Tuberculosis in voles
2. *M. paratuberculosis* – Enteritis in cattle and sheep (Johne's bacillus)
3. *M. lepraemurium* – Causes rat leprosy

MYCOBACTERIUM TUBERCULOSIS

Habitat : The main reservoirs of *M. tuberculosis* are infected persons, also occasionally present as pathogens in animals.

Pathogenesis

Tuberculosis is a slowly progressive, chronic granulomatous infection. *Mycobacterium tuberculosis* is the main causative agent and less often *Mycobacterium bovis*. Clinically tuberculosis is seen in two forms : *primary* and *post-primary* infections.

I. Primary infection : Primary infection may occur in any organ such as lung, tonsils, intestine or skin, but in children the usual site is lung and is called *primary complex*.

Primary complex : This consists of (i) a small local lesion as peripheral or subpleural focus of tuberculosis pneumonia in the lung parenchyma *(Ghon focus)*, (ii) enlargement of the regional hilar lymph nodes, and (iii) lymphangitis of the draining lymph vessel. In most cases the primary complex heals spontaneously. It may, however, progress to tuberculous bronchopneumonia, miliary tuberculosis, tuberculous meningitis, bone and joint tuberculosis and genitourinary tuberculosis (renal, endometrial, epididymis).

II. Post-primary infection : The lesions, characteristically more localised and fibrotic, are modified by the development of hypersensitivity by the host.

Source :

(i) *Endogenous* : Mainly due to *reactivation* of primary lesion.

(ii) *Exogenous* : Reinfection by bacilli newly inhaled or ingested from the environment.

Lesions : It most often involves the lung with lesions in the apical region. In untreated case, chronic progressive disease develops with tubercle formation, caseation, cavitation and shedding of bacilli.

Immunocompromised patients (ICP)

ICPs, especially those with HIV infection, are extremely susceptible to tuberculosis. The infection may be rapid and overwhelming with depression of delayed hypersensitivity.

Laboratory diagnosis

Specimen :

1. *Sputum* – concentrate prepared.

2. *Urine* – 3 consecutive morning samples used, concentrate prepared.

3. *CSF* – centrifuged aseptically before culture.

4. *Bone, joint, endometrium samples* — disrupted in a sterile grinder before culture and concentrate prepared.

Microscopy : Slender, 2-3 × 0.2–0.4 μm, non-sporing, beaded bacilli. Smear is stained by Ziehl-Neelsen stain. Heat-fixed smears are treated with concentrated carbol fuchsin, mordanted by heating and then decolourised with 20% sulphuric acid and alcohol and counter stained by methylene blue. The bacilli retain bright red colour of carbol fuchsin against the background of counter stain. For positive microscopic finding, there should be at least 20,000 bacilli per ml of sputum.

Nowadays, AFB are usually detected in Western countries by fluorescent microscopy with auramine stain. It facilitates rapid diagnosis and is useful in mass screening.

Culture : *M. tuberculosis* is an obligate aerobe and does not grow on ordinary media. It grows luxuriantly *(eugonic growth)* on Löwenstein-Jensen medium which contains egg, asparagine, glycerol and malachite green. Glycerol augments growth of *M. tuberculosis* and inhibits that of *M. bovis*. The malachite green inhibits contaminants, but contaminated specimens such as sputum, laryngeal swabs, gastric juice, pooled specimens of urine and pus from secondarily infected wounds require decontamination and concentration of the specimen before culture. For routine purposes, sodium hydroxide (4% W/V) is an effective decontaminant.

Concentration of specimen : Concentration method not only increases the organismal population per unit volume of sample but also kills the contaminated organisms other than mycobacteria. Concentrate of specimen is used for smear, culture and animal inoculation. Culture is a more sensitive method for detection of bacilli, moreover, it is necessary for drug sensitivity.

1. ***Petroff's method*** : About an hour before culturing, mix equal volumes of sputum and 4% sodium hydroxide and incubate at 37°C for 20-30 minutes. Shake at intervals to homogenise the sputum. After centrifugation at 3,000 rpm for 15-20 minutes, it is neutralised with 8% hydrochloric acid in presence of phenol red indicator. A "wide range indicator paper" may be used. After neutralisation, the deposit is again washed with sterile normal saline. The supernatant is thrown-off.

2. ***Acid homogenisation method*** : Equal volumes of specimen and 6% sulphuric acid are mixed. The mixture is then centrifuged. The deposit is washed three times with sterile normal saline.

3. ***NALC method*** : 0.5G N-acetyl-L cysteine (NALC) in 50 ml 1 N (4%) NaOH and 50 ml 0.1 M (2.94%) trisodium citrate, 3 H2O digestant is mixed (by vortexing) to sputum in equal volume (sputum : digestant = 1 : 1) and allowed to act for 20 minutes followed by addition of 0.67 M phosphate buffer (pH 6.8) in excess amount. The whole thing is centrifuged. The deposit is resuspended in 1 ml of phosphate buffer (pH 6.8) with bovine serum albumin (BSA). This resuspended material is used for culture and smear preparation.

The concentrate of specimen thus prepared is utilised for preparation of ZN stained smear and also for culture. By this technique, larger number of cases of tuberculosis can be detected. Smear examination sensitivity is 6000-10,000 bacilli/ml.

Inoculation and incubation : Concentrate of sputum, urine, tissue and deposit of CSF are cultured in two bottles of Löwenstein-Jensen medium and incubated at 37°C in dark and light up to 8 weeks. Cultures are examined first after 4 days for rapid growing mycobacteria and then weekly till 8 weeks. Tubercle bacilli usually grow in 2-8 weeks. Longer incubation up to 12 weeks may be necessary for strains originating from treated patients.

M. tuberculosis often grows as twisted rope-like colonies in liquid culture medium which are called serpentine cords. This cording of the organism is not specific for *M. tuberculosis* and may occur to a lesser extent with other *Mycobacterium species*.

Identification of M.tuberculosis cultures :

1. *Colonies* : Dry raised, yellowish colonies in LJ medium, often described as "rough, tough and buff".

2. *Morphology* : ZN stained smear of culture shows slender, beaded, acid and alcohol-fast bacilli. Many *M. tuberculosis* strains show cording (serpentine cords). See Table 3.1.

3. *Niacin test* : *M. tuberculosis* is niacin positive.

Animal Inoculation

Part of the concentrated material (0.3 ml) or 0.5 ml of culture suspension is inoculated intramuscularly into thigh of a tuberculin negative 12-week-old healthy guinea pig. The animal develops disseminated disease in 4-8 weeks and becomes tuberculin positive. Postmortem findings include caseous lesion

Table 3.1 : Distinguishing points between *M. tuberculosis* and *M. bovis*

Test	*M. tuberculosis*	*M. bovis*
1. Morphology	Slender, long and usually curved	Stout, short and straight.
2. Staining	Barred or beaded	Uniform
3. Growth	Eugonic	Dysgonic
4. Action of glycerol in media	Growth enhanced	Growth inhibited
5. Colony	Dry, rough, raised and wrinkled; consistency tough, tenacious and difficult to emulsify; colour-creamy white or buff coloured.	Moist smooth and flat; consistency friable; white.
6. Biochemical reaction :		
(a) Niacin production	+	–
(b) Nitrate reduction	+	–
(c) TCH selective action	–	+ (No growth)
7. Animal pathogenecity :		
(a) Progressive disease in rabbit	– or mild lesion	+ (generalised lesion)
(b) In guineapig	+ (Progressive and ultimately fatal disease)	+ (Similar action)

at inoculation site, caseous draining lymph node, tubercles in lungs, spleen and kidney. *M. tuberculosis* is virtually non-pathogenic for rabbits.

Nucleic acid amplification : Molecular techniques like genetic probes and PCR are now increasingly used in developed countries for rapid diagnosis of tuberculosis. The sensitivity of the test ranges from 75-100%.

Atypical mycobacteria : Several species of mycobacteria other than *Mycobacterium tuberculosis* (MOTT) can infect humans (Table 3.2).

Vaccine : Bacille Calmette-Guerin (BCG) vaccine,

Table 3.2 : Atypical mycobacteria and diseases produced by them

Runyon Group	Name	Sepcies	Disease produced in man
I	Photochromogens	*M. kansasii*, *M.simiae*	Pulmonary disease
		M. marinum	Swimming pool granuloma
II	Scotochromogens	*M. scrofulaceum*, *M. gordonae*, *M. szulgai*	Lymphadenitis in children
III	Non-chromogens	*M.avium**, *M. intracellulare*, *M. xenopi*	Pulmonary disease in immunocompromised
		M. ulcerans	Buruli ulcer/Lupus vulgaris
		M. malmoense, *M. terrae***	Pulmonary disease and lymphadenitis
IV	Rapid growers	*M. chelonae****, *M. fortuitum*, *M. abscessus*, *M. mucogenicum*, *M. peregrinum*	Superficial and systemic disease

* = Also grouped together with *M. intracellulare* as *M. avium-intracellulare* complex.

** = Includes *M. nonchromogenicum* and *M. trivale*.

*** = Previously spelt as *M. cholonei*.

an alternated strain of *M. bovis*, when injected intradermally, it confers tuberculin hypersensitivity and enhanced activity to macrophages that kill the pathogen. It is about 80% protective in serious forms of tuberculosis such as meningitis in children as has been used in mass immunisation by WHO.

Test your knowledge on Ziehl-Neelsen (ZN) Staining

QUESTIONS

1. What is the primary dye in ZN stain?

2. What is the role of phenol in carbol-fuchsin solution?

3. What makes a mycobacterium acid fast?

4. What are different decolourisers commonly used in acid-fast staining method?

5. Enumerate the acid fast objects in microscopy?

6. Why hot and steaming carbol fuchsin is used to stain Mycobacterium?

7. Briefly describe Kinyoun's modification of acid-fast staining method.

8. What is the decolouriser used to stain **M. leprae**?

9. In cold abscess, does smear examination shows acid-fast bacillus?

10. How sensitive is Z.N. stained smear examination to detect A.F.B. in sputum?

11. How can you increase the sensitivity of detection of A.F.B. by Z.N. stain in sputum sample?

12. What is the alternative better method of Z.N. stain?

13. How can you grade the AFB positivity of a smear (or what is bacteriological index)?

14. What is morphological index of AFB in smear examination?

15. How can you assess the progress of antituberculosis treatment by sputum smear examination?

16. Briefly describe the steps of Rhodamine-Auramine method of staining and examination of sputum smear from a case of pulmonary tuberculosis. Why it is superior to Z.N. stain?

17. Name the solid media used for isolation of *Mycobacterium*?

18. Name the liquid media used for isolation of *Mycobacterium*?

19. What is the generation time of *M. tuberculosis*?

20. How long it takes to appear visible growth on L. J. medium by slow growing *Mycobacterium*?

21. How long it takes to appear visible colonies on L. J. medium by rapid growing *Mycobacterium*?

22. What is the composition of L.J. medium? Mention the role of each component.

23. How L. J. medium is solidified and sterilised?

24. Why 'L.J. medium' or 'Dorset Egg' medium for growth of *M. tuberculosis* is prepared in McCartney's bottle?

25. What is the colony character of *M. tuberculosis* and *M. bovis* on L.J. medium?

26. Name two non-fastidious pathogenic *Mycobacterium* which grow on nutrient agar?

27. Name some photochromogenic *Mycobacterium*.

28. Name some scotochromogenic Mycobacterium.

29. Name some rapid grower *Mycobacterium*.

30. Name the tests employed for identification of *M. tuberculosis complex*.

31. How biochemically identity of *M. tuberculosis* and *M. bovis*, is established?

32. Name the battery of tests employed to identify the human pathogenic mycobacteriae.

33. What is the importance of heat resistant catalase test?

34. Name the different methods for decontamination, homogenisation and concentration of *Mycobacterium* in a sputum sample.

35. For microscopical examination only, which is the preferred method of concentration for sputum?

36. What is the advantage of NALC method over Petroff method.

37. How will you tutor patients, who are suspected to be suffering from pulmonary and renal tuberculosis for collection of specimen?

38. Mention the stepwise work-up to establish *Mycobacterium spp* as the aetiology in a sample.

39. How do you suspect the presence of *Mycobacterium* in a sample of C.S.F. by physical examination?

40. Narrate in short the method to isolate *Mycobacterium* from pleural effusion fluid.

41. Why animal inoculation with suspected clinical sample is avoided nowadays for primary isolation of *Mycobacterium*?

42. Stepwise narrate the animal inoculation procedure.

43. How does *M. bovis* differ from *M. tuberculosis* as regards *in vivo* experiment for pathogenicity?

44. How will you differentiate between *M. bovis* and *M. tuberculosis*?

45. Name the principles of rapid methods of culture for *M. tuberculosis* isolation.

46. Name the molecular methods available for detection of M. tuberculosis in clinical sample.

47. What is the antigen used for skin test (tuberculin test) for tuberculosis? What is the dose and procedure?

48. How do you interpret the tuberculin test result?

49. Does a positive tuberculin test indicates protective cell mediated immunity (CMI)?

50. Enumerate the conditions influencing Mantoux test result by producing false positive and false negative reaction.

51. Once negative, is it wise to recommend a second test within one month to verify the first result?

52. What is new tuberculin?

53. How CMI against tuberculosis can be assessed?

54. State briefly the events of Koch's phenomenon? Does any clinical condition mimic it?

55. Is there any vaccine against tuberculosis? Does it give full protection?

56. Name the conditions when B.C.G. vaccination may cause disseminated infection.

57. What is the latest development of vaccine against tuberculosis?

58. State the Runyon's classifcation of Mycobacterium with examples in each group.

59. Enumerate the common diseases produced by MOTT bacillus.

ANSWERS

1. Basic Fuchsin.

2. Phenol helps in penetration of the dye.

3. High content of mycolic acid in cell wall prevents the access of mineral acid decolouriser inside the cell causing retention of primary dye, or in otherwards imparts acid fastness to the bacteria.

4. 20% H_2SO_4 for staining most of the species of *Mycobacterium*. 5% H_2SO_4 for staining *M. leprae*. 3% Acid Alcohol for staining *Isospora, Cryptosporidium, Cyclospora* oocysts in stool. 0.5% H_2SO_4 for staining bacterial spores. 1% H_2SO_4 for *Nocardia*.

5. All *Mycobacterium spp, Nocardia,* peripheral part of granules of mycetoma caused of Actinomycetes, bacterial spores and oocytes of *Isospora, Cryptosporidium, Cyclospora* and many artefacts in stool are acid fast.

6. Mycolic acid and other waxes in the cell wall of *Mycobacterium* makes it difficult to stain. For better penetration hot and steaming carbol fuchsin is used.

7. Composition of Kinyoun's Carbol Fuchsin :

Basic Fuchsin – 4G, liquefied phenol – 8 ml, 95% ethyl alcohol – 20 ml and distilled water upto 100 ml.

Preparation of stain :

Basic fuchsin is dissolved in alcohol while grinding in mortar and pestle. Water is added slowly with constant mixing. Then 8 ml liquefied phenol is added. Prepared stain is filtered before use.

Staining method :

- Heat fixed slide is flooded with Kinyoun Carbol Fuchsin stain and allowed 5 minutes contact at room temperature. If regular carbol fuchsin of Z.N. stain is used, contact period is 30 minutes at room temperature.
- Drain the stain, wash with deionised water.
- Decolourise with 3% acid-alcohol (conc HCl 3 ml and absolute alcohol 97 ml) for oocysts of protozoa, or 1% H_2SO_4 for *Nocardia*.
- Wash
- Counterstain with Löeffler's methylene blue (methylene blue 0.24G, Rectified spirit 10 ml, Distilled water 90 ml). Wash and air dry.
- Examine under oil-immersion lens.

8. See answer to Q. 4.

9. It is very rare to demonstrate AFB in cold abscess, although the aetiology is *Mycobacterium tuberculosis complex*.

10. Sensitivity is low in direct smear examination. It is estimated that at least 10,000 bacillus/ml requires to be present to detect by Z.N. stained smear examination.

11. By concentrating the bacilli in the sample the sensitivity could be increased to 6000 baillus/ml.

12. Auramine-Rhodamine Fluorochrome stain.

13. Bacteriological index (according to C.D.C. Atlanta) :

1–2 bacillius/300 field	—	Doubtful
1–9/100 field	—	1+
1–9/10 field	—	2+
1–9/field	—	3+
> 9/field	—	4+

14. Morphological index is the percentage of solid (viable) bacillus.

15. Progress is indicated by decrease in bacteriological index in smear.

16. Staining method :

- Heat fix the slide at 80 °C for 15 minutes.
- Stain for 15-20 minutes at room temperature by auramine-rhodamine staining reagent.
- Drain the stain and wash with deionised water.
- Decolourise with 0.5% conc. HCl in 70% Alcohol for 2-3 minutes.
- Wash
- Counterstain with 0.5% potassium permanganate for 2-4 min.
- Wash and air dry.

Superiority —

Stained fluorescent bacilli stand out brightly, so fields could be examined under low power magnification. Thus sensitivity is more (about 3000 bacillus/ml) than conventional Z.N. stain method.

17. Egg based : Löwenstein-Jensen medium (LJ), LJ Gruft, LJ with pyruvic acid, LJ with iron,
Dorset egg medium.

Agar based : Middle brook 7-H-10, MB 7-H-10 selective.
Middle brook 7-H-11, MB 7-H-11 selective.

18. Middle brook 7-H-9 broth, Kirschner medium, BACTEC 12B medium, Septi-Chek AFB.

19. It is a slow growing bacteria. Doubling time is about 18 hours.

20. Minimum period – 4 weeks. Usually 6 weeks.

21. Within 7 days.

22. Composition : See chapter 19.

23. By inspissation :

1st day at 85°C for 1 hour. Keep overnight at room temperature. 2nd and 3rd day at 85°C for 30 minutes.

24. Screw capped bottles prevent drying of medium during long incubation.

25. *M. tuberculosis* —dry, rough, tough and buff coloured.

M. bovis— flat, smooth, moist and white, breaking up easily when touched. *M bovis* is sparsely grown (dysgonic growth) as compared to a luxuriant growth (eugonic growth) of *M. tuberculosis*.

26. *Mycobacterium chelonae* and *M. fortuitum*.

27. *M.kansasii, M. asiaticum, M. marinum, M simiae.*

28. *M. scrofulaceum, M. gordonae, M. szulgai.*

29. *M. fortuitum, M. chelonae, M. smegmatis, M. abscessus.*

30. Tests performed : Ability to grow at 37°, Rate of growth (all slow growth), colony type, Niacin test, growth on TCH (10 μg/mL), Nitratase test.

31. *M. tuberculosis* is positive in Niacin test, Nitratatase test and resistant TCH. *M. bovis* produce *opposite* result.

32. Optimal temperature of growth (37°C, 22°C, 42°C), rate of growth (slow growth/rapid grower), pigment production (in light and dark), catalase test at 68°C, Niacin test, Aryl-sulphatase test in 3 days, Nitratase test, urease test, growth on MacConkey's agar, pyrazinamidase in 4 days, Tween 80 hydrolysis.

33. Normally *M. tuberculosis complex* shows negative result. But INH resistant strains show + ve in the test.

34. *Methods* : (a) For sputum, urine and wound:

(i) Petroff's method (NaOH method), (ii) N-acetyl-L-cysteine (NALC)–NaOH method and (iii) Zephiran-trisodium phosphate method.

(b) Faecal specimen — NALC-NaOH, or 5% oxalic acid methods.

35. 10% Na (OCl) Cl [sodium hypochlorite or liquid bleach] method — which liquefies as well as kills the bacteria.

36. 4% NaOH in Petroff's method is very corrosive and kills a large percentage of *Mycobacteria* present in sample too. In NALC-NaOH, NaOH used is 2% and contact time is 15 minutes, thus reducing the deleterious effect of NaOH. Moreover, use of buffer and bovine serum albumin as neutralising agents, protect live *Mycobacterium*.

37. (a) Collection of sputum — Patient is to be insisted on collection of whole of first morning samples of real coughed up material unmixed with saliva for 3 consecutive days or in a scheme of spot - morning-spot samples.

(b) Collection of urine — In sterile containers, 3 consecutive whole of first morning samples are to be collected.

38. Steps : (i) Collection, preservation (if required in refrigerator at 8°C) and transport to the laboratory. (ii) Decontamination, liquefaction and concentration of sample. (iii) Concentrated material is used for microscopy (by Z.N. or fluorochrome staining) and culture in both liquid and solid medium made selective using a cocktail of antibiotics. (iv) Incubation is done at 37°C, 22°C and 41°C in dark and light. (v) Any growth appear, is confirmed by Z.N. stained morphology and identification tests (see Ans. to Q. 32).

39. On standing in a test tube, C.S.F. sample may show a cob-web.

40. Collection — About 250 ml fluid is collected aseptically using 1 mg/mL EDTA or 0.1 mg/mL heparin. Medium and inoculation — whole material is inoculated in double strength Sula's or Dubo's medium. After enrichment for 4 weeks, the whole material is centrifuged and the deposit is used for growth on solid medium.

41. Reasons : (i) Animal ethical committee forbids animal experiment, where alternative methods are available. (ii) Use of BACTEC or Septi-chek method greatly improved culture procedures. (iii) Indirect method by molecular techniques (eg. INNO-LiPA) are also available for detection of *Mycobacterium* in clinical sample. (iv) Animal experiment is a threat to biosafety unless done under proper containment measures.

42. Animal model : 12 weeks old healthy guinea pig. Weigh first.

Inoculum size : 0.5 ml of bacterial suspension in normal saline.

Site of inoculation : Intramuscularly over the innerside of thigh.

Observation : Take weight at weekly interval. Tuberculin test to be done after 3-4 weeks and autopsy after 6 weeks. Animal become positive to tuberculin test and shows progressive loss of weight.

Autopsy finding (after death or at 6 weeks) : At the site — caseation. Draining lymph nodes — caseation. Other organs like lung, spleen, peritoneum may show tubercles.

43. *M. tuberculosis* show progressive and fatal disease in guinea pig but no or mild lesion in rabbit, whereas, *M. bovis* is fatal for both.

44. See text page 406 (Table 40.5).

45. (a) *BACTEC 460 TB System* — Here the liquid medium contains ^{14}C-labelled palmitic acid. Multiplying bacteria releases $^{14}CO_2$, which is measured by scintillating counter. Radioactive index or growth index $\geq$ 10 developed slowly is considered positive.

(b) *Septi-Chek AFB system* — A biphasic medium. Liquid part is Middlebrook 7H9 broth-in a bottle. 3 sided paddle holding modified 7H11 Agar, chocolate agar and L.J. medium — hangs from the lid. Inoculation is done in liquid medium. The bottle is inverted regularly to inoculate the solid medium.

(c) *Mycobacteria Growth Indicator Tube (MGIT)* — A fluorescent compound embedded in a silicone sensor placed in selective MB 7H9 broth. As the bacteria multiplies and respires, O_2 tends to diminish. Lowered O_2 level increases fluorescence emission, indicating growth of bacteria.

46. Nucleic acid amplification technique proved its usefulness to identify *Mycobacterium* in clinical sample showing smear positivity. In smear negative samples molecular method is still not a promising one. Methods available —

(a) P.C.R. to detect *Mycobacterium* in respiratory specimen (e.g. Amplicor *Mycobacterium tuberculosis* test by Roche).

(b) P.C.R. to amplify rRNA (e.g. Amplified Mycobacterium Tuberculosis Direct Test by Gen-Probe).

(c) Reverse hybridisation line probe assay P.C.R. to detect and enumerate **IS 6110**.

47. Purified Protein Derivative (PPD), obtained from Seibert's strain of *Mycobacterium tuberculosis* is the Ag used for tuberculin skin test.

Dose : For India, recommended dose is 0.1 ml containing 1 U of PPD.

For Europe and USA — the dose is 0.1 ml containing 5 U of PPD.

For immunosuppressed patients (e.g. AIDS) the dose is 10 U of PPD.

Method of inoculation : Intracutaneously in 0.1 ml over the volar aspect of forearm. A bleb formation with orange peel like pitted appearance indicate right procedure.

Reading : After 48 hours diameter of induration and erythema is measured in two opposite direction.

Inference : Induration of more than 10 mm diameter is considered as positive.

48. See inference of 47.

49. No. It indicates that patient's active immune response was exposed to Mycobacterium Ag and he is primed to it and showing type IV hypersensitivity.

50. False positive result may be encountered in cases of non-tubercular mycobacterium infection or colonisation. False negative result (previously +ve, now turned –ve) may be found in miliary tuberculosis, Hodgkin's lymphoma, histoplasmosis, HIV (when 1U of PPD is used).

51. Within one month second test is not recommended. It should be deferred to 6 months.

52. See Textbook P. 402.

53. CMI is assessed by challenge using killed *M. tuberculosis* in : (i) Lymphocyte migration inhibition test, (ii) protective cytokine response by macrophage.

54. Koch's phenomenon — If an animal previously infected with tuberculosis bacteria is reinfected intracutaneously, a local inflammatory reaction marked by necrotic lesions will develop rapidly and heal quickly.

55. Yes, BCG. See text.

56. When BCG is administered in acute tuberculous infections and in AIDS. Hence it is advisable to administer BCG vaccine only in tuberculin negative individuals.

57. See textbook p. 408.

58. See Table 3.2.

59. See Table 3.2.

STAINING BLOOD FILM

Blood parasites such as plasmodia etc. are studied by Leishman's stain and Giemsa's stain.

Leishman's stain

Stain may be purchased ready for use (0.15 G of Leishman's powder dissolved in 100 ml of pure aldehyde-free methyl alcohol).

Staining techniquue :

Pour undiluted stain on air dried unfixed blood film and allow to act for one minute. Then add double the volume of distilled water on the slide by means of a pipette, mix and leave for 10 minutes. Wash slide gently with water and dry. Examine under oil immersion lens. Malaria parasites are demonstrated by this method.

Giemsa's stain

Stain is prepared by mixing different proportions of methylene blue and eosin. Ready-made stain is commercially available. It is a useful stain to demonstrate malaria parasites, Schuffner's dots and Trypanosomes.

Staining techniquue :

(1) Fix films in methyl alcohol for 3 minutes.

(2) Stain in a mixture of 1 part stain and 10 parts buffer solution pH 7.2 for one hour.

(3) Wash with buffer solution, allowing the preparation to differentiate for 30 seconds.

(4) Blot and dry in the air.

Culture Media : Identification

4

INTRODUCTION

Most culture media commonly used in the laboratory for isolation of bacteria are : **Solid** and **liquid** media (Tables 4.1 and 4.2).

Table 4.1 : Solid media and their use

Type of medium	*Name of medium*	*Composition and appearance*	*Laboratory use*
SOLID **A. Simple**	Nutrient agar	Nutrient broth + Agar – 2-3% It is semi-transparent and pale yellow in colour.	Routine culture
B. Complex (a) **Enriched** (i) General purpose	Blood agar	Nutrient agar + 5-10% sheep blood or horse blood. Two layers are present, one above the other. The lower layer consists of nutrient agar and upper layer of sheep blood. The medium is opaque.	General culture, *Streptococcus;* Most widely used medium.
(ii) Special purpose	1. Chocolate agar	Heated blood agar (75°C × 10 minutes)	*Culture of H. influenzae, N. gonorrhoeae.*
	2. Loeffler's serum	Nutrient broth, Glucose, horse or sheep serum.	Culture of *C. diphtheriae.*
(b) **Selective**	1. MacConkey agar	Peptone water, agar, bile salt 0.5%, lactose – 1%, neutral red. The medium is transparent. When finger is placed outside below the culture plate it can be seen through the medium as it is clearly visible, while the finger cannot be seen through the blood agar medium.	Enterobacteria, lactose fermenters produce pink colonies.
	2. Deoxycholate citrate agar	Nutrient agar, sodium deoxycholate, sodium citrate, lactose, neutral red.	Selective medium for *Salmonella* and *Shigella.*
(c) **Myco-bacterial culture**	3. Lowenstein Jensen	Mineral salt solution, glycerol, malachite green, whole egg.	Culture of M. tuberculosis.

Table 4.2 : Liquid media and their use

Type of medium	*Name of medium*	*Composition and appearance*	*Laboratory use*
LIQUID	1. Peptone water	Peptone — 1%, NaCl – 0.5%, water — 100 ml (pH – 7.4) It is colourless or slightly yellowish	Routine culture, basal medium for sugar fermentation tests
	2. Nutrient broth	Peptone water + meat extract – 1%.	Routine culture.
	3. Glucose broth	Nutrient broth + 0.5% glucose. It is yellowish in colour.	Blood culture, culture of delicate organisms.
	4. Robertson's cooked meat broth	Nutrient broth + glucose – 0.5% cooked meat medium	Culture of anaerobic bacteria and delicate organisms.

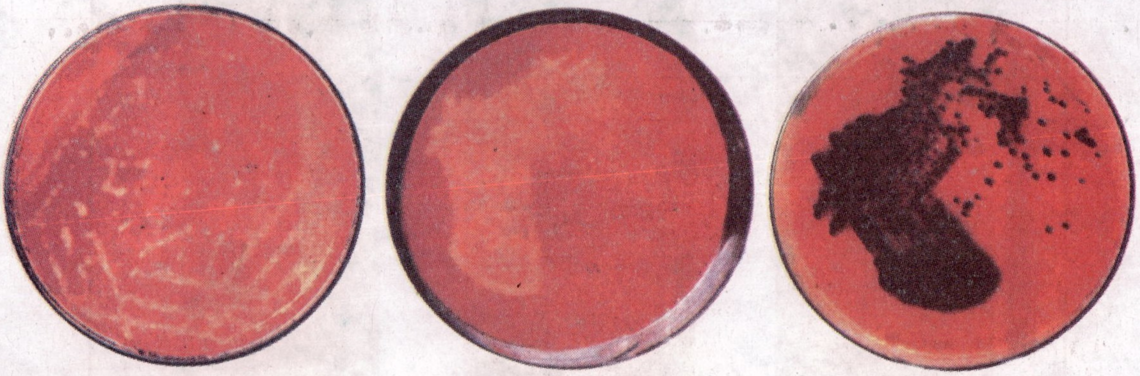

A. Blood agar medium with colonies of *Streptococcus pyogenes* (showing beta haemolysis)

B. Blood agar. Viridans streptococci (alpha haemolytic colony)

C. Colonies of diphtheria bacilli in blood tellurite agar

Figs. 4.1. A–B : Blood agar media with colonies of streptococci; C : Blood tellurite agar medium with colonies of diphtheria bacilli

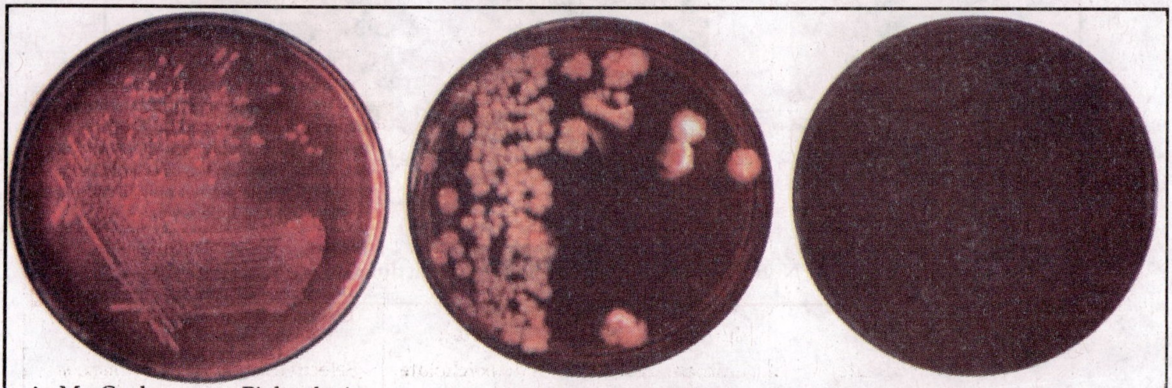

A. MacConkey agar : Pink colonies of *E. coli*

B. MacConkey agar with typical mucoid colonies of *Klebsiella pneumoniae*

C. Colonies of *Vibrio parahaemolyticus* on TCBS agar illustrating characteristic semitranslucent, green-gray appearance

Fig. 4.2. A to B : MacConkey agar with lactose fermenting bacterial colonies; C : TCBS agar with green colonies of *Vibrio parahaemolyticus*

Table 4.3 : Differentiating features of three solid media

Character	Nutrient agar	Blood agar	MacConkey's agar
1. Colour	Pale yellow in colour	Bright red (like blood) in colour	Pink red in colour
2. Opacity	Semi-transparent	Opaque	Transparent
3. Two layers in the medium	Absent	Present	Absent.

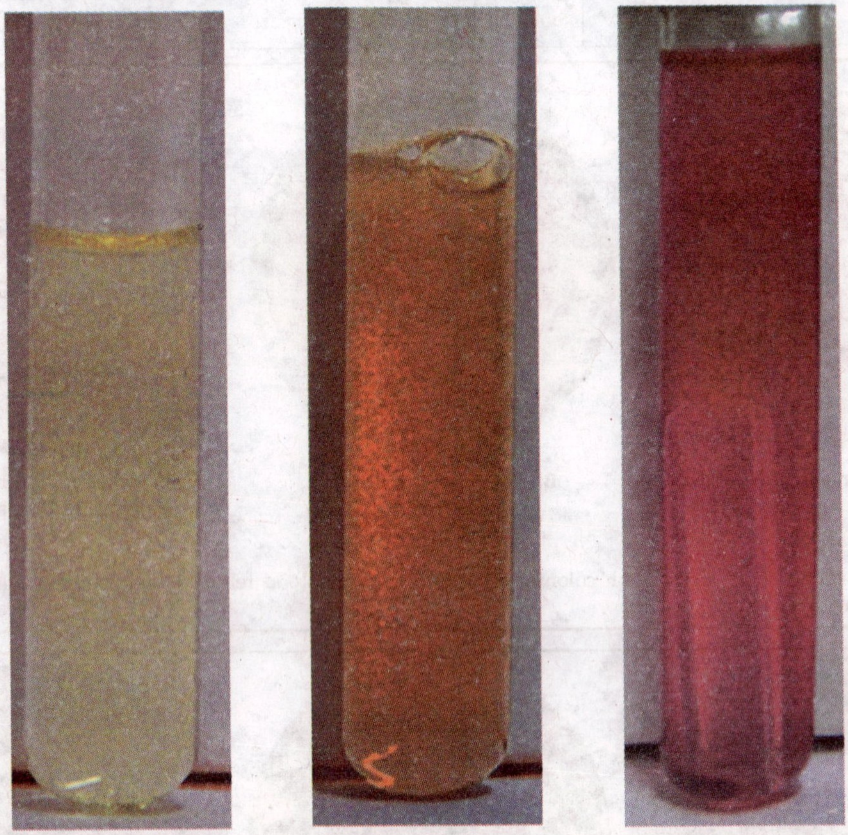

Fig. 4.3 : Peptone water, Nutrient growth and Glucose broth with different types of reactions

Laboratory Diagnosis of Bacterial Disease

5

INTRODUCTION

Laboratory diagnosis of infectious diseases involves the following steps :

1. *Specimen* : To be collected aseptically, at a proper time, inproper manner.
2. *Demonstration* of bacteria (in stained smear and motility preparation) and their products. (antigen, signature sequence of DNA).
3. *Isolation* : Culture.
4. *Identification* : Morphology, growth character, biochemical, agglutination tests and others.
5. *Animal inoculation* test.
6. *Serology* : Detection of specific antigen in sample and antibody titre in serum.
7. Molecular biological tests.

The laboratory reagents and procedure undertaken should be subjected to regular quality control tests.

Specimens reaching the laboratory should be properly collected, well-chosen and of good quality. They must be accurately labelled. If there is any special risk of infection associated with handling of the specimen, this must be indicated on the label (e.g. ***Hepatitis B*** or ***HIV infection***).

Transport of specimens to the laboratory should be made without delay. Some specimens (e.g. urine, CSF, sputum etc) provide a good growth medium for the *commensals* and *non-fastidious* bacteria and the latter outgrow the pathogens, particularly gram-negative bacilli. Non-sporing anaerobic bacilli and *Neisseria* species survive poorly during transport. These specimens are to be inoculated in relevant culture media immediately after collection. If delay is inevitable, specimens are to be collected in *transport media* or a special container to maintain anaerobiasis during transit. **Storage at 4°C** may be made when delay is inevitable and bacterial overgrowth is the main problem (e.g. urine). However, low temperatures kill some bacteria, e.g. *N. meningitidis* in C.S.F. Specimens required for different bacteriological tests and relevant transport media are listed in Table 5.1.

Culture and Isolation of Organisms

Bacterial culture provides isolation and identification of bacterial strains from patients' specimens, and also for assessing antimicrobial sensitivity. Cultures require a minimum of 12-18 hours of incubation before reports are made.

A. Culture media : Culture media employed for the isolation of common bacteria are shown in Table 5.2.

1. ***General purpose media*** : Blood agar is the most widely used media, and chocolate agar are used in special cases. Both media support the growth of most organisms. Colonial morphology, haemolysis, pigmentation can be determined from the bacterial colonies in blood agar.

2. ***Special media*** : Use of **enriched medium** (e.g. chocolate agar) facilitates the growth of some organisms (e.g. *H. influenzae*), **selective medium** (Thayer-Martin agar) for *Neisseria gonorrhoeae*, and **differential** media (e.g. MacConkey's agar) for culture of gram-negative enteric bacilli.

3. ***Anaerobic*** culture media (Robertson's cooked meat medium) are nutritionally enriched and pre-reduced of molecular oxygen to enhance recovery of anaerobic organisms (Clostridium) from specimens of patients and environment. RCM does not support growth of Non Clostridium anaerobes, which requires pre-reduced laked blood agar supplemented with vit K_1, haemin cystein.

Table 5.1 : Type of specimens to be collected and their storage

Specimen	Collection	Storage and transport
Urine (pyogenic organisms)	Mid-stream specimen.	Fresh sample is preferable. If delay is inevitable, to store at 4°C, slide coated with solid medium (e.g. MacConkey agar) is dipped in urine and placed in a sterile container for transport.
Urine (AFB)	First morning samples on three consecutive days	Refrigeration
Faeces (bacillary dysentery)	In sterile glass or plastic container, fresh sample is to be collected	Fresh sample should be plated without delay. If it is impossible, faeces or mucus to be collected into a 30% buffered glycerol saline solution in suspected case of bacillary dysentery.
Faeces (cholera)	Rectal swab or faecal swab is collected	When sample is to be transported in laboratory at a distant place, specimen to be transported in alkaline peptone water, or Venkatraman-Ramakrishnan medium. Swab is transported in Cary-Blair transport medium.
Sputum (pyogens)	Morning sample in a wide-mouthed sterile container	Specimen to be freshly plated after liquefaction by freshly prepared dithiothreitol (1%) solution followed by dilution in normal saline (1 : 10, 1 : 100, 1 : 1000).
Sputum (AFB)	Specimen collected on 3 consecutive days, morning samples	Specimen is concentrated before culture by Petroff or N.A.L.C. method.
Serous fluids (pleural, synovial, ascitic)	Fresh sample in sterile container	Citrate may be added to prevent clotting. For culture centrifuged deposit of 250 ml sample is used as inoculum in cases of pleural or peritoneal fluid.
CSF	Collected by lumbar puncture into a sterile container	Fresh sample is preferred. If storage is required, it is kept at 37°C in incubator.
Blood culture	6-10 ml blood aseptically collected	Specimen after collection is injected into each of two screwcapped bottles with a perforation in the cap to allow injection through the rubber liner; one bottle of 50 ml heart infusion broth for aerobic culture, other anaerobic media, prereduced brucella broth with haemin and vit. k.
Pus, swab from throat or wound	Specimen collected by sterile cotton wool swab	Specimen to be inoculated without delay. When delay is unavoidable, Stuart's transport medium (a sloppy agar containing a salt with reducing agent and sometimes charcoal) may be used with swabs. Swabs of specimen are placed in the tubes with medium. Delicate bacteria are preserved.

Table 5.2 : Culture media for common bacteria

Medium	Type	Application	Important constituents
Blood agar	General purpose routine culture media	Most widely used	Nutrient agar + 5-10% sheep blood.
Chocolate agar	Special purpose enriched	*Haemophilus influenzae*, *Neisseria* spp.	Lysed sheep blood haemoglobin.
MacConkey agar	Selective (Gram-negative bacilli); differential (lactose fermenters)	Enterobacteriaceae	Bile salts and crystal violet inhibit gram-negative bacteria; neutral red serves as an indicator of lactose fermentation.
Thayer-Martin agar	Selective	*Neisseria gonorrhoeae* *Neisseria meningitidis*	Haemoglobin enhances growth, four antimicrobial agents added to inhibit contaminants.
Charcoal yeast extract agar	Enriched	*Legionella*	Charcoal, buffering agents, and three antibiotics for inhibition of contaminants.
Löwenstein-Jensen agar	Enriched, selective	*Mycobacterium*	Egg enhance growth, malachite green inhibits contaminants.

Identification: The isolated organism is identified by :

(a) Presumptive identification by *growth characteristics* in media, gram stained morphology and motility test, oxidase test and catalase tests.

(b) Results of *biochemical tests* (carbohydrate utilisation, indole production, urease production, phenylalanine production, and nitrate reduction). Test media are inoculated with bacterial culture and incubated for 18-24 hours.

  (i) End products of fermentation (acid, gas production) vary with different species of bacteria.

  (ii) End products can also be studied by gas-liquid chromatography for identification of non-clostridium anaerobes and mycobacterium.

(c) Slide agglutination test with high titre sera.

(d) Test for toxin production.

B. Antimicrobial susceptibility testing: The isolated organism is tested for antimicrobial susceptibility testing for which the organism must be isolated in pure culture.

Microscopic examination

A. Unstained preparation: Unstained preparations (**wet mounts**) are useful in motility study of bacteria, examinations of deposits of urine, cerebrospinal fluid, faeces and vaginal secretions.

B. Stained smears/sections: Staining is the classic approach for making rapid presumptive diagnosis :

1. ***Common stains*** include *Gram* and *Ziehl-Neelsen* stains, and sometimes *Giemsa* and *Methenamine silver-staining.*

2. ***Fluorescent dyes*** (fluorochromes) : Bacteria stained with fluorescent dye become visible as a bright object against dark background when examined in UV light under a fluorescent microscope.

   (a) *Commonly used fluorochromes* :

   (i) Auramine rhodamine, that binds mycolic acid in mycobacterial cell walls.

   (ii) *Acridine orange*, which binds nucleic acid in bacteria and yeast.

   (iii) *Calcofluor white*, which binds cellulose fungal cell walls.

   (b) *Counter–staining* : When examination of stained smear it is necessary.

Stain	Counter stain
1. Auramine rhodamine	Pot. permanganate
2. Acridine orange	Pot. permanganate
3. Gram	Safranin, Acid-fuchsin, Dil (1:20) Carbol fuchsin
4. Z. N.	Methylene blue, Malachite green

C. Dark ground illumination (DGI): DGI, also called darkfield microscopy, uses a dark ground condenser on a microscope that illuminates the object. Bacteria is illuminated over a dark background.

Uses: This method is extensively used to identify spirochaetes in wet mount, which are too thin to be seen in 1000 x magnification (resolution < 200 nm).

D. Direct immunofluorescence (DIF) : To a tissue or cell suspension, fluorescein-labelled monoclonal or polyclonal antibodies against specific microbial antigens are added and allowed sometime for reaction to occur to be followed by washing with phosphate buffer. Antigen-antibody complex fluoresces when viewed under fluorescent microscope.

E. Culture, growth character, biochemical tests—are discussed in chapter 6 and 7.

Detection of pathogen-specific molecules

A. Detection of bacterial antigens are done by

1. ***Enzyme-linked immunosorbent assay (ELISA) (Fig. 5.3)***: ELISA kits are now commercially available and most tests use antibodies absorbed or cross-linked to a solid phase (e.g. a microtitre polyvinyl plate, polystyrene tube, a bead or a membrane) that captures antigen in a liquid specimen. The solution to be tested for antigen is placed on the antibody-coated well (or membrane) and incubated. After the antigen has been bound by the immobilised antibody, an enzyme-linked antibody of the same specificity is added to the mixture and incubated. The antigen, in positive case, is thus sandwiched between the first antibody and the enzyme-linked antibody. Then a specific substrate is added, which produces a visible (coloured) product if the first antibody has successfully captured the antigen.

Uses: ELISA kits are available for streptococcal antigens, HCG (pregnancy test), toxins (*Cl. difficile*),

C. trachomatis and many viruses. These rapid tests require only 10 minutes to 1 hour for completion and easy to perform. Their sensitivity is excellent (greater than 95%).

2. ***Particle agglutination*** : These agglutination tests use antibody-coated latex particles, which are stable for long periods of time. Soluble antigens in the specimen react with antibody-coated particles in the form of cross-linking resulting into visible aggregates.

The **Fc regions** of IgG antibodies are bound by latex particles or by protein A in killed *Staphylococcus aureus*, so that the **Fab** regions remain available for the antigens. These rapid tests are easy to perform and require only 10 minutes to 1 hour for completion. Agglutination assays can be performed with tubes or slides.

Clinical uses

(i) Latex agglutination test kits are now routinely used for detection of soluble antigens in urine, CSF and serum from patients with infections due to *Streptococcus pneumoniae. Haemophilus influenzae*, group A, and group B streptococci, *Neisseria meningitidis*, and *Cryptococcus neoformans*.

(ii) Slide agglutination tests are also done for rapid identification of organisms grown in culture.

B. Antibody detection in serum : Qualitative and quantitative Ab titre is detected by whole bacterial agglutination (eg. Widal test, Weil-Felix reaction, Brucella agglutination test), Latex agglutination test (eg. A.S.O. titre detection), Microscopic Agglutination Test (MAT in leptospirosis), ELISA (e.g. in leptospirosis, Vi-Ag detection), Slide flocculation test (e.g. VDRL test in syphilis), Ag coated R.B.C. agglutination (e.g. T.P.H.A. in syphilis), etc.

C. Molecular detection of microorganisms involve DNA probes and PCR.

1. ***Nucleic acid probe tests*** : Every species of living being has on its chromosome a unique DNA sequence that distinguishes it from every other species. **Gene probes** are cloned fragments of DNA that recognise complementary sequences of nucleic acid of microorganisms. These are biochemically synthesised or obtained by cloning specific genomic fragments into bacterial vectors (plasmids).

Bacterial restriction endonucleases cleave double-stranded DNA at specific oligonucleotide sequences and produce discrete fragments. These fragments are further separated to single-stranded fragment by electrophoresis.

Tagging probe with marker : The gene probe thus prepared is tagged or labelled either with radio-isotopes (e.g. ^{32}P), or an enzyme that gives colour reaction (e.g. alkaline phosphatase) after reacting with substrate. The single-stranded DNA probe recognises a complementary strand with which it hybridises under controlled conditions. An instrument that measures chemiluminescence emitted by a molecule attached to the probe is used to detect the probe-target hybrid.

Procedure : In the detection of an unknown micro-organism, its nucleic acid needs to be extracted before they can be hybridised with the probes. The target DNA is readily extracted with the help of NaOH.

There are three formats of nucleic acid hybridisation : *liquid phase* (hybridisation reaction in solution), *solid phase* (hybridisation in a fixed support such as nitrocellulose or nylon filter, e.g., colony hybridisation), or *spot blots, dot blots,* or *slot blots.*

Hybridisation in *liquid phase* is widely used. When a probe is mixed with test sample, it seeps out and binds to its complementary nucleic acid sequence. The double-stranded nucleic acid thus formed (capture hybrids) (Fig. 5.1) then gets separated from the rest of the sample. Multiple alkaline-phosphatase conjugates bind to the hybrid amplifying the signal. A chemiluminescent substrate emits light which is measured with a luminometer.

Clinical applications (Table 5.3) : A number of commercially prepared DNA probes for the identification of infectious agents are now available.

Table 5.3 : Diagnostic DNA probes available commercially

Group	Diseases
Bacterial	*L. pneumophila, Mycoplasma pneumoniae, Campylobacter jejuni, Helicobacter pylori, M. tuberculosis, M. avium, M. intracellulare, E. coli* (ST and LT toxins)
Viral	HSV types 1 and 2, HBV, Rotavirus type A, HIV 1 and 2

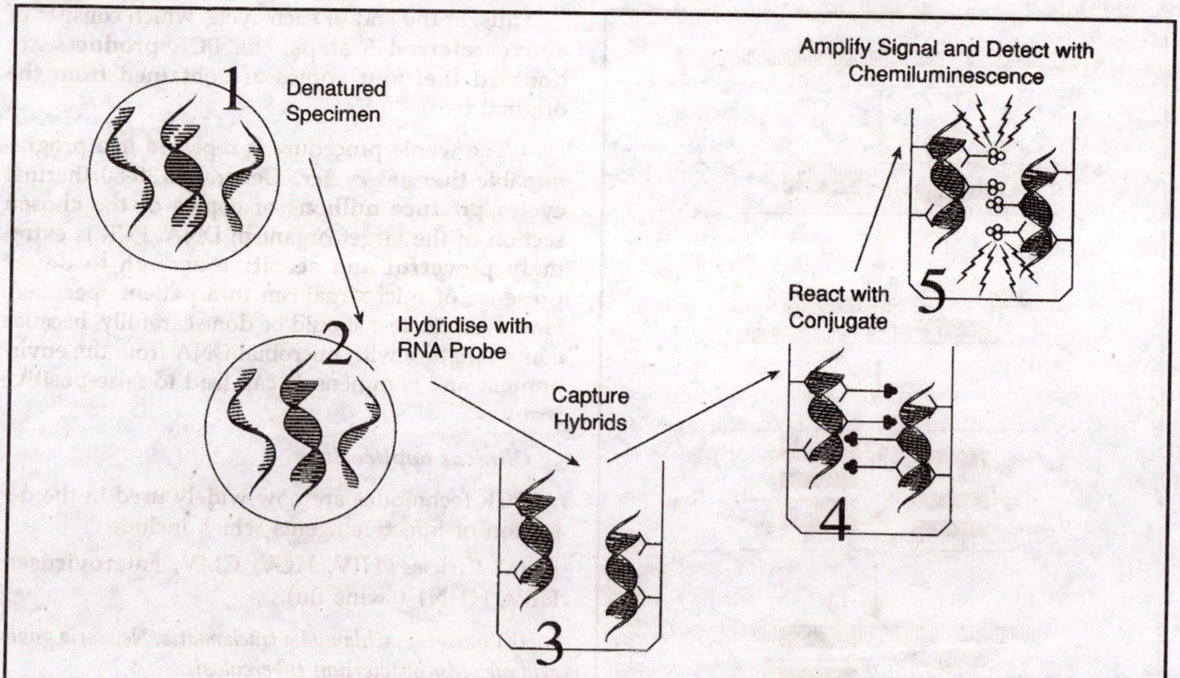

Fig. 5.1 : Digene hybrid capture system. Step 1, patient's specimen is denatured; Step 2, hybridisation of denatured specimen with RNA probe; Step 3, resulting RNA-DNA hybrid (in positive case) is captured by an antibody specific for RNA-DNA hybrids; Step 4, multiple alkaline phosphatase conjugates bind to the hybrid amplifying the signal; Step 5, a chemiluminescent substrate emits light that is measured with a luminometer.

(a) DNA probes permit rapid identification of bacteria in patient specimens where reliable culture systems are not practical, such as HPV, hepatitis B virus (HBV), Epstein-Barr virus, *N. gonorrhoeae* and *C. trachomatis.*

(b) These are useful culture confirmation probes in problematic cases, such as *Histoplasma capsulatum, Coccidioides immitis, Blastomyces dermatitidis,* and *Cryptococcus neoformans, Mycobacterium tuberculosis* etc.

Other uses of gene cloning: (a) Production of mammalian proteins, e.g. *stomatostatin, human growth hormone, insulin,* several *interferons,* and tissue plasminogen activator. (b) Preparation of **vaccines**, e.g. HBV, Rabies, *B. pertussis* and malaria.

2. ***Polymerase chain reaction (PCR)***: PCR has dramatically changed the technique of detection and characterisation of nucleic acids. The credit for development of this new technology in 1985 goes to its inventor Kary B Mullis (and associates) working at the Cetus Corporation and the Department of Human Genetics, Emerysville, California. For this discovery, Mullis was awarded the Nobel Prize for Medicine in 1993.

Principle : PCR is based on the ability of DNA polymerase to synthesise a large amount of specific DNA signature sequence from a single large piece of DNA. Primers required for PCR are usually synthesised using a nucleotide synthesiser.

Technique (Fig. 5.2)

1. Two short DNA primers, which are themselves short complementary oligonucleotides, are selected, which flank the portion of the DNA segment one wishes to identify. A heat-resistant polymerase (*taq* polymerase, extracted from thermophilic bacterium *Thermus aquaticus*), and free nucleotides are mixed together. The primers and nucleotides are present in excess.

2. The entire mixture is put into a special heating block (thermocycler), which raises and lowers the temperature to permit and regulate the three steps of PCR.

(a) *DNA denaturation step* : Two double-stranded DNA is dissociated to a single-stranded DNA at a denaturing temperature between 90°-95°C.

(b) *Primer annealing step* : As the mixture cools to approximately 50°-60°C, the primers will anneal

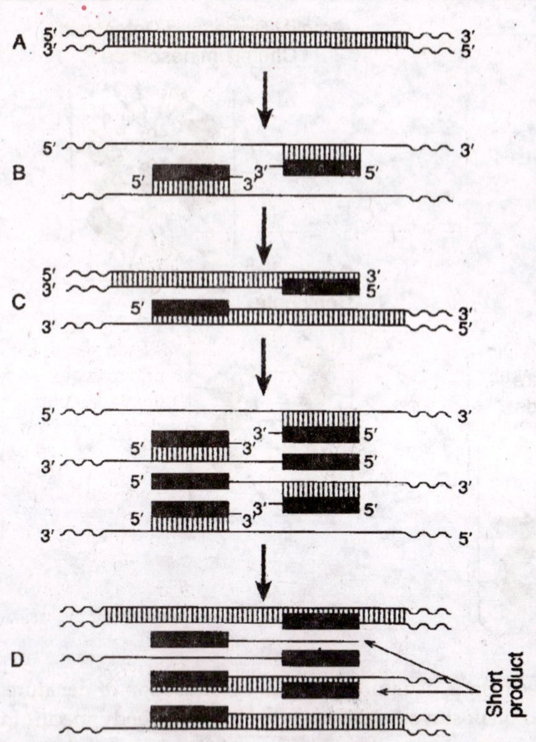

Fig. 5.2: PCR, *First cycle*: **A.** double-stranded DNA target sequence is used as template; **B.** two strands are separated by heat denaturation, and synthetic primers (solid bars) anneal to their respective recognition sequences in both the 5' and 3' directions (note the 3' end of the primers are facing each other); **C.** a thermostable DNA polymerase initiates synthesis at the 3' end of the primers. Extension of primer via DNA synthesis results in new primer binding sites. Net result is that the PCR product is doubled, i.e. two ragged copies of the original target DNA molecule; **D.** in the second cycle each of the four DNA strands in panel C anneals to primers (present in excess) to initiate a new round of DNA synthesis.

wherever they complement the target DNA strands (annealing temperature 50°-70°C). Their presence in large numbers ensures that hybridisation with primers will take precedence over hybridisation with homologous strand.

(c) *An extension reaction step*: In this step, temperature rises to 72°C (polymerisation temp.), the Taq polymerase adds exogenous nucleotides to the primers, which have hybridised with each original strand. Elongation — the addition of nucleotides in both the 5' direction of longer target strand DNA and 3' direction of short primer— results in the duplication of the target sequence in each chromosome.

Thus, at the end of each cycle, which consists of above referred 3 steps, the PCR products are doubled (i.e. four copies are obtained from the original two).

3. The whole procedure is repeated in a programmable **thermal cycler**. Generally, 30-50 thermal cycles produce millions of copies of the chosen section of the target organism DNA. PCR is extremely powerful and sensitive enough to detect presence of microorganism in a patient specimen. However, the test should be done carefully, because contamination with microbial DNA from the environment and commensals can lead to false-positive results.

Clinical applications

PCR techniques are now widely used in the detection of infective agents which include:

(a) *Viruses*: HIV, HCV, CMV, enteroviruses, HBV, H1 N1 (swine flu).

(b) *Bacteria*: *Chlamydia trachomatis, Neisseria gonorrhoeae, Mycobacterium tuberculosis.*

RT-PCR: Reverse transcriptase (RT)-PCR is a variation of the PCR, and it involves the use of reverse transcriptase of retroviruses to convert viral RNA or messenger RNA to DNA before PCR amplification. It has been successfully done with *Hantavirus* sequences as primers for RT-PCR to detect the agent responsible for an outbreak of haemorrhagic fever in New Mexico. The infectious agent was found to be a *Hantavirus*.

Detection of proteins: Some viruses and certain other infectious agents have been identified on the basis of certain characteristic enzymes or specific proteins, e.g. presence of reverse transcriptase enzyme in a specimen (serum, body fluid) or culture indicates the presence of retrovirus. Using sodium dodecyl sulphate-polyacrylamide gel electrophoresis (SDS-PAGE), different strains of virus of bacteria can be distinguished by the pattern of proteins of the concerned species of virus or bacteria. For example, the electrophoretically separated proteins of HSV will help to distinguish different types and strains of HSV 1 and HSV 2. Specific antibody to the electrophoretically separated proteins can be used in SDS-PAGE using a **Western blot technique**.

Serologic testing

In general, diagnosis of infectious diseases is made on the basis of detection of specific antibody to the infectious agent. The antibody titre reaches detect-

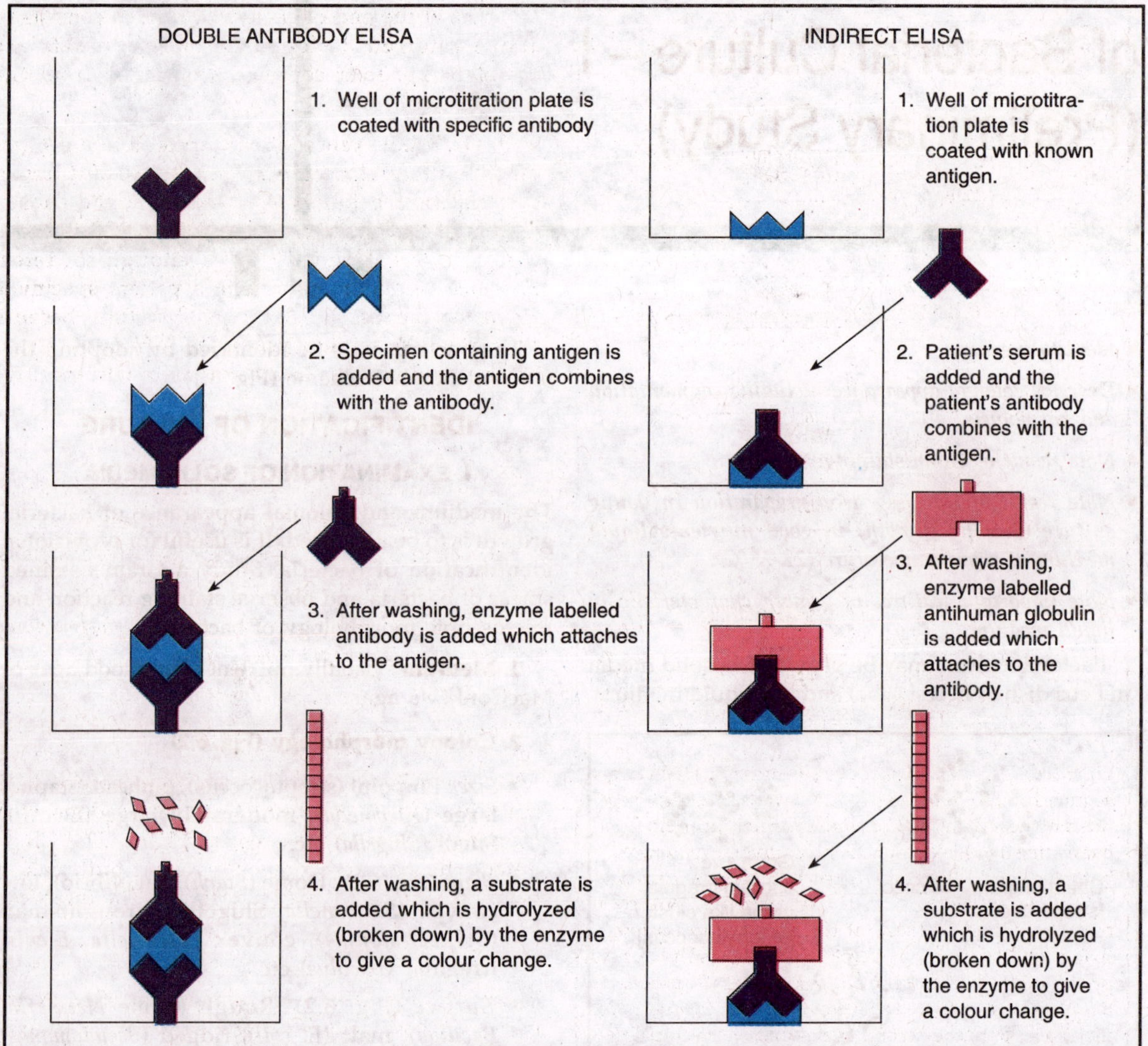

Fig. 5.3 : Enzyme-linked immunosorbent assay (ELISA test). This technique can measure serum Abs (A) or Ag (B) and depends on the ability of certain plastics (polystyrene, polyvinyl) to absorb proteins (Ags, Abs) strongly. Only the component added in step 1 is bound to the plastic, which is then coated with unrelated protein to make sure that the substances added subsequently stick only specifically to reactants rather than non-specifically to the plastic. This figure shows the EIA procedure for detection of antibodies against HIV-1.

able level usually after one week of onset of infection and then the titre rises. IgM antibody appears first and IgG antibody appears later. The following tests are most commonly employed :

1. *Agglutination test,* e.g. Widal in enteric fever, latex agglutination test in rheumatoid arthritis.

2. *Complement fixation test.*

3. *Flocculation tests,* e.g. VDRL and RPR test, routine screening tests for syphilis.

4. *ELISA.*

5. *Indirect immunofluorescence tests,* a fluorescein-labelled anti-human immunoglobulin is used to detect specific human antibodies bound to a known antigen, e.g. :

(a) Fluorescent treponemal antibody absorption test (**FTA-ABS**) in diagnosis of syphilis.

(b) Other commercially available indirect fluorescent antibody (IFA) test kits include *L. pneumophila, Mycoplasma pneumoniae, Borrelia burgdorferi.*

6. *Immunodiffusion* assays are mainly used for detection of fungal antibodies.

Procedure for Identification of Bacterial Culture – I (Preliminary Study)

6

- *Identify medium.*
- *Describe colonial appearance including pigmentation and haemolysis.*
- *Note result of Gram-staining.*
- *Note result of Hanging drop preparation in young culture (3-6 hrs growth) in good nutrients liquid medium at room temperature (22-25°C).*
- *Note important features of growth characteristic in liquid medium.*

Bacterial culture may be provided in solid media (in Petri dish or in test tube) and in a liquid medium.

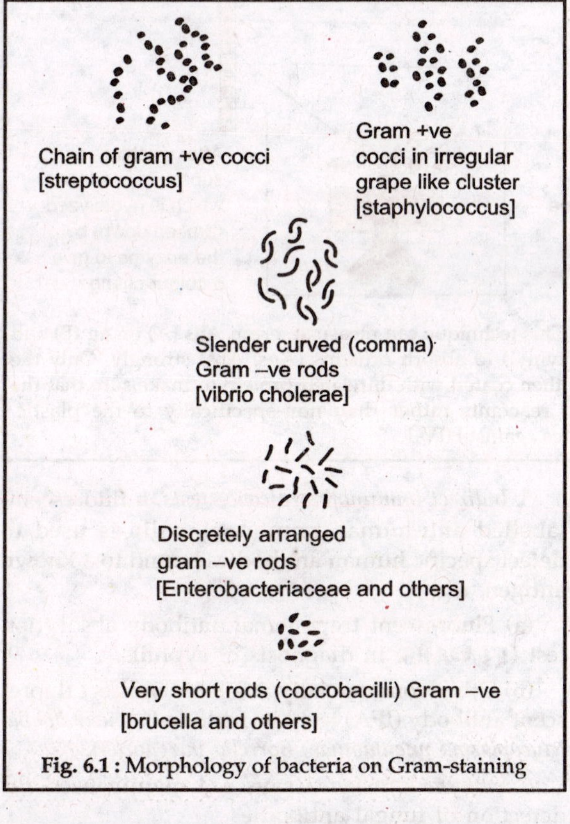

Fig. 6.1 : Morphology of bacteria on Gram-staining

The bacteria is to be identified by adopting the undermentioned scheme (Fig. 6.1).

IDENTIFICATION OF CULTURE

I. EXAMINATION OF SOLID MEDIA

The medium and colonial appearance of bacterial growth is to be identified. It is useful for provisional identification of bacteria. Study a Gram's-stained smear of bacteria and observe staining reaction and microscopic morphology of bacteria.

1. Medium : Usually nutrient agar, blood agar or MacConkey's agar.

2. Colony morphology (Fig. 6.2)

- *Size* : Pinpoint (streptococcus), pinhead (staph.), large (*Klebsiella*), moderately large (*E. coli*), Small (*Shigella*) etc.
- *Shape* (Fig. 6.2) : Dome (*Staph*), flat (vibrio), low convex (*Salmonella*, Shigella), droughtsman (*S. pneumoniae*), convex (*Klebsiella*, *E.coli*) irregular (*Bacillus*) etc.
- *Surface* (Fig. 6.2) : Rough (Some *Neisseria*, *Bacillus*), matt (*E. coli*), ridged (*Pseudomonas*) smooth (*Salmonella*) etc.
- *Margin* (Fig. 6.2) : Entire (*Salmonella*), irregular (*Pseudomonas*), crenated (*Bacillus*), spreading (*Proteus*) etc.
- *Translucency* : Opaque (*Staph*), transparent (*Vibrio*), semitranslucent (*Salmonella*).
- *Pigment* — Golden yellow (*Staph aureus*), bluish-green (*Pseudomonas*), brick-red (*Serratia marcescens*).
- *Pigment restricted to colony — Staph, Micrococcus, Serratia.*
- *Pigment diffused in medium — Pseudomonas.*
- *Haemolysis* — Beta haemolysis (*S. pyogenes*), alfa haemolysis (*S. pneumoniae*).

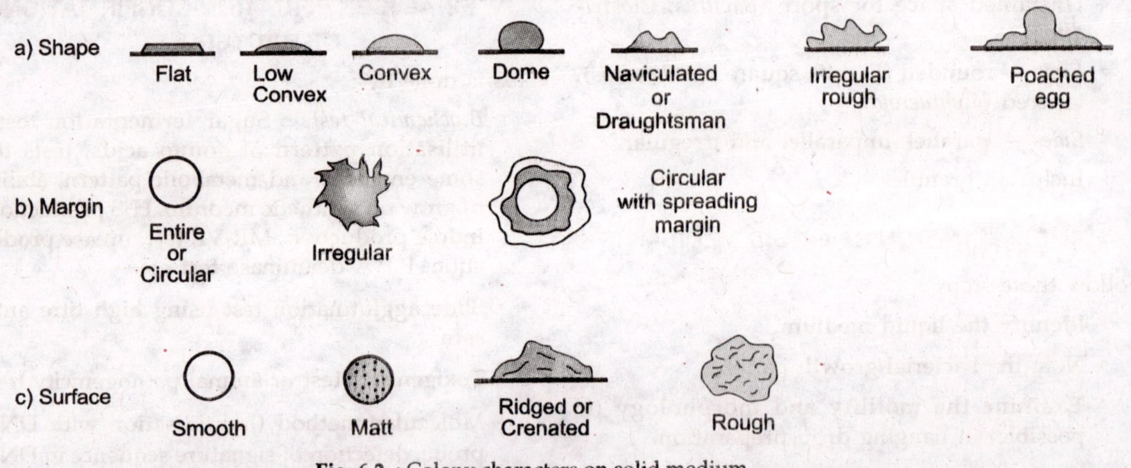

Fig. 6.2. : Colony characters on solid medium

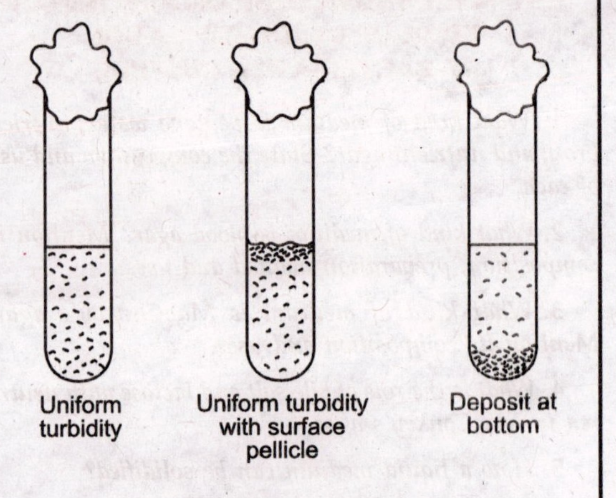

Fig. 6.3 : Growth in liquid medium

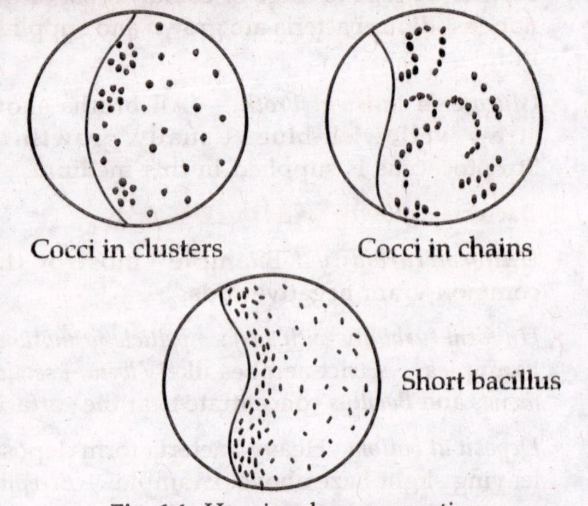

Fig. 6.4 : Hanging drop preparation

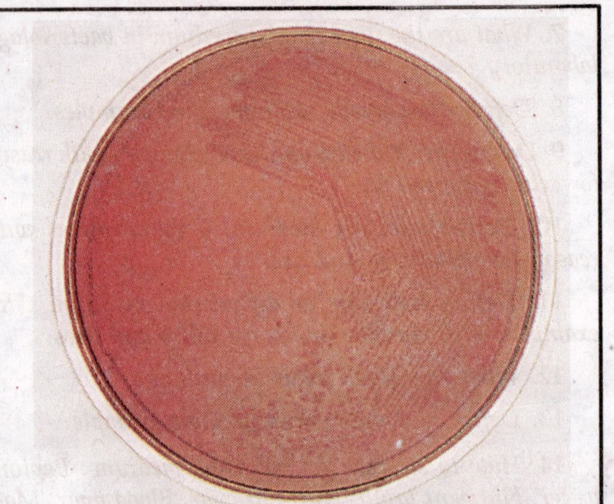

Fig. 6.5 : NLF in MacConkey agar

- *Haemodigestion* — *Proteus, Pseudomonas* etc.
- *Consistency* — Mucoid (*Klebsiella*), butyrous (*Staph*), friable (*some Neisseriae*), firm (*Bacillus*), Sticky (*V. parahaemolyticus*).

3. Gram stained smear examination

(i) *Staining reaction* : Gram-positive / Gram-negative / Gram-variable.

(ii) *Microscopic morphology* (Fig. 6.1) — Note the following :

- *Shape* — rod (*E. coli* etc.), spherical or cocci (*Staph* etc.), coccobacilli (*Brucella* etc.), comma (*Vibrio*).
- *Length/Size*— long (*E. coli*), short (*Klebsiella* etc.), large (*Micrococcus*), small (*Streptococcus*) etc.
- *Width* — stout (*E. coli, Bacillus*), slender (*Salmonella*) etc.

- Unstained space for spore (*Bacillus, Clostridium*).
- *Ends* — rounded (*E. coli*), square cut (*bacillus*), tapered (*diphtheroid*).
- *Sides* — parallel, unparallel and irregular.
- Inclusion granules.

II. EXAMINATION OF LIQUID MEDIUM

Follow these steps :

- Identify the liquid medium.
- Note the bacterial growth pattern.
- Examine the motility and morphology (if possible) in hanging drop preparation.

1. Identification of liquid culture medium

- *Peptone water* : No tinge of colour. Most of the non-fastidious bacteria are grown and supplied in it.
- *Glucose in nutrient broth* — All broths show straw/yellowish-blue. Usually growth of Streptococcus is supplied in this medium.

2. Bacterial growth pattern (Fig. 6.3)

- *Uniform turbidity* : Example – most of the common gram negative rods.
- *Uniform turbidity with surface pellicle formation* : Examples — Strict aerobes like *Vibrio, Pseudomonas* and *Bacillus* concentrate near the surface.
- *Deposit at bottom* : Heavy bacteria form deposit leaving slight haze above. Example — *Streptococcus*.

3. Hanging drop preparation

Note :

- True/active motility or non-propagative brownian movement.
- If motile, characteristic of motility (eg, darting and fish in stream by *Vibrio cholerae*, tumbling motility by *Y. enterocolitica* etc.)
- Morphology — rods are identifiable but cocci in cluster, discrete or in short chain are difficult to visualise (Fig. 6.4).

III. PRIMARY DIAGNOSIS

Colony character, medium on which growth appeared, pattern of growth in liquid medium, gram stained morphology and motility study generate clues for primary diagnosis and help to formulate scheme for confirmatory or final diagnosis.

IV. FINAL IDENTIFICATION/CONFIRMATION OF BACTERIA

This is done by :

- *Biochemical tests* : Sugar fermentation tests, utilisation pattern of amino acids, tests for some enzymes and metabolic pattern, ability to grow on synthetic medium, H_2S production, indole production, MR-VP test, urease production, P.P.A deaminase test etc.
- Slide agglutination test using high titre antisera.
- Toxigenicity test or animal pathogenicity test.
- Molecular method (hybridisation with DNA probe, detection of signature sequence in DNA and in 16S rRNA).

TEST YOUR KNOWLEDGE ON PRELIMINARY WORK-UP OF IDENTIFICATION OF BACTERIA IN A CULTURE

1. *What kind of medium is peptone water, nutrient broth and nutrient agar? State the composition and uses of each.*
2. *What kind of medium is blood agar? Mention its composition, preparation method and uses.*
3. *What kind of medium is MacConkey's agar? Mention its composition and uses.*
4. *What is the role of bile salt and lactose with neutral red in MacConkey's agar.*
5. *How a liquid medium can be solidified?*
6. *What are the uses of liquid medium in bacteriology laboratory?*
7. *What are the uses of solid medium in bacteriology laboratory ?*
8. *Define enrichment medium. Give examples.*
9. *Define enriched medium. Give examples with reason for selectivity and use.*
10. *Define selective medium. Give examples with reason for selectivity and use.*
11. *Define indicator or differential medium. Give examples with reasons for its speciality and uses.*
12. *What role NaCl plays in medium?*
13. *Define halophilic bacteria. Give example.*
14. *How to sterilise the following medium : Peptone water, Nutrient broth, Nutrient agar, Blood agar, MacConkey's agar, Müeller Hinton agar, Löeffler serum slope, Dorset egg medium, L.J. medium.*

15. *How to make a good smear of bacteria for gram stain morphological study?*

16. *What counterstains could be used in gram staining?*

17. *Define resolution power of a microscope. On what factors the resolution depends? Give the formula to calculate the resolution.*

18. *What is the resolution power of a light microscope using × 100 lens. What is the role of oil here?*

19. *What roles are played by Crystal-violet/Methyl-violet/Gentian-violet and iodine in gram staining?*

20. *What makes a gram +ve bacteria to retain primary stain and gram –ve bacteria to loss it when treated with acetone/acetone-alcohol.*

21. *How a smear of staphylococcus colony becomes false gram-negative or gram-variable?*

22. *How does cell wall of a gram +ve bacteria differ from gram –ve bacteria.*

23. *How many ways the motility of bacteria could be detected?*

24. *How to grow bacteria for demonstration of motility?*

25. *What is the organ of motility? How can it be demonstrated.*

26. *How examination of flagella help to establish identity of a bacterium.*

27. *Name some motile bacteria showing characteristic motility.*

28. *Mention the reasons for non-motility of a known motile bacterium.*

29. *What is the organ of locomotion of spirochaetes?*

30. *How can you differentiate between true motility and brownian movement in hanging drop preparation.*

31. *Enumerate the motile gram –ve rods.*

32. *Name the motile gram +ve rods.*

33. *Name the non-motile Enterobacteriaceae.*

ANSWERS

1. All three media are simple and basal medium. Compositions :

	Peptone water	Nutrient broth	Nutrient agar
NaCl	0.5%	0.5%	0.5%
Peptone	1%	1%	1%
Beef extract	Nil	1%	1%
Agar Agar	Nil	Nil	1.5–2%
pH	7.4-7.6	7.4-7.6	7.4–7.6
Sterilisation	Autoclave 15 Lbs; 15 min	Autoclave 15 Lbs; 15 min	Autoclave 15 Lbs; 15 min
Uses :	1. Basal medium for preparation of nutrient broth and nutrient agar. 2. To grow non fastidious bacteria for inoculum preparation.	1. Basal medium for preparation of nutrient agar. 2. To grow bacteria for motility test and tube coagulase test.	1. To grow bacteria to note pigment production. 2. Basal medium for preparation of blood agar medium.

2. Blood agar is an enriched (because of presence of blood) and indicator (indicates haemolysis and its patterns) medium.

Composition : *Nutrient* agar with 5-10% defibrinated sheep blood. Method of preparation : Nutrient agar is prepared first and the temperature is brought to 55C° by keeping it in water bath. Then aseptically 5-10% defibrinated sheep blood is added and plates are poured.

Use : (i) *To* isolate streptococcus and some other fastidious bacteria from throat swab, CSF, sputum, pus etc, (ii) to note haemolysin production of an isolate, (iii) to note pattern of haemolysis.

3. MacConkey's agar is a selective and indicator medium. It is selective for the presence of bile salt inhibiting all coliforms except Salmonella and Shigella. Lactose and neutral red is the indicator system in the medium; the lactose fermenting bacteria produce pink colour colonies and non lactose fermenter produce pale colonies.

Composition : *Peptone* 2G, NaCl 0.5G, Bile salt 0.5 G, Lactose 1 G, Agar agar 1.5 G, 1 ml of 1% Neutral red solution in 100 ml distilled water.

Uses : Or*igin*ally Mac-Conkey's agar was used to select out growth of Salmonella and Shigella from stool. Traditionally it is still used for urine culture when CLED is unavailable.

4. See answer in '3'.

5. A liquid medium is solidified by addition of (i) Agar agar, (ii) Egg fluid and (iii) Serum. Egg and serum needs inspissation.

6. Uses of liquid medium : (i) to grow bacteria for motility test, (ii) to grow bacteria for inoculum production for antibiogram, (iii) to note growth pattern of a bacteria for identification, (iv) to revive a bacteria from lyophilised or stock culture, (v) to study metabolism, toxin and enzyme production, (vi) for enrichment and transport of clinical material.

7. Uses of solid medium : (i) to study colony character, haemolysin production, antibiogram (by disc diffusion), (ii) to isolate causative bacteria from clinical material, (iii) to study pigment and bacteriocin production.

8. Enrichment medium is a liquid medium, which contains in its composition agent(s) which prevents growth of undesired bacteria present in a mixture of bacteria and allows or facilitates growth of desired bacterium, thus enriching the number of latter.

Example : (i) Alkaline Peptone Water — enriches the number of Vibrio and prevents the growth of coliforms in stool. (ii) Selenite-F broth — enriches the number of Salmonella in stool.

9. Enriched medium is the basal medium, fortified with blood or serum or egg fluid or yeast extract or special organic materials like 'V'-factor, 'X'-factor, haemin, Vit K_1, etc.

Use : Enriched medium is needed for growth of nutritionally exacting fastidious bacteria like Streptococcus, Neisseria, Haemophilus, Corynebacterium, Mycobacterium etc.

10. A selective medium is a solid medium which contains agent(s) to inhibit growth of undesired bacteria in a sample containing varieties of genera and thus selects out growth of the desired bacterium.

Example	Reason of selectivity	Use
1. MacConkey's agar	Presence of bile salt	To isolate salmonella and shigella from stool.
2. Salmonella-Shigella agar (S.S.A)	Bile salt, Sodium citrate, Sodium thiosulphate.	—do—
3. Thiosulphate Citrate Bile Salt Sucrose agar (TCBS agar)	—do—	To isolate vibrio from stool.

11. An indicator medium contain indicator system for indicating growth of certain bacteria.

Example	Reason for indication	Use
MacConkey's agar	Lactose and neutral red is the indicator system. Lactose fermenter-pink colony. Lactose non-fermenter pale colony.	Identification of LF & NLF colonies isolated from urine and stool.
Blood agar	RBC in medium is lysed by haemolysin producing bacteria.	Identification of haemolytic colonies of streptococcus, staphylococcus, Bacillus etc.
S.S. agar	(i) Lactose and neutral red — indicates lactose fermentation. (ii) Sodium thiosulphate and Ferric citrate — indicates H_2S production.	To note NLF colonies of salmonella and shigella. Salmonella produce H_2S too → indicated by black centered colonies.

12. NaCl in medium provides isotonic environment for bacterial growth.

13. Helophilic bacteria fails to growth in NaCl free medium, although it is isotonic or a solid medium. Usually a helophilic bacteria grows at or above 2% NaCl concentration in medium.

14.

Medium	*Sterilisation*
(a) Peptone water, Nutrient Broth, Nutrient Agar, Müeller Hinton agar.	(a) Sterilised by autoclaving at 121°C (i.e., 15 Lb pressure) for 15 minutes.
(b) Mac-Conkey's agar	(b) Except lactose & neutral red, all ingredients are sterilised by autoclaving at 121°C for 15 minutes. Then aseptically lactose and neutral red is added and the final composition is sterilised by steaming at 100°C for 1 hour.
(c) Löeffler's serum slope, Dorset egg and Löwenstein Jensen medium.	(c) All these solid media contain protein, so sterilised by inspissation.

15. • Place a drop of sterile normal saline on a clean grease free slide.

- Pick up a small amount of bacteria by touching the tip of an isolated colony.
- Emulsify the bacteria in saline drop with spreading the margin. Thus make a small (1/2" diameter), uniformly spread, not too thick nor too thin film.
- Air dry. Fix it by passing over the flame few times, taking care not to overheat to prevent charring.

16. Counter stains in gram method :

- Safranin 1% solution.
- Acid Fuchsin 1% solution.
- Carbol-Fuchsin solution diluted 1 : 20 in distilled water (it stains *Vibrio, Haemophilus, Brucella* better).

17. Resolution of a microscope is defined as the capacity, expressed quantitatively, to distinguish two very closely placed points as separate entities.

Factors influencing resolution :

(i) Wave length of light (λ)

(ii) Numerical aperture (NA) of objective

Resolution (r) is calculated by the following formula :

$$r = \frac{0.61 \times \lambda \text{ (wave length of light used)}}{NA}$$

18. Formula of NA = n Sin u (n = refractive index of the medium between object & objective, eg. air = 1, cedar wood oil = 1.5).

2 u = Angle of aperture

Theoretical limit of ∠ DAC = 180°C (Fig. 6.6)

∴ For oil immersion lens,

n Sin u = 1.5 × Sin 90° = 1.5 × 1 = 1.5

In practice it is 1.4.

$$\therefore \text{Resolution} = \frac{0.61 \times 0.55 \times 10^{-4}}{1.4} \text{ (cm)}$$

(λ of green light = 0.55×10^{-4}) = 240 nanometer

In practical situation < DAC cannot be 180°C. Therefore theoretical limit of resolution comes down from 240 nm to below 200 nm. In most of the commercially available microscope it is 180 nm.

Role of oil is to prevent divergence of light from objective.

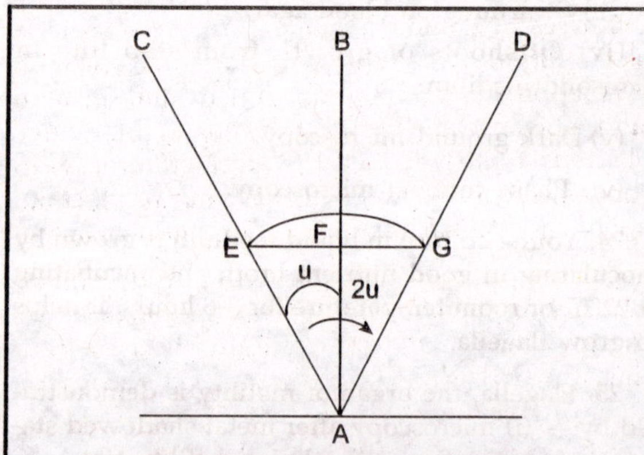

Fig. 6.6

19. Crystal violet/Methyl violet/Gentian violet – stains the cytoplasm of the bacteria. Iodine acts as mordant in the staining.

20. Knowledge about mechanism is still nebulous. There are more than one theories :

(i) Thick peptidoglycan cell wall of gram +ve bacteria prevents entry of decolouriser.

(ii) Gm +ve bacterial cytoplasm is more acidic one due to abundant mRNA to retain basic dye.

(iii) Dye-iodine complex actively blocks the pores of cell wall of gram +ve bacteria, preventing entry of decolouriser.

21. In old culture of staphylococcus, some of the bacteria might be dead or cell wall undergoing degradation. On the other hand, if staphylococcus is grown in presence of cell wall inhibiting agent, L-form may arise. In both these situations, primary dye cannot be retained properly when treated with decolouriser, resulting gram –ve or gram variable cocci.

22.

	Gm +ve	*Gm –ve*
• Structural complexity	Less	More
• Peptidoglycan	Thick (80 nm)	Thin
• Periplasmic space	Nil	Present
• Outer membrane of phospholipid bilayer	Nil	Present
• LPS in outer membrane	Nil	Present
• Ribitol-Teichoic acid in Peptidoglycan matrix	Present	Absent

23. Methods of motility test :

(i) Hanging drop preparation,

(ii) Craigie's tube method,

(iii) Swarming on blood agar,

(iv) Offshoots of growth from stab line in semisolid medium.

(v) Dark ground microscopy.

(vi) Phase contrast microscopy.

24. Young culture in liquid medium is grown by inoculating in good nutrient broth and incubating at 22°C, or room temperature for 3-6 hours. It helps to grow flagella.

25. Flagella, the organ of motility is demonstrated by — (i) microscopy after metal shadowed staining of smear, (ii) indirectly by motility test.

26. (i) Presence of flagella or motility is the morphological character of some bacteria, (ii) number of flagella, position, wave length are characteristics of many bacteria.

27. • Darting motility — V. cholerae

• Tumbling motility — Listeria

• Cork Screw with slow gliding — Treponema

• Spiral with sudden bending — Leptospira

28. • Growing the bacteria in solid medium

• Growing the bacteria in Phenol agar medium

• Growing the bacteria at 37°C

29. Axial filaments

30. True motility shows wide displacement having a direction. Brownian movement is to and fro movement without any direction and significant displacement.

31. *E. coli, Proteus, Providencia, Morganella, Salmonella, Citrobacter, Pseudomonas, Vibrio, Aeromonas, Plesiomonas, Enterobacter Alcaligenes faecalis* etc.

32. Clostridium tetani (except serotype 6), *Bacillus Spp* (except *B. anthracis*).

33. *Shigella, Klebsiella.*

Procedure for Identification of Bacterial Culture – II (Growth Specific Study)

7

Usually nutrient agar or blood agar or MacConkey's agar media with bacterial growth (Table 7.1) are supplied to students for identification.

Table 7.1 : Showing the common media with bacterial growth supplied to students for identification

Medium	Probable organism
(1) Nutrient agar *(Basal medium)*	(i) *Pseudomonas spp.* (ii) *Staphylococcus spp.* (iii) *Bacillus spp.* (iv) *Others*
(2) Blood agar *(Enriched and indicator medium)*	(i) *Staphylococcus spp.* (ii) *Streptococcus spp.* (iii) *Proteus spp.* (iv) *Others*
(3) MacConkey's agar *(Selective and indicator medium)*	**(A) Lactose fermenters** (i) *Esch. coli* (ii) *Klebsiella spp.* (iii) *Others* **(B) Non-lactose fermenters** (i) *Salmonella spp.* (ii) *Shigella spp.* (iii) *Others*

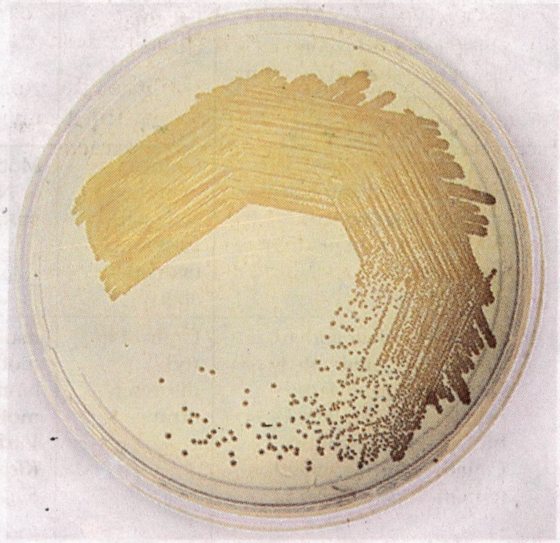

Fig. 7.1 : *Staphylococcus spp.* on Nutrient agar

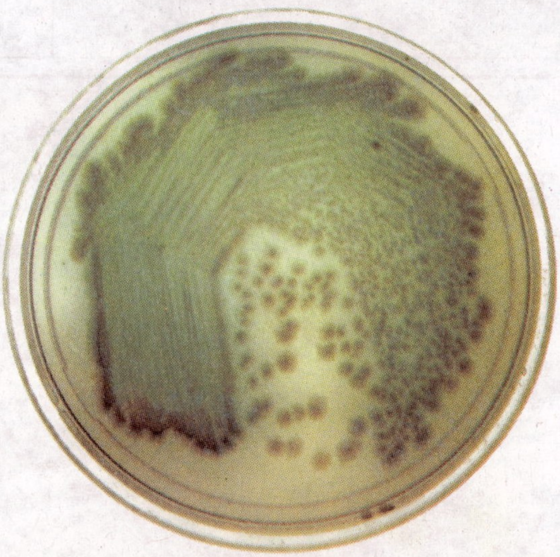

Fig. 7.2 : *Pseudomonas spp.* on Nutrient agar

Diagnostic methods used for the identification of specific organisms are described here. Students are provided with the bacterial growth on one of the solid media mentioned above as well as in the liquid medium such as peptone water or glucose broth.

I. GROWTH ON NUTRIENT AGAR (Table 7.2)

Steps to be adopted :

1. **Observe and record the morphology** of colony and pigment production in nutrient agar plate or tube. To identify a bacteria by its colonial morphology only, may not be enough. So a battery of other relevant tests are to be undertaken.

Table 7.2 : Growths on nutrient agar (aerobic incubator at 37°C)

Colony character	Morphology	Motility	Prov Diag	Further tests required
1. Bluish or yellowish green pigment diffused into medium. Margin-irregular. Surface-Smooth or crenated or rugosed. Semitranslucent. Fruity smell. Raised colony. In liquid medium-surface pellicle.	Gram –ve slender short rods, discretely arranged	Motile	*Pseudomonas Spp.*	Oxidase, OF or Glucose fermentation, Extractibility of pigment with water (*aerogenes*) or both with water and chloroform (fluorescein). Confirmatory test for *Pseudomonas* — vide Table A.
2. Dome shaped, butyrous, opaque, 2-3 mm diameter, golden yellow or white or non-pigmented colony. Pigment restricted to colony. In liquid medium uniform turbidity with deposit.	Gram +ve cocci in irregular cluster.	Non-motile	* *Staphylococcus Spp.*	Tests to differentiate the bacteria from *Micrococcus* and tests for species identification — vide Table B.
3. Large opaque, raised, irregular surfaced and margined, non-pigmented colony. In liquid medium form pellicle.	Gram +ve stout long rods with unstained endospore space.	Motile or Non-motile	* *Bacillus Spp.*	Follow the scheme of table 'C' to confirm two pathogenic species *B. anthracis* and *B. cereus*.
4. Flat or raised, or convex colony. Size moderate to large, smooth surfaced colony. Translucency — transparent to opaque. Usually non-pigmented (except *S. marcescens*).	Gram –ve rods, discretely arranged.	usually motile. Non-motile *Variants*: *Kleb, Shigella*	*Family* : • Enterobacteriaceae → • Vibrionaceae → • Afermentative Gram –ve rods → • *Stenotrophomonas* • *Burkholderia* • Pigmented *Pseudomonas* • *P. stutzeri* (these four →)	*O.F* / *Oxidase* / *Nitrate* / *Follow* F / (–) / + / Table D F / + / + / Table E No reaction / +/– / +/– / Table F O / + (except *P. maltophila*) / + / Table A

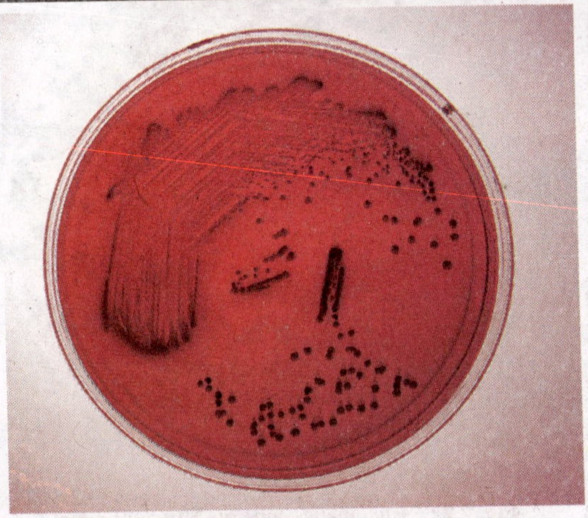

Fig. 7.3 : Lactose fermenters (non-mucoid colony) on MacConkey agar

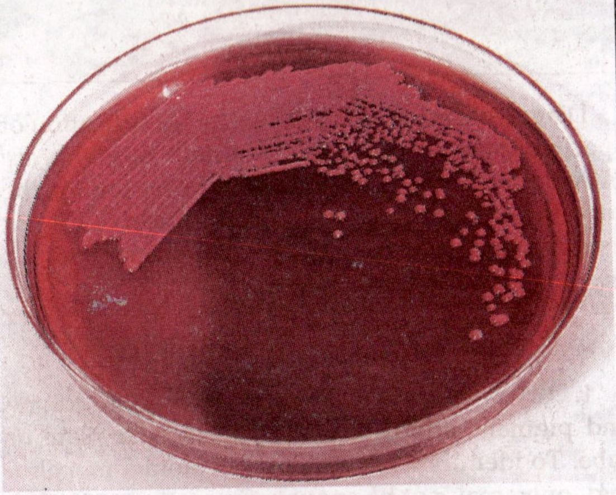

Fig. 7.4 : Lactose fermenters (mucoid colony) on MacConkey agar

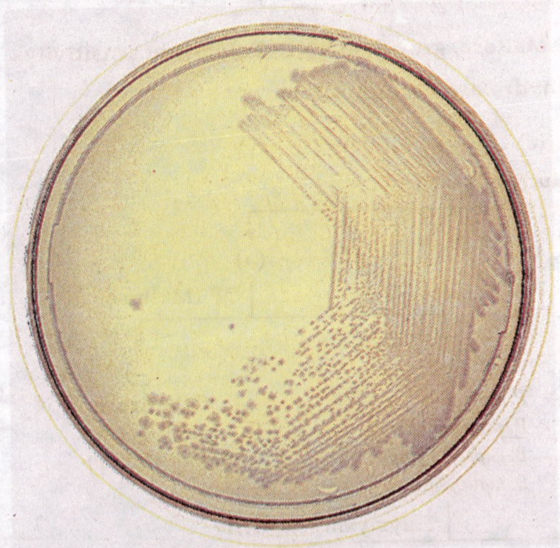

Fig. 7.5 : Non-lactose fermenters colony on MacConkey agar

However, pigment production, if present, may give some clue. Generally, bacterial growth with green pigment on nutrient agar is supplied. Pigment is diffusible in the medium in case of pigmented *Pseudomonas* (Fig. 7.2) whereas Staphylococcal pigment remains localised within the bacterial colony (Fig. 7.1), e.g. golden-yellow pigment in *Staph. aureus* and white pigment in *Staph. epidermidis*.

In ***liquid medium*** like peptone water, greenish pigment may also be present with surface pellicle formation. Surface pellicle (e.g. in cases of vibrio and Bacillus) indicates strong aerobic nature of bacteria as more oxygen is available near surface.

2. **Examine Gram's stained** smear and **hanging drop preparation**. Record your findings :

(i) ***Gram staining***: (a) Gram-negative rods

(b) Gram-positive cocci in clusters (Staphylococci)

(c) Gram-positive rods with or without spore

(ii) ***Hanging drop***: (a) Motile rods

(b) Non-motile cocci rod

Findings : The findings are recorded and Tables 7.3, B, C, G & H are followed to arrive at identity.

Table 7.3 : Identification scheme for bluish or yellowish-green pigmented colony on nutrient agar showing oxidase +ve

Test	Result	Inference
O.F./H.L. test	O	*Genus Pseudomonas*
Oxidase	+	
Extractibility of pigment with :		
Alcohol	–	*P. fluorescein*
Water	+	
Alcohol	+	*P. aeruginosa*
Water	+	

* For details of identification of *Pseudomonads* follow Table H.

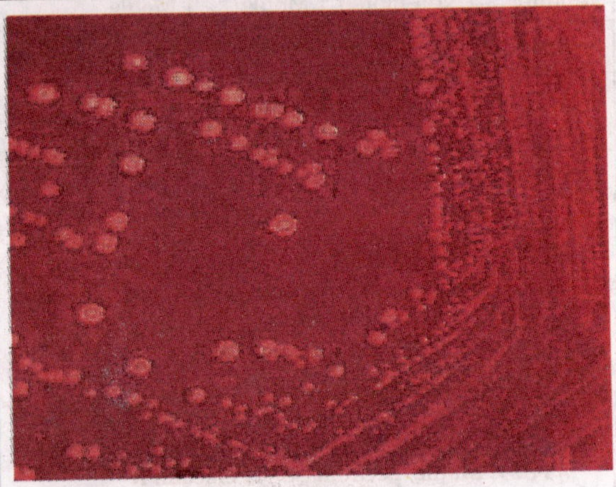

Fig. 7.6 (a) : Growth of *Staphylococcus aureus* showing beta haemolysis and golden pigment on blood agar

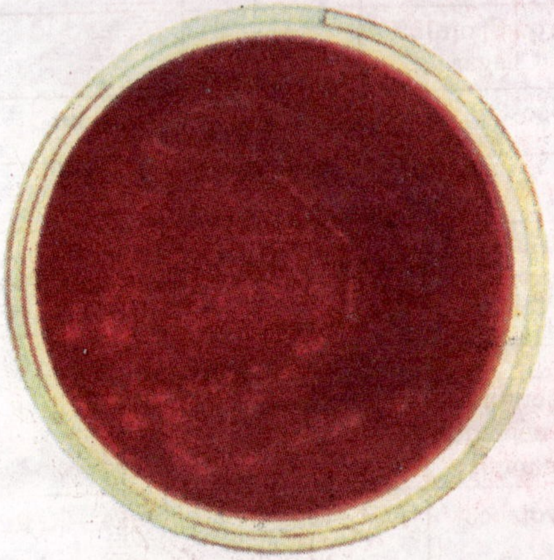

Fig. 7.6 (b) : Growth of *Streptococcus pyogenes* showing beta haemolysis on blood agar

TABLE — A : Identification scheme of *Pseudomonads*

(a) Tests to be done : Pigment production, OF-Lactose, OF-Maltose, growth at 42°C, Polymyxin sensitivity, Gelatin hydrolysis, Arginine dihydrolase. (b) Algorithm

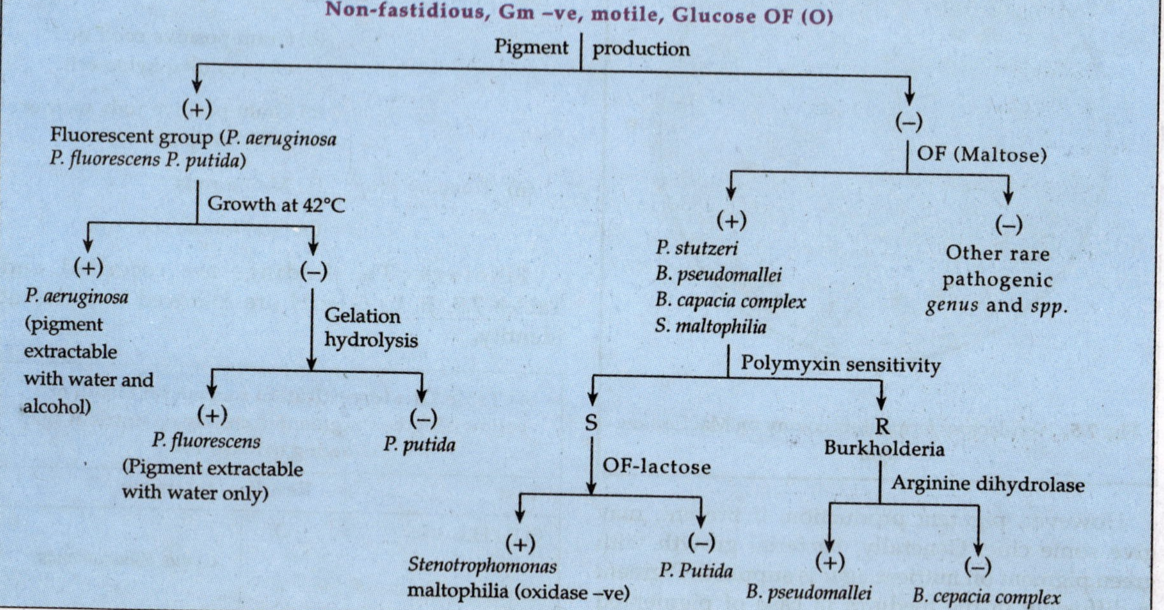

Table B

(a) Tests for differentiation of gm +ve cluster forming cocci grown on nutrient agar

Test	*Staph*	*Micrococcus*
1. Cluster pattern in smear	Irregular grape like	Packet of four
2. Size	Smaller 0.5–1 μ	> 1 μ
3. Growth on 15% NaCl agar	+	–
4. Lysostaphin	Sensitive	Resistant

(b) Tests to identify species of *Staphylococcus*

Test	*aureus*	*epidermidis*	*saprophyticus*
• Coagulase	+	–	–
• Phosphatase	+	+	–
• Anaerobic Fermentation of manitol	+	–	+
• Novobiocin (5 μg) sensitivity	S	S	R
• DNase	+	–	–

Table C

Identification tests for aerobic spore bearing gram +ve rods, grown on nutrient agar

Tests to differentiate pathogenic from non-pathogenic spp :

Test	B. anthracis	B. cereus	Non-pathogenic Bacillus Spp.
Motility	Non-motile	Motile	Motile
Growth on Egg yolk agar	No or weak precipitate	Wider zone of precipi-tation	No precipitation

Confirmatory tests :

- B. anthracis —
  1. Spore +, Non-motile
  2. Capsule +ve by Macfadyean stain — capsule + in clinical material and culture
  3. Ascoli's thermoprecipitation test +ve
  4. Penicillin – sensitive
- B. cereus —

  Spore +, Motile, Lecithinase +, Penicillin R

Table D : Identification Scheme of Enterobacteriaceae

(a) **Tests for family identity** —

1. Morphology — Gram negative aerobic rods.
2. Growth — Non- fastidious. Form characteristic colonies on nutrient and MacConkey's agar. In peptone water — uniform turbidity.
3. Motility — Motile or non-motile. Aerobic and facultative anaerobic.
4. Catalase + 5. Oxidase – 6. OF – Fermentative 7. Nitratase – Positive.

(b) **Tests for identification of common enterobacteriaceae** —

(i) Biochemical tests : Carbohydrate fermentation (glucose, lactose, sucrose, mannitol), H_2S production, urease, P.P.A, growth on Simmon's citrate, Indole production, V.P., ONPG.

(ii) Algorithm for identification :

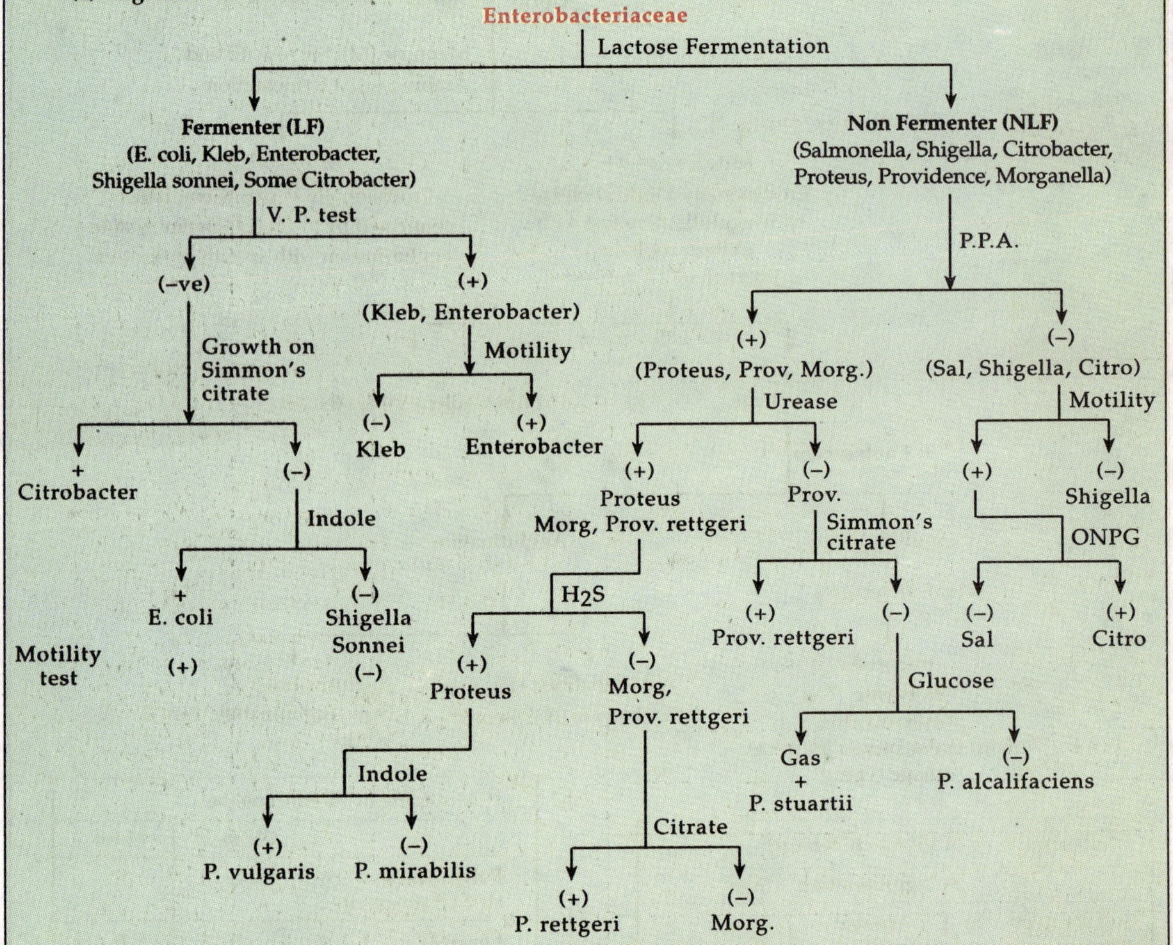

(iii) Further biochemical tests may be required for species level identification (see text book).

(iv) Serotyping, serovar identity and Spp of Shigella and Salmonella are identified by slide agglutination test using specific antisera. For *S. enterica*, Serovar Typhi and *S. Sonnei*, bacteriophage typing and bacteriocin typing are done for epidemiological typing. Serotyping, toxigenicity test (in vivo and vitro) of E. coli is needed for isolates from stool.

(v) For serovar identification of Salmonella follow table 7.6.

(vi) For species identification of Shigella follow table 7.7.

Table E : Identification scheme of Vibrionaceae

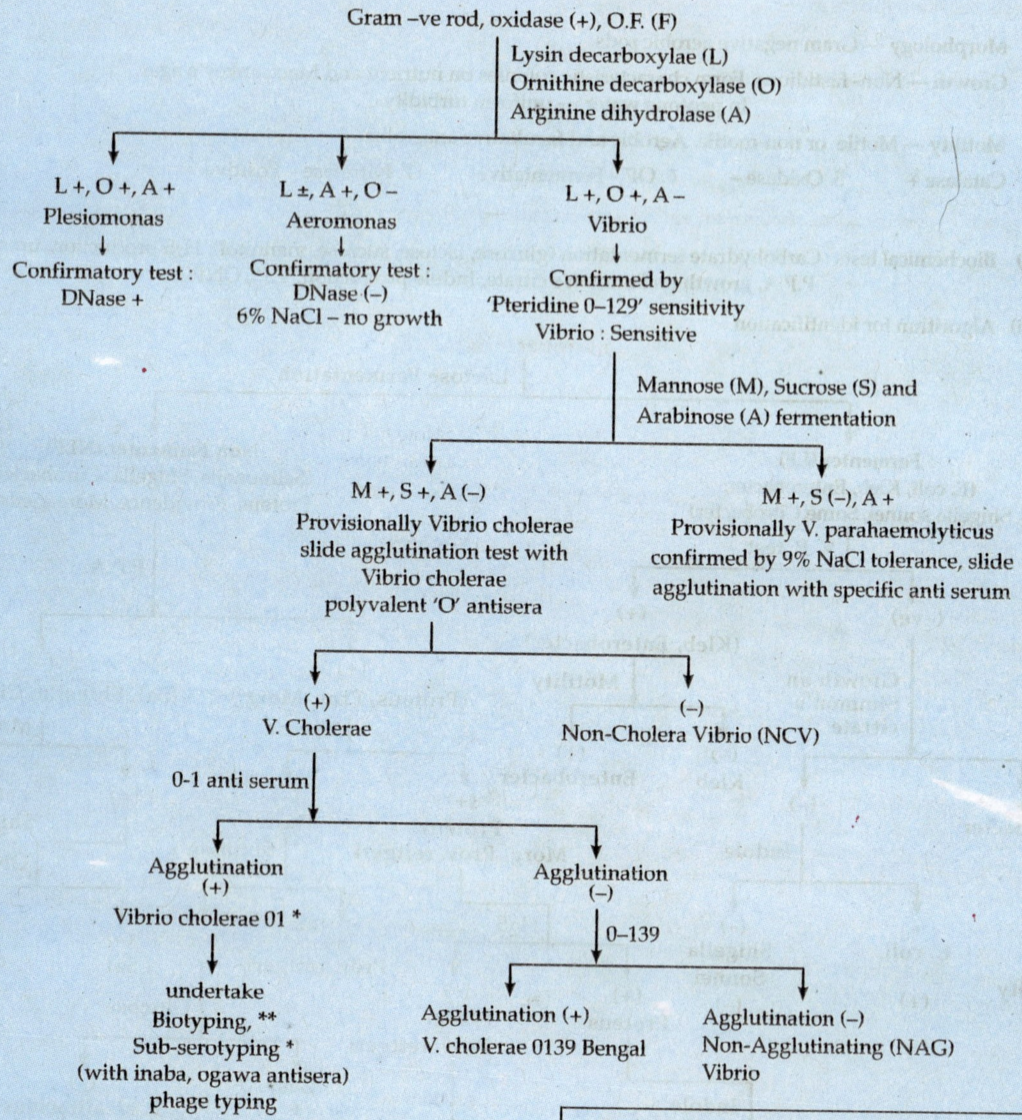

* Sub-serotyping of Vibrio cholerae 01

Sub-serotype	Agglutinating Sera: Inaba	Ogawa
Inaba	+	–
Ogawa	–	+
Hikojima	+	+

** Biotyping of Vibrio cholerae

	Classical	El-tor
Polymyxin B (100 U) sensitivity	S	R
Phage IV	S	R
Phage V	R	S
Chick RBC agglutination	–	+
Sheep RBC haemolysis‡	–	+
VP	–	±

‡ *By Filey-Pittman method*

Table F : Afermentative, Gm –ve rod (*Moraxella, Alkaligenes, Acinetobacter* and similar bacteria)

Oxidase test
- (+) *Moraxella, Alkaligenes*
  - Urease
    - (+) *Alkaligenes*
    - (–) *Moraxella*
- (–) *Acinetobacter baumannii* & similar others

Table G

(a) Test to differentiate *Streptococcus* and *Enterococcus* from other cocci :

Catalase test — Streptococcus and Enterococcus are catalase –ve . All other cocci are +ve.

(b) Tests for species identification of *Streptococci* and *Enterococci*. Note haemolytic character on sheep or horse blood agar, ability to grow on MacConkey's agar and 6.5% on NaCl agar, bacitracin (0.04 U/disc) sensitivity, perform CAMP test, bile aesculin reduction test and Lancefield grouping. Then follow this algorithm :

Gram +ve cocci in chain or pair

Ability to grow on MacConkey's agar
- No growth
  - Haemolytic pattern
    - Complete (β)
      - Bacitracin Sensitivity
        - S: *S. pyogenes* (Gr. A) Confirm by Lancefield grouping
        - R
          - CAMP
            - +: *S. agalactiae* (Gr. B) Confirm by Lancefield grouping
            - (–) Strepto GrC or Gr. G: Carbohydrate Ag extraction and Lancefield grouping by (any one) :
              - Capillary precipitation
              - Staph co-agglutination
              - Sensitised Latex agglutination
    - Incomplete (α) → see table below
    - No (γ) haemolysis viridans strepto
- Growth +ve by Gr. D Strepts
  - 6.5% NaCl agar
    - Growth +ive: *Enterococci*
    - Growth –ve: *Non-Enterococci*

	E. faecalis	*E. faecium*
(1) Hippurate hydrolysis	+	–
(2) Arabinose	–	+

Confirmation by :
- Hydrolysis of aesculin fermentation in presence of 40% bile
- PYR production

	S. pneumoniae	*Viridans Strepto*
Optochin (10 μg)	S	R
Bile salt solubility (40%)	Soluble	Insoluble
Inulin hydrolysis	+	–
Capsule	+	–
Mice pathogenicity	±	–

S = Sensitive R = Resistant

Table 7.4 : Growth on blood agar (aerobic incubaction at 37°C)

Colony character	Morphology by Gram stain	Motility	Provisional diagnosis	Further tests for confirmation
(a) Dome shaped, moderate sized (3-4 mm), smooth opaque, butyrous with non-diffusible golden yellow or white pigment. Beta haemolysis may be present.	Gram +ve cocci in irregular grape like cluster	Non-motile	*Staphylococcus Spp.*	Catalase +ve Follow table 'B'.
(b) Small (0.5-1 mm) pin-point, convex transparent or semi-transparent, colony with β, α or no haemolysis. Corresponding liquid medium shows deposit at bottom.	Gram +ve cocci in short or long chains or in pairs.	Non-motile	*Streptococcus Spp.*	Catalase (–) Follow table 'G'
(c) Colonies of wide range of sizes and shapes.There may swarming, haemolysis or haemodigestion.	Gram –ve rods	Motile or non-motile	• Enterobacteriaceae • Pseudomonads • Afermentative gram negative rods	→ Follow table D → Follow table A → Follow table F

Table 7.5 : Growth on MacConkey's agar with or without NaCl (aerobic incubation, at 37°C)

Colony character	Morphology	Motility	Provisional identity	Further test for confirmation
1. Moderately large, convex lactose fermenting (LF) pink colonies. Surface smooth or matt. Margin — entire or irregular. Usually non-mucoid.	Gram –ve stout long rods, arranged discretely	Motile	*E. coli*	Follow-D. Indole +ve MR +ve Simmon citrate –ve H_2S –ve
2. Large, convex, mucoid LF (pink), smooth surfaced, entire marginal colony.	Small, plump gram -ve rod, arranged discretely.	Non-motile	*Klebsiella pneumoniae Spp*	Follow – D. Indole –ve, VP +ve Simmon citrate +ve urease +, starch hydrolysis (–)
		Motile	*Enterobacter*	Follow – D. Indole –ve VP +ve Simmon citrate +ve urease + starch hydrolysis (+)

Table 7.5 contd. next page

Table 7.5 : Growth on MacConkey's agar with or without NaCl (aerobic incubation, at 37°C) contd. from previous page

Colony character	Morphology	Motility	Provisional identity	Further test for confirmation
3. Non-lactose fermenting (NLF), low convex or raised, semitransparent, very small (> 2 mm) to small (2-3 mm) colonies.	Small gram –ve slender rods.	Non-motile	Shigella	Follow-D
		Motile	*Salmonella* *Proteus* *Providencia* *Morganella* *Citrobacter*	Follow – D
4. Pinpoint (< 1 mm), Convex, LF, opaque colonies.	Gram +ve cocci in short chain	Non-motile	*Enterococcus*	Follow Table - H

Table 7.6 : Tests to distinguish of *Salmonella* serovars

Test	*Typhi*	*Paratyphi A*	*Paratyphi B*	*Paratyphi C*
1. Sugar fermentation • *Glucose*	A	AG	AG	AG
2. Simmon's Citrate	–	–	Growth +	+
3. H_2S production in TSI	+	–	+	+
4. Agglutinating factor serum	9	2	4	6, 7

+ = Positive; – = Negative; A = Acid; AG = Acid and gas

Table 7.7 : Tests to distinguish *Shigella* species

Test	*Sh. dysenteriae*	*Sh. flexneri*	*Sh. boydii*	*Sh. sonnei*
1. *Glucose fermentation*	A	A	A	A
2. *Lactose fermentation*	–	–	–	A →
3. *Mannitol fermentation*	–	A	A	A
4. *Sucrose fermentation*	–	–	–	A
5. *Ornithine decarboxylase*	–	–	–	+
6. *Indole*	Variable	Variable	Variable	–
7. *Serogroup*	A	B	C	D

+ = Positive; – = Negative; A = Acid only, no gas; → = Late fermenter

GROWTH ON ANY OTHER SPECIAL (SELECTIVE/INHIBITORY/INDICATOR) MEDIUM

Any growth on special selective/indicator/ inhibitory medium is to be identified by undertaking the following steps :

1. Identify the medium and think the bacteria which grows on it.
2. Note the colony character and any indicator of growth for any special genus, eg, sucrose fermenting flat yellow colony on T.C.B.S. agar indicates growth of vibrio.
3. Perform morphological study by gram stain or any special stain (eg. capsule staining, spore staining, Wayson's staining for *Y. pestis* etc.).

4. Perform motility.
6. Go for biochemical tests.
7. Tests for enzyme and toxin production.
8. Antigen detection by slide agglutination or capsule swelling using specific high titre sera (HTS).

PSEUDOMONAS AERUGINOSA

Pathogenicity

The organisms produce blue pus and pyocyanea literally means "blue pus". *Ps. aeruginosa* is an important cause of hospital-acquired infection. Most infections occur in patients with serious underlying diseases like burns and malignancy or as a result of therapeutic procedures (catheterisation, cystoscopy). Prior treatment with antimicrobials favour pseudomonas infection.

1. **Skin infections** especially in wound, pressure sores and burns.

2. **Urinary infection**, usually following catheterisation or in chronic infections.

3. **Respiratory infections**, especially in immunosuppression and cystic fibrosis.

4. **Ear infections**, e.g. chronic otitis media and otitis externa.

5. **Eye infections**, usually hospital acquired.

6. **Septicaemia** may develop in neonates and old debilitated persons, particularly in patients receiving cytotoxic drug or irradiation.

7. **Acute necrotising vasculitis** which leads to haemorrhagic infarction of skin (*ecthyma gangrenosa*) and of internal organs (liver and kidney).

Laboratory diagnosis

Specimens : Pus, wound swab, mid-stream specimen of urine, CSF, sputum or blood.

Culture : On MacConkey's agar they show pale, flat colonies with a spreading border. In nutrient agar or Mueller-Hinton agar there is diffuse bluish, greenish or reddish brown pigments, and a grape-like or fruit-like odour. Selective media such as cetrimide agar is useful for isolation of the organism from faeces or other samples contaminated with mixed flora.

Identification is made based on :

1. Characteristic colony morphology and gram-film appearance.
2. Grape-like or fruit-like odour of the colony.
3. Mucoid colony variants are particularly prevalent in respiratory tract specimens.
4. Biochemically, *P. aeruginosa* is confidently identified based on the following features :
   (a) Positive oxidase test (Table 7.10).
   (b) Triple sugar iron (TSI) agar reaction of alkaline over no change.
   (c) Bright green diffusible pigments on Mueller-Hinton or other non-dye-containing agars (e.g. N. agar).
   (d) Growth at 42°C.

Occasional strains of *P. aeruginosa* produce only pyoverdin, which would not differentiate them from *P. fluorescens* or *P. putida*. These latter species fail to grow at 42°C, while *P. aeruginosa* grows at 42°C.

STAPHYLOCOCCUS (S.aureus)

Pathogenicity

S. aureus is an important pyogenic organism and Box 1 shows the important diseases produced by the same.

Box – 1 : Infections caused by *Staph. aureus*

Group	Lesions
Superficial infections :	
Skin	Folliculitis, boil, impetigo, carbuncle, abscess, styes, pemphigus neonatorum, sepsis in wounds and burns.
Deep infections :	
Bone and joint	Osteomyelitis, septic arthritis.
Respiratory	Tonsillitis, pneumonia, lung abscess, empyema.
Intestinal	Enterocolitis.
Cardiac	Endocarditis, pericarditis.
CNS	Meningitis, brain abscess.
Blood stream	Septicaemia, pyaemic abscesses.
Toxin-mediated :	
Toxic food poisoning	Results from ingestion of preformed toxin with food.
Skin exfoliation	Stripping of superficial layers of skin from underlying tissue by exfoliative (epidermolytic) toxin.
Toxic shock syndrome (TSS)	TSS is a syndrome caused by enterotoxin F produced by some strain of *S. aureus*.

Table 7.8 : Some properties of *Pseudomonas* species

Organism	Oxidation of				Pyocyanin production	Lysine decarboxylase	Arginine dihydrolase	Oxidase
	Glucose	Maltose	Lactose	Mannitol				
P. aeruginosa	+	–	–	+	+/–	–	+	+
P. putida	+	–	–	–	–	–	+	+
B. pseudomallei	+	+	+	+	–	–	+	+
B. mallei	+	–	–	–	–	–	+	+/–
B. cepacia	+	+	+	+	–	±	–	+
S. multophilia	+/–	+	+	–	–	+	–	–

Laboratory diagnosis

Specimens : These are to be collected depending on the nature of lesion, pus from suppurative lesions, CSF from meningitis, blood from septicaemia, sputum from respiratory infection and suspected food, vomit or faeces from food poisoning.

1. **Smear** : Examination of a Gram-stained smear of pus and other specimens shows Gram-positive cocci in clusters with some single and paired cocci.

2. **Culture** : (a) Specimens are inoculated on blood agar or selective agar medium with 7% sodium chloride which inhibits the growth of most organisms other than staphylococci.

(b) Mannitol salt agar is selective and differential media for staphylococci. Mannitol is fermented by *S. aureus* but not most other staphylococci.

3. **Identification** : (a) *Coagulase test* : *S. aureus* is coagulase positive.

(b) Antibiotic susceptibility tests, biochemical profiles (biotyping), phage typing, nucleic acid analysis may be done for the intraspecies identification of the organism for epidemiological study to trace the source of staphylococcal infections.

BACILLUS

Members of the genus *Bacillus* are aerobic, spore-bearing, gram-positive bacilli arranged in chain. The spores are refractile, oval and central in position and its diameter is the same as the width of the bacteria.

Bacillus anthracis

Species

I. **Pathogenic** : (a) *B. anthracis* — causative agent of anthrax.

(b) *B. cereus* — cause food poisoning.

II. **Non-pathogenic** (saprophytes)

(1) Large-celled : *B. megaterium*, *B. cereus*

(2) Small-celled : *B. subtilis*, *B. stearothermophilus*

Pathogenicity

Anthrax is a zoonosis, humans are occasionally secondarily infected from diseased animal or animal products. Anthrax is of 4 clinical types :

(1) **Cutaneous anthrax** : Spores enter the skin most commonly through abraded skin, crusts or hair follicles and usually produce a single painless blister, often called 'malignant pustule'.

(2) **Intestinal anthrax** : Ingestion of contaminated meat results in severe and often fatal form of gastroenteritis which is far less common than cutaneous form.

(3) **Pulmonary anthrax** : It is often referred to as 'wool-sorter's disease' and is caused by inhalation of large number of spores and is usually fatal. It is a rare form of anthrax in developing countries.

(4) **Septicaemia anthrax** : Cutaneous intestinal and pulmonary anthrax, if not treated in time, progress into septicaemia and death occurs from overwhelming infection.

Laboratory diagnosis

Specimens : Pus, fluid, sputum or blood depending on the type of lesion. Specimen must be labelled "High Risk".

Microscopy

B. anthracis is capsulated, non-motile, large (5-8/1.5 μm), gram-positive rod with square ends (Fig. 7.30). Spore forms never occur in tissues but develop after the organism is shed or if it is grown on artificial media. Spores can be stained by modified Ziehl-

Neelsen's method. Capsules are formed in the tissues but are usually lacking in culture.

McFadyean's reaction : When *B. anthracis* in blood of animals in a heat fixed film is stained with polychrome methylene blue for 10-20 seconds, disintegrated capsular material appears amorphous and purplish around the bacilli.

Culture

B. anthracis is aerobe and facultative anaerobe, grows readily on ordinary media over a wide-range of temperature (25°-30°C), optimum 35°C. Colonies are 2-5 mm in diameter, dense, grey-white; they are composed of parallel chains of cells producing wavy margin of the colony, the so-called 'Medusa head' or 'curled hair lock' appearance.

1. **Blood agar** : Colonies are non-haemolytic or only slightly haemolytic (saprophytic *Bacilli* species are markedly haemolytic).

2. **Nutrient broth** : Growth is not usually turbid but forms a thick pellicle on the surface.

3. **Gelatin stab culture** : Growth occurs along the tract of inoculating wire with lateral spikes, widest near the surface — the "inverted fir tree" appearance, but the liquefaction is late.

Animal inoculation

When white mouse or guinea pig is intra-peritoneally inoculated with a small amount of exudate or, culture, the animal dies in 36-48 hours. Heart blood and sputum shows *B. anthracis*.

Bacillus subtilis

It is a non-pathogenic saprophyte and appear as common contaminant of specimen and laboratory media.

Laboratory diagnosis

Culture : Nutrient agar shows dry, 2-3 mm greyish-white opaque colonies. In nutrient broth, there is uniform turbidity.

Gram-staining : Gram-positive bacilli with subterminal spore.

Animal pathogenicity : Non-pathogenic to laboratory animals. They also differ from *B. anthracis* in producing β-lactamase which is different from that produced by staphylococci and are motile.

STREPTOCOCCUS

Streptococcus is a gram-positive coccus arranged in chain.

Classification

A. **Haemolytic classification** : Preliminary classification of streptococci is made based on the type of haemolysis produced on blood agar plates.

(i) *β-haemolytic streptococci* : They produce a wide (2-4 mm wide) clear zone of complete haemolysis around the colony (Fig. 7.8).

(ii) *α-haemolytic streptococci* : They produce a partial haemolysis (1-2 mm wide) with greenish discolouration. Some unhaemolysed RBCs are detectable in the haemolytic zone. Alpha haemolysis is seen in pneumococcus and viridans streptococci.

(iii) *γ-haemolytic streptococci* : They produce no haemolysis and *Streptococcus faecalis* is a typical member.

B. **Serological classification** (Lancefield and Griffith classification) : The β-haemolytic streptococci are classified by Lancefield (1933) serologically into a number of broad groups on the basis of group specific polysaccharide antigen of cell wall. To date, 20 Lancefield groups have been identified, numbered A-V (without I and J) by precipitation reaction with appropriate sera. Majority of the human pathogens belong to group A which are also called *Streptococcus pyogenes*.

The strains of group A streptococci are further subdivided by type specific antisera into 80 Griffith serotypes (type 1, type 2, etc.) according to their surface proteins (M, T and R). M protein is most important type specific antigen which exists in approximately 80 antigenic forms, each of which is present in a different serotype of *S. pyogenes*.

Streptococcus pyogenes

Pathogenicity

Box 2 shows the important lesions produced by different species of streptococci.

Box 2 : Streptococcal lesions

Group	Lesions
S. pyogenes	
Suppurative lesions	
Respiratory tract infections	Acute sore throat and tonsillitis, scarlet fever.
Skin and soft tissue infections	Impetigo, erysipelas, infection of wound, burns and chronic skin lesions (eczema), psoriasis.

Box 2 contd. next page

Box 2 contd. from previous page

Genital infections	Puerperal sepsis.
Deep infections	Bone and joint infections lymphadenitis, septicaemia, acute endocarditis, abscess in internal organs.
Non-suppurative complications	
Heart	Rheumatic fever.
Kidney	Acute glomerulonephritis.
S. faecalis (*Enterococcus*)	Endocarditis, urinary tract infection.
Viridans streptococci (*S. mitis, S. sanguis, S. mutans, S. salivarius*)	Endocarditis
Group B streptococci (*S. agalactiae*)	Neonatal infections (pneumonia, meningitis), septic abortion, puerperal sepsis.

Laboratory diagnosis

A. Acute suppurative infections

Specimen is collected from the site of lesion such as swab, pus or blood depending on the nature of infection, such as swabs taken from throat, vagina or purulent lesion of patients and from the throat and nose of suspected carriers.

1. **Smears** : Microscopy of smears of pus showing Gram-positive spherical or oval cocci in chains or pairs in association with pus cells suggests the presence of streptococci (Fig. 7.7). Non-viable organisms are gram-variable.

2. **Culture** : Specimen should be inoculated immediately or sent to the laboratory in *Pike's transport* medium (blood agar containing 1 in 1,000,000 crystal violet and 1 in 16,000 sodium azide).

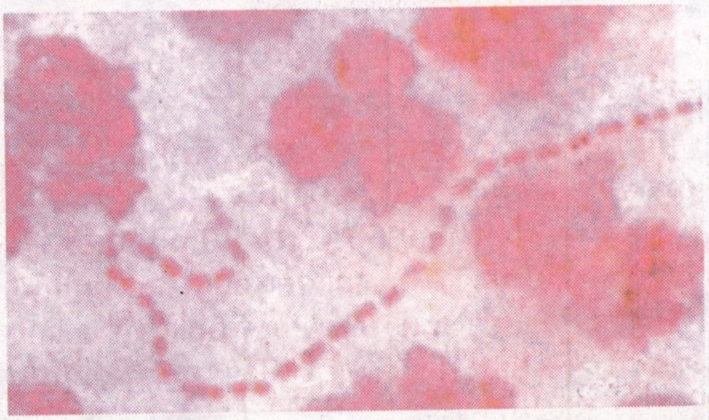

Fig. 7.7 : Gram-staining of pus showing pus cells and Gram-positive streptococci

Specimen is inoculated in blood agar medium and incubated at 37°C overnight. Haemolysis develops better under anaerobic conditions or under 5-10% carbon dioxide. Sheep blood agar is preferable as human blood may contain inhibitors. The bacterial colonies are small, typically matt or dry and surrounded by β-haemolysis. Haemophilus haemolyticus produces colonies resembling those of β-haemolytic streptococci but their haemolysis is inhibited by sheep blood. Hence primary isolation should be done in sheep blood agar.

Serological testing for determination of **Lancefield group** and **Griffith type** of haemolytic streptococci is done when needed for definite classification and for epidemiological study. A simple technique of detection of *S. pyogenes* (group A) is done by agar plate test using paper discs impregnated with bacitracin. *S. pyogenes* is more sensitive to bacitracin than other streptococci.

Selective media like crystal violet blood agar that inhibits throat commensals and may facilitate the detection of small numbers of *S. pyogenes* in throat swabs, but are rarely used in routine culture.

3. **Antigen detection tests** : Commercial test kits of ELISA, and agglutination tests are now available to demonstrate group A streptococcal antigen from throat swabs which are 75-80% sensitive.

Commercial test kit of a nucleic acid probe-based test for direct detection of group A streptococci in throat swabs is available.

4. **Serological tests** : Although antibodies to most toxins and enzymes of group A streptococci are produced, these antibodies appear late, hence test for antibodies is not helpful in diagnosing acute infection. They are more commonly used to diagnose non-suppurative complications.

B. Non-suppurative complication

Culture of throat swab or pus from skin lesions helpful for checking the continuing presence of *S. pyogenes* in throat or impetigo. Serological tests provide evidence of recent streptococcal infection. A rising titre of antibodies to group A streptococcal antigens are usually detectable. ASO titre of 200 units or more is significant in rheumatic fever. ASO titre is usually found in high levels in respiratory disease and rheumatic fever; but in streptococcal skin infections and acute glomerulonephritis, ASO titre tends to be low and DNase-B test is more reliable. Complement (C3) level is also reduced in serum in acute post-streptococcal glomerulonephritis.

PROTEUS, MORGANELLA, PROVIDENCIA

Classification

Genus	Species	Incidence
Proteus	*P. mirabilis* *P. vulgaris*	Frequent Occasional
Morganella	*M. morganii*	Occasional
Providencia	*P. alcalifaciens* *P. rettgeri* *P. stuartii*	Occasional Occasional Occasional

Habitat

Human and animal intestine. Some species are saprophytes and are found in soil, sewage and water.

Pathogenicity

P. mirabilis is the most important, other species are occasionally encountered in human lesions.

1. *Urinary tract infection*, especially following catheterisation or cystoscopy.

2. *Sepsis* : Abdominal, wound and middle ear infections. The organisms are generally low grade pathogens and often are secondary invader of ulcers, pressure sores, burns and damaged tissues.

3. *Septicaemia*.

Laboratory diagnosis

Specimen

Depending on the site of infection, which include urine, pus, blood.

Microscopy

These are actively motile, non-capsulate, gram-negative pleomorphic bacilli.

Culture

Proteus species grow well on routine media (nutrient agar, blood agar) with a swarming type of growth. This makes the isolation of other bacteria difficult in mixed cultures because swarming from a single colony of *Proteus* may cover the whole plate culture. However, swarming is inhibited in media containing bile salts, sewage. MacConkey agar, DCA and XLD agar. Swarming is also inhibited by increasing agar concentration (2%), chloral hydrate (1:500) and boric acid (1:1000) by incorporating in the media.

Colonies

Colourless, non-lactose fermenting on MacConkey agar. Proteus cultures have a distinctive smell (fishy/seminal).

In a mixed culture, pathogen can be separated from *Proteus* contaminated plate by subculturing in MacConkey agar. Swarming is not exhibited by the *Morganella* and *Providencia*.

Biochemical reaction

Table 7.9 shows the distinctive biochemical characters of the three genera.

Table 7.9 : Different properties of *Proteus, M. morgagnii* and *Providencia*

Species	*Urea*	*Citrate*	*Indole*	*Sucrose*	H_2S	*PPA*	*Gas from glucose*
P. mirabilis	+ (4 h)	d	–	–	+	+	+
P. vulgaris	+ (4 h)	d	+	+	+	+	d
M. morganii	+ (8 h)	–	+	–	–	+	d
Prov. alcalifaciens	–	+	+	+ (slow)	–	+	d
Prov. rettgeri	+ (4 h)	+	+	+ (slow)	–	d	–
Prov. stuartii	–	+	+	+ (slow)	–	+	–

d = some strains show positive reaction

1. Lactose is not fermented by any of the three genera, hence colonies are pale on MacConkey or DCA.

2. All produce indole except *P. mirabilis*, and only two members (*P. mirabilis* and *P. vulgaris*) produce H_2S.

3. All members produce *phenylalanine deaminase* and deaminate phenylalanine to phenyl pyruvic acid (PPA).

4. Production of *urease* and hydrolysis of urea is another characteristic of all members of the group except *P. stuartii* which is urease-negative.

Differentiation from the common pale colonies of pathogens isolated on lactose containing media is made by testing urease activity. *Shigella* and *Salmonella* do not produce urease.

Serology

Certain antigens (alkali-stable fraction O) of *Proteus* strains (0 × 19, 0 × K and 0 × 2) are common to *Rickettsial prowazekii* and agglutinate with sera from patients with rickettsial disease. This antigen sharing forms the basis of Weil-Felix reaction (heterophile agglutination test).

CITROBACTER, ENTEROBACTER, SERRATIA

Citrobacter, *Enterobacter* and *Serratia* species are Gram-negative motile rods and opportunistic pathogens.

Habitat : They are found in intestinal tract of man and animal, and in soil, sewage and water.

Culture : These members grow well on routine media such as MacConkey agar, blood agar and nutrient agar.

Biochemical tests : Citrobacters are late or non-lactose fermenters and enterobacters are lactose fermenters. Serratia is a non-lactose fermenting organism. Some strains of *Serratia* produce red pigment.

Medically important species include *C. freundii*, *E. aerogenes*, *E. cloacae* and *S. marcescens*.

Pathogenicity

1. Urinary tract infection.

2. Wounds, skin lesions and respiratory infections in hospitalised patients.

3. Septicaemia : Some are responsible for outbreaks of infection in nursery, ICU and burns units. They are often multi-drug resistant.

ENTEROBACTERIACEAE

Classification

The classification of *Enterobacteriaceae* is complex and controversial. There has been successive changes in the nomenclature of taxonomy with DNA homology studies. More than 30 genera and 120 species or groups have been defined, about 96% of the medically important isolates belong to 14 genera and constitute 38 species.

Tribe	Genera
Tribe I : *Escherichiae*	1. Escherichia 2. Edwardsiella 3. Citrobacter 4. Salmonella 5. Shigella
Tribe II : *Klebsielleae*	1. Klebsiella 2. Enterobacter 3. Hafnia 4. Serratia
Tribe III : *Proteae*	1. Proteus 2. Morganella 3. Providencia
Tribe IV : *Erwinieae*	1. Erwinia
Tribe V : *Yersinieae*	1. Yersinia

The oldest method of classification of enteric bacilli is based on **lactose fermentation** and members fermenting lactose are called lactose fermenters or **coliforms** and their differential properties are shown in Table 7.15.

ESCHERICHIA COLI

The main species of medical importance is *Escherichia coli* which are gram-negative motile bacilli.

Habitat

E. coli is a normal inhabitant of intestinal tract of humans and animals.

Pathogenicity

I. *Sepsis* : UTI, wound infection, peritonitis, biliary tract infection, septicaemia, neonatal meningitis.

II. *Diarrhoea* : Infant gastroenteritis (EPEC),

travellers' diarrhoea (ETEC), haemorrhagic diarrhoea (VTEC) (haemorrhagic colitis, haemolytic uraemic syndrome).

I. Sepsis

E. coli is an important cause of sepsis:

(a) Urinary tract infection including cystitis, pyelitis and pyelonephritis.

(b) Wound infections, appendicitis, peritonitis, biliary tract infection.

(c) Septicaemia.

(d) Neonatal meningitis.

II. Diarrhoea

Despite being a normal gut flora, four pathogenic groups of *E. coli* are recognised that cause diarrhoea.

(a) *Enterotoxigenic E. coli* (ETEC) : *E. coli* produces either one or two plasmid mediated enterotoxins, heat-labile enterotoxin (LT) and heat-stable enterotoxin (ST).

LT stimulate adenyl cyclase in mucosal cells of small intestine, which, in turn, activates cyclic adenosine monophosphate (cAMP) that causes hypersecretion of fluid and electrolytes into the intestinal lumen and produces watery diarrhoea. In contrast, ST appears to activate guanylate cyclase and cause diarrhoea.

(b) *Enteroinvasive E. coli* (EIEC) : The EIEC are far less pathogenic than ETEC and invade the mucosa of colon and cause a dysentery like shigella dysentery in all age groups. They are non-motile and resemble shigella strains in their biochemical reaction (NLF). Important serogroups are O 124 and O 164.

(c) *Enteropathogenic E. coli* (EPEC) : EPEC is an important cause of outbreak of infantile gastroenteritis in developed countries.

(d) *Verocytotoxigenic E. coli* (VTEC) : VTEC are named so because of the cytopathic effect of their toxins on vero-monkey kidney cells. There are two antigenically distinct *verocytotoxins* — VT-1 and VT-2. Commonest VTEC is a serogroup O 157 that causes *haemorrhagic colitis* and *haemolytic uraemic syndrome* in children.

Laboratory diagnosis

Specimens : Depending on the site of infection specimens are collected which include urine, pus, blood and stool. In case of diarrhoeal diseases, faeces may be examined for toxin detection.

Microscopy

E. coli is a gram-negative motile rod. A few strains are non-motile (formerly referred to as *Alkalescens dispar* group). Some *E. coli* strains are capsulated.

Culture

Specimen is inoculated on MacConkey agar and blood agar plates and incubated at 37°C for overnight.

Colonies : The colonies are 1-4 mm in diameter, pink, circular, convex, smooth and usually non-viscous in MacConkey agar (Fig. 7.8).

Blood agar : Colonies may be haemolytic.

Growth on other media : Most strains do not grow or markedly inhibited in xylose-lysine-deoxycholate (XLD), DCA and SS agar.

Gram-stain : Gram-negative bacilli.

Motility study : Most strains are motile.

Biochemical reaction

IMViC reactions with *Esch. coli* are : Indole positive methyl red positive, VP negative and Simmon's citrate negative (IMViC^{++--}).

	Motility	Indole	MR	VP	Urease	Citrate
E. coli	+	+	+	–	–	–
Klebsiella	–	–	–	+	+	+
Enterobacter	+	–	–	+	–	+
Citrobacter	+	–	+	–	–	+

Serology

The isolated organism is confirmed by agglutination test, first with polyvalent and then by individual specific O antisera. More than 164 *E. coli*

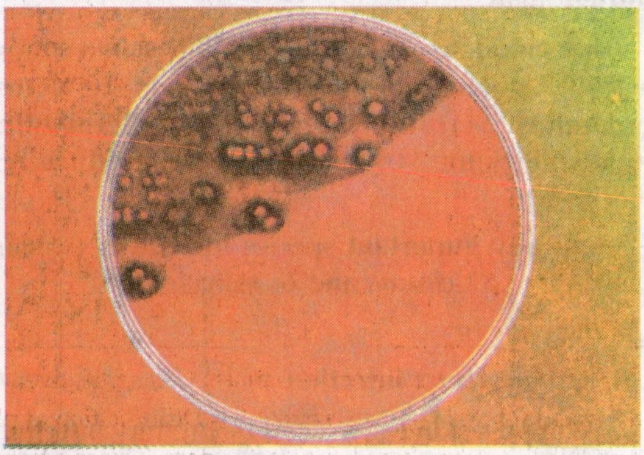

Fig. 7.8 : MacConkey agar with 24 hour growth of red lactose-fermenting colonies (*E. coli*)

serogroups are identified. H and K antigens of many of these serogroups have been identified.

Bacterial count in bacteriuria

In urinary tract infection, sample of unspun mid-stream urine is inoculated in MacConkey's agar and blood agar and incubated for overnight at 37°C. An estimate of the number of organism per ml of unspun urine sample is made by counting the number of colonies formed. The loop of an inoculation wire is made such that a loopful amount of sample equals a volume of 0.01 ml. As each bacterial colony represents progeny of a single bacterium, the colony count in the plate when multiplied by 100 gives the bacterial count per ml sample. When bacterial count is 10^5 (100,000) or more per ml of urine in untreated cases of UTI, it is called significant bacteriuria. When bacterial count is between 10,000 to 100,000 per ml, the culture may be repeated. Counts of 10,000 or less per ml are due to contamination during voiding and are insignificant. However, bacterial count in UTI may be lower than 100,000 per ml. in certain conditions, e.g. when the patient is on antibiotic therapy and in coccal infections (*S. aureus, S. faecalis*).

KLEBSIELLA

It is a non-motile, capsulated gram-negative rod and produces mucoid colony in solid media.

Habitat

They are widely distributed in nature occurring both as commensals in human and animal mouth, upper respiratory tract and intestine, as well as saprophytes in soil, water and vegetation.

Classification

Biochemically and antigenically, *Klebsiella* is classified as :

1. *K. pneumoniae* — also called *K. aerogenes.*
2. *K. rhinoscleromatis.*
3. *K. ozaenae.*

Pathogenicity

(a) *K. pneumoniae*

1. *Urinary tract infection*, particularly those that are hospital acquired.

2. *Respiratory tract infection* : Occasionally it causes pneumonia.

Table 7.10 : Differential properties of important genera of enteric bacteria

Test	*Escherichia*	*Salmonella*	*Shigella*	*Klebsiella*	*Enterobacter* [a]	*Proteus*	*Providencia*	*Citrobacter*	*Yersinia*	*Serratia*	*Hafnia*
Gas in glucose	V	V	–	+/V	+	+	V	+	–	–	+
Acid in lactose	+	–	–	+	+	–	–	+	–	+	+
PPA test[b]	–	–	–	–	–	+	+	–	–	–	–
Gluconate oxidation	–	–	–	+	+	–	–	–	–	–	–
Citrate utilisation	–	+	–	+	+	d	+	+	–	+	+
Lysine decarboxylase	+	+	–	+	V	–	–	–	–	–	+
ONPG test[c]	+	–	V	+	+	–	–	+	+	–	–
Urease production	–	–	–	V	–	+	–	–	+	+/–	–
Indole formation	+	–	V	–	–	V	+	V	–	+	–
Motility	+	+	–	–	+	+	+	+	V	+	+
H_2S	–	+/–	–	–	–	+	–	+	–	–	–

+ = most strains positive; – = most strains negative; V = variable (some strains positive, others negative)
a = including the genus *Serratia* • b = Deamination of phenylalanine to phenylpyruvic acid
c = ONPC, o-nitrophenyl, β-galactosidase. This is a test for β-galactosidase activity
d = Result different in different species or strains

3. *Septicaemia.*

4. *Meningitis* (especially in neonates).

5. Rarely abscesses, endocarditis, peritonitis and other lesions.

(b) *K. rhinoscleromatis* : It causes *rhinoscleroma*, a chronic granulomatous growth of nose and pharynx.

(c) *K. ozaenae* : It causes ozena in nasal mucosa, a disease characterised by foul-smelling nasal discharge with progressive atrophy of mucosal membranes.

Laboratory diagnosis

Specimens : Urine, sputum, pus and infected tissue depending upon site of lesion.

Microscopy

Gram-negative, non-motile, capsulated rods.

Culture

Large and usually mucoid colonies (due to production of extracellular slime) on MacConkey agar and blood agar. Majority of the stains produce pink colonies and MacConkey's medium due to lactose fermentation.

Biochemical reaction

Lactose fermenter, indole negative and citrate positive (see *Escherichia coli*). IMViC reactions are $IMViC^{--++}$. Majority of *Klebsiella* strains are urease-producers but much slower and less intense in this regard than the *Proteus* strains.

Serology

More than 80 capsular types have been identified. Identification by Quellung reaction is recommended.

Urinary tract infection

Causative agents

1. *E. coli*
2. *Klebsiella* spp.
3. *Proteus* spp, especially *P. mirabilis.*
4. *Enterococcus.*
5. Occasionally *Enterobacter*, *Citrobacter*, *Ps. aeruginosa* and *Serratia.*
6. *Staph. aureus.*
7. *Staph. epidermidis.*

Significant bacteriuria

When bacterial count is 10^5 (100,000) or more per ml of unspun urine sample in untreated cases of UTI, it is called significant bacteriuria.

A standard calibrated loop of 3 mm internal diameter that can hold 1/300 ml urine is used for transferring undiluted urine sample for inoculation into MacConkey agar and blood agar and then the plates are incubated overnight.

Bacterial count :

1. No colonies < 30 = < 10^4 organisms/ml → not significant

2. No colonies 30-300 = 10^4 organisms/ml →doubtful significance

3. No colonies > 300 = 10^5 organisms/ml → significant

SALMONELLA

Habitat

Most salmonellae are found in the gut of animals especially of pigs, cows, goats, sheeps, rodents, hens, ducks and other poultry. They are pathogenic for their hosts and also cause disease in man. *S. typhi* and *S. paratyphi* differ from other salmonellae, in that man is the only natural host.

Classification

Salmonellae produce 3 main types of lesions but mixed forms are common.

(a) *Enteric fevers*

1. Typhoid fever — *S. typhi.*
2. Paratyphoid fever — *S. paratyphi* A, B and C.

(b) *Food poisoning* (gastroenteritis)

1. *S. typhimurium.*
2. *S. enteritidis* phase type 4.
3. *S. dublin.*

Box 3 : Differentiating biochemical properties of *S. typhi* and *S. paratyphi* A or B

Organisms	*Lactose*	*Glucose*	*Mannitol*	*Sucrose*	*Indole*	*MR*	*VP*	*Citrate*
S. typhi	–	A	A	–	–	+	–	–
S. paratyphi A or B	–	AG	AG	–	–	+	–	±

(c) *Septicaemia with or without local suppurative lesion*

1. *S. choleraesuis*. 2. *S. dublin*.

3. *S. virchow*.

1. Typhoid fever

(a) *Incubation stage* : *S. typhi* is ingested with contaminated food and water. The organisms then pass from small intestine into blood (transient bacteraemia) via mesenteric lymph nodes and thoracic duct. Blood stream is rapidly cleared by mononuclear phagocytic system in the liver, spleen and gallbladder.

(b) *Symptomatic stage* : From the gallbladder the organisms invade the Peyer's patches of intestine causing inflammation and ulceration. The bacilli then pass into blood leading to bacteraemia and generalised infection. Organisms are excreted in faeces and urine in third and fourth week.

2. Paratyphoid fever

Clinically, the disease is generally milder than typhoid fever with shorter duration and incubation. *S. paratyphi* A and C infections are more common in tropical countries.

S. paratyphi C : It mainly causes septicaemia and important lesions caused by the organism include formation of abscess, arthritis and inflammation of gallbladder.

3. Food poisoning (enterocolitis)

Salmonella food-poisoning is caused by ingestion of contaminated food like meat, egg and milk with *S. typhimurium* and *S. enteritidis*. Symptoms occur within 10-30 hours. Food-poisoning strains can also cause septicaemia, inflammation of gallbladder and osteitis.

Salmonellae causing septicaemia occasionally cause localised pyogenic lesions, such as, osteomyelitis, meningitis and deep abscesses.

Laboratory diagnosis

Culture and isolation of salmonellae are essential to confirm a diagnosis. Identification of the isolate is based on biochemical characteristics and serology. The optimal specimen for culture varies with presentation.

(a) In a classic case of salmonella gastroenteritis faecal sample is best. Patients' vomitus and suspected foodstuffs are also useful.

(b) In a suspected case of enteric fever, blood culture or bone marrow aspirate is most likely to yield positive results. Later, with intestinal and renal involvement, culture of faeces and urine is indicated.

The specimens to be tested at different stages of enteric fever and the percentage of positivity are shown in Fig. 7.9 and Table 7.11. General blood picture in enteric fever may show leucopenia (leucocyte count, 2,000–2,500 cumm) with relative lymphocytosis.

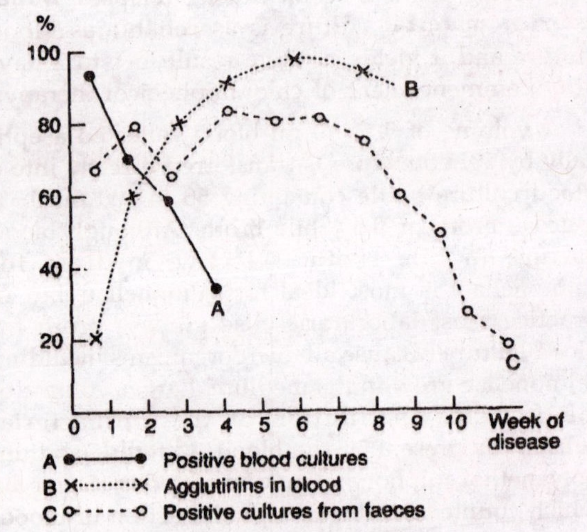

Fig. 7.9 : Data on bacteriological findings in typhoid fever

Table 7.11 : Show materials for examination at different phases of enteric fever

Stage	Examination	Result (% positive)
1st week	Blood culture	95
	Blood picture	Leucopenia with relative lymphocytosis
2nd week	Blood culture	40-50
	Widal test	Low titre antibody
3rd week	Widal test	100
	Blood culture	15-20
	Stool and urine culture	80
4th week	Widal test	100
	Stool and urine culture	90
	Blood culture	5-10

Isolation of the organism

1. ***Culture*** : Specimens of blood or bone marrow in enteric fever; faeces, vomitus or suspected food in gastroenteritis should be collected before starting treatment.

As there is transient bacteraemia, there are small number of organisms in blood. Repeated culture with larger volume (5-10 ml) of blood is necessary. **Blood culture** is positive in 80-90% patients in first week and up to 10 days of fever. The chances of positive culture progressively diminishes with increase in duration of illness (Fig. 7.9). Blood culture also yields positive result during relapses. **Bone-marrow material** culture is as reliable as blood culture and it yields positive result in 1 to 2 days after commencement of chloramphenicol therapy.

A volume of 5 to 10 ml blood collected aseptically by venepuncture is transferred directly into a blood culture bottle containing 50 to 100 ml 0.5% glucose broth or 0.5% bile broth. Although blood culture in bile broth (selective medium for salmonellae) is most ideal for salmonellae, but in practice most laboratories use glucose broth for blood culture because all microorganisms including salmonellae grow in the medium. Larger volume of media helps in dilution of the antibacterial substances present in the blood. **Liquoid** (sodium polyanethol sulphonate) may be added in the media which counteracts the bactericidal action of blood.

Alternatively, 5 ml venous blood, collected aseptically, is allowed to clot in a sterile screw-capped universal container. After removing serum, 15 ml bile salt streptokinase broth streptokinase, 100 units per ml) is added aseptically to each bottle. The streptokinase digests the clot causing its lysis and thereby the bacteria are released from the clot. The separated serum is utilised for **Widal** test. **Clot culture** offers a higher rate of isolation than blood culture as the bactericidal activity of serum is obviated in the technique.

After incubation overnight at 37°C , **subculturing** is done on MacConkey agar or DCA. Subculturing is economically carried out by spreading a loopful of broth over a sector of solid media, one-fourth of an 8.5 cm Petri dish and incubated for 24-48 hours. Colourless colonies (NLF) appear. Cultures may be discarded as negative after 10 days.

As growth may be delayed and also to eliminate the risk of introducing contamination during repeated subcultures, **Castaneda's** method of blood culture may be adopted, which provides both liquid (liver infusion broth) and solid media (3% nutrient agar slope) in one bottle. It is a diphasic medium, the broth has an agar slant on one side.

2. ***Stool and urine culture*** : Culture of faeces and urine are always positive during 3rd and 4th week of enteric fever. Repeated cultures are required for positive result. Stool culture is mainly done for detecting the **carriers**.

3. ***Duodenal juice or bile culture*** : Bile is cultured to detect ***chronic carriers*** in whom the organisms are present in the biliary tract.

Identification

In MacConkey's agar or DCA, salmonellae grow as nonlactose fermenters which are further studied by *Gram's staining, motility preparation* and *biochemical reactions* in different sugar media. Subculture from the colonies is made in nutrient agar to be utilised for *agglutination test*.

Slide agglutination test : A loopful of isolated organism (unknown culture) from the colony in agar is emulsified in a drop of saline on a microscopic slide without spreading the drop. The emulsion must be absolutely smooth and of medium opacity. One small loopful of specific antiserum is added and then mixed by tilting the slide. In the same way, a control of bacterial suspension in normal saline is prepared on another slide and to which no specific serum is added. Clumping of bacteria in test slide occurs within a few minutes if the antigen-antibody reaction is specific. Control saline emulsion of bacteria does not show any change.

Biochemically positive strains (Box 3) are first tested with polyvalent O serum, which reacts with salmonella strains in groups A to G, provided agglutination is not blocked by Vi antigen, which can be checked by testing all negative strains using *S. typhi* Vi serum. Positive results with polyvalent O serum indicates a *Salmonella* strain. In the next step, the strain is tested with sera prepared against O antigens of the individual salmonella groups. The following are the most useful sera which react with factor 2, Group A factors 4 and 5, group B; with 6 and 7, group C1; with 8, group C2; with 9, group D; and with 3, 10, 15 and 19, group E.

When the strain is positive with individual salmonella O serum, and biochemically it is typically *S. typhi*, the strain is tested against *S. typhi* O serum, factor 9. Prompt agglutination indicates that the microorganism belongs to *Salmonella* group D. Its identity is established as *S. typhi* by agglutination with salmonella H specific serum which reacts with flagellar antigen d.

In a non-typhoid salmonella, the strain is tested for agglutination with O and H sera for groups A, B and C. When unusual serotypes are encountered, the same should be referred to the National Salmonella Reference Centre (Central Research Institute, Kasauli, for human strain, and Indian Veterinary Research Institute, Izatnagar, for salmonella of animal origin).

Subtyping : Subtyping methods are frequently used for the common serotypes *(S. typhi, S. typhimurium* and *S. enteritidis)* which include phage typing, biotyping, and more recently introduced genotyping methods (plasmid finger printing). These techniques are employed in CDC for subtyping within serotypes of *Salmonella*.

Serological test

1. **Widal test**: It is an agglutination test which detects presence of *serum agglutinins (H and O)* in patient's serum with typhoid and paratyphoid fever. Salmonella antibody starts appearing in serum at the end of first week (Fig. 7.33) and rises sharply during the 3rd week of enteric fever. It is preferable to test two specimens of sera at an interval of 7 to 10 days to demonstrate a rising antibody titre.

Convalescent sera from salmonella gastroenteritis cases often agglutinate a suspension of the causal serotype which helps in retrospective diagnosis.

Procedure: In Widal test, two types of tubes were originally used : (1) Dreyer's tube (narrow tube with conical bottom) for H agglutination, and (ii) Felix tube (short round-bottomed tube) for O agglutination. Nowadays 3 × 0.5 ml Kahn tubes are used for both types of agglutination.

A serial two fold dilution of patient's serum in normal saline (1 : 20, 1 : 40 and so on up to 1,280 or more) is prepared in 8 small (3 × 0.5 ml) test tubes for each series; 7 for serum dilutions and 8th for a non-serum control. To the diluted serum and control saline equal volume (0.4 cc) of antigen suspensions (TH, TO, AH and BH) are added and mixed thoroughly by shaking the rack and then the mixtures are incubated at 37°C for 4 hours and read after overnight refrigeration at 4°C. Some workers recommended incubation in a water bath at 37°C overnight.

Observation: Loose and cotton-woolly clumps are formed in *H agglutination* and a disc-like granular deposit in *O agglutination* at the botton of tube. Control tube shows a compact deposit. The **Maximum dilution** of serum at which agglutination occurs indicate the titre of antibodies. The routinely used antigens are H and O of *S. typhi, H* of *S. paratyphi* A and B. As paratyphoid O antigen cross reacts with typhoid O antigen due to the sharing of factor 12 by them, paratyphoid O antigens are not used.

Preparation of Widal antigen : *H suspension* of bacteria is prepared by adding 0.1% formalin to a 24 hours broth culture or saline suspension of an agar culture. For preparation of *O suspension* of bacteria, the organisms are cultured on phenol agar (1 : 800). Standard smooth strains of the organism are used; *S. typhi* 901, O and H strains are employed for this purpose.

Interpretation of Widal test

1. *Agglutinin* starts appearing in serum by the end of 1st week with sharp rise in 2nd and 3rd weeks and the titre remains steady till the 4th week after which it declines.

2. *Rising titre* : Demonstration of *rising titre* of four-fold or greater of both H and O agglutinins at an interval of 4 to 7 days is the most important diagnostic criterion.

3. In a *single test*, a titre of 100 of O or more and a titre of 200 of H agglutinins signifies presence of active infection, but that has to be interpreted taking into consideration the following factors :

(i) *Local titre* : Due to sub-clinical infection of salmonellosis in endemic area, low titre of agglutinins is present in the serum of normal individuals, which may cause positive reaction. This is known as *local titre.* Local titre is up to 80 in Kolkata and 60 in Siliguri.

(ii) *Immunisation* : In immunisation with TAB vaccine, vaccinated individuals may show high titres of antibody (H antibody titre 160 or more) to each of the salmonellae.

(iii) *Anamnestic reaction* : Persons who had past enteric infection or who have been vaccinated may develop transient fever like malaria, influenza etc.

(iv) *Non-specific antigens* (e.g. fimbrial antigen) may produce false positive result.

(v) *Antibiotic treatment* : When treatment with chloramphenicol is started before the appearance of agglutinins, they are unlikely to appear subsequently; if the antibody is already present, no further rise in titre is expected.

(vi) *Carriers* : Widal tests may be negative in many healthy carriers and some have to be detected by Vi agglutination test.

2. **Other serological tests** : ELISA is sensitive method of measuring antibody against the lipopolysaccharide of *Salmonellae,* titre of IgM antibody corresponds fairly well with the Widal O titre. ELISA in vertical flow membrane format (Typhi-DOT) detects Vi Ag in blood/serum at an early stage of the disease.

SHIGELLA

Habitat : *Shigella* species are exclusively parasites of human and other primates and cause bacillary dysentery in man.

Classification : Shigellae are gram-negative non-motile bacilli. Antigenically, shigellae are divided into four groups (A, B, C, D) based on specificity of O antigen. These groups are differentiated by a combination of biochemical reactions and antigenic structure (Table 7.14). Mannitol fermentation reactions are important, group A is mannitol negative and the rest are mannitol positive.

Pathogenesis

Shigella species cause bacillary dysentery (shigellosis). Infection is transmitted by faecal-oral route. *S. dysenteriae* type 1 *(S. shiga)* produces exotoxins that causes most severe form of disease. *S. flexneri* and *S. boydii* cause less severe dysentery and are prevalent in tropical countries including India. *S. sonnei* is the cause of most dysentery in Britain.

The organisms are taken up by the epithelial cells of distal parts of the colon with necrosis of surface epithelial cells leading to an acute inflammation in lamina propria and submucosa. Necrotic epithelia sloughs forming superficial ulcers which leads to bleeding mucosa.

Table 7.12 : Classification of *shigella*

Group	*Species*	*Serotype*	*Synonyms*
Mannitol negative			
A	*S. dysenteriae*	1-12	A1-*S. shiga* A2–*S. schmitzi*
Mannitol positive			
B	*S. flexneri*	1-6 X and Y variants	1-5–*S: paradysenteriae*
C	*S. boydii*	1–18	*S. paradysenteriae*
D	*S, sonnei*	1	

Laboratory diagnosis

To confirm diagnosis, *shigella* must be isolated in pure culture from an adequate sample. Specimens include fresh stool, mucous flakes, and rectal swabs.

A. Microscopical examination of stool

Cover slip preparation in saline and iodine shows large number of pus cells (neutrophils) with degenerated nuclei, RBC, and macrophages. The presence of protozoa, cysts or helminthic ova is excluded. The normal bacterial flora is considerably diminished. Fluorescent antibody technique is of some help in rapid diagnosis of a case but it is not usually practised.

B. Bacteriological examination

I. *Culture*

Media : MacConkey's agar, DCA, S-S agar, Selenite F broth.

A loopful of material is inoculated on selective media like MacConkey's agar or SS agar media.

Selenite-F broth (0.4%) is used as enrichment and transport medium which permits rapid growth of enteric pathogens while temporarily (for 9-12 hours) inhibiting the growth of *E. coli*. Organisms from selenite-F broth are subcultured in MacConkey's agar after 24 hours incubation at 37°C.

Colourless colonies appear on MacConkey's agar medium after 12 to 18 hours incubation which are further tested by *smear* examination, *motility* preparation and *biochemical* reactions. Shigellae are Gram-negative non-motile bacilli.

II. *Biochemical reactions*

Urease, citrate, H_2S and KCN negative; indole and M R positive Gram-negative non-sporing bacillus is suggestive of a shigella strain (Fig. 7.10, Table 7.15). *S. sonnei* is a late lactose fermenter.

III. *Slide agglutination test*

It is done by using polyvalent antisera of three groups (A, B and C) of shigella and antiserum of group D (*S. sonnei*), one by one against the isolate. Monovalent antisera are used for the group for which agglutination has occurred with polyvalent antisera. Then type specific antisera for strains belonging to Group A, B or C is used for agglutination test.

Occasionally, agglutination may not occur due to masking of O antigen by K antigen, which can be

Table 7.13 : Biochemical characteristics of genus *shigella*

Subgroup (species)	Gas from Glucose	Acid from			Indole	Lysine	Ornithine	Catalase	ONPG test
		Lactose	Mannitol	Sucrose					
S. dysenteriae 1	–	–	–	–	–	–	–	–	+
S. dysenteriae 2-10	–	–	–	–	V	–	–	+	V
S. flexneri 1-5	–	–	+	–	V	–	–	+	–
S. flexneri 6	V	–	+	–	–	–	–	+	–
S. boydii	–	–	+	–	V	–	–	+	–
S. sonnei	–	(+)	+	(+)	–	–	–	+	+

KEY : V = variable; (+) = delayed positive (after prolonged incubation); ONPG = o-nitrophenyl β-galactoside.

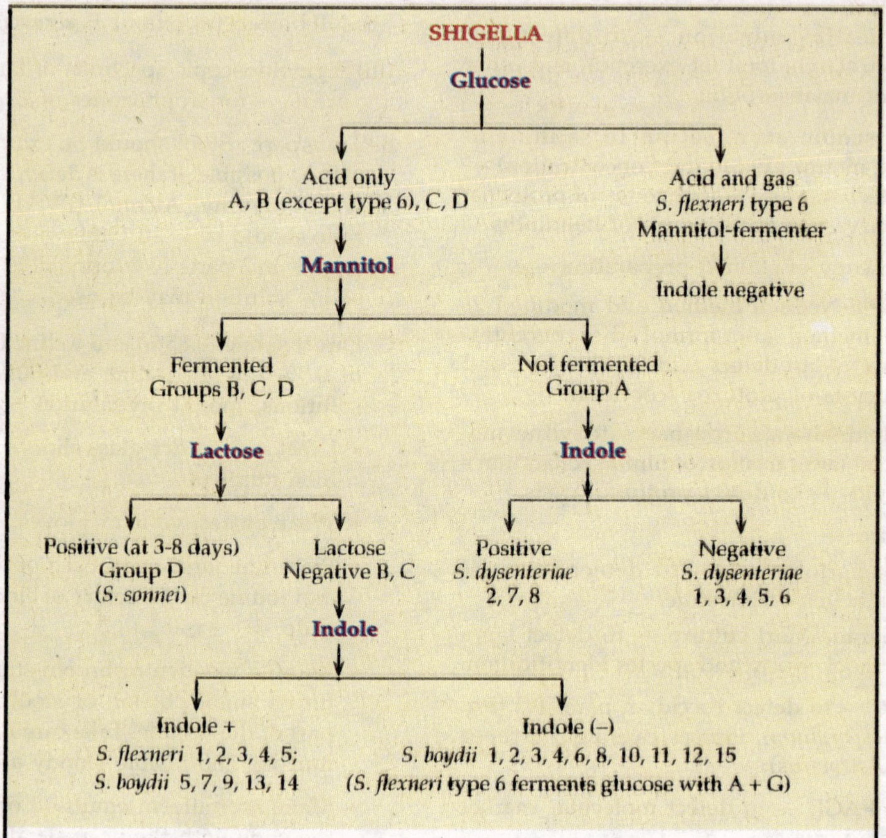

Fig. 7.10 : Biochemical reactions of Shigella species

removed by boiling the bacterial suspension at 100°C for 60 minutes.

IV. *Colicin typing* : It is done for group D strains.

V. *Sereny test* may be done to confirm the invasiveness of the isolated strain of shigella, although, it is seldom practised.

8

Stool Examination

Examination of stool in laboratory consists of :

(i) Naked eye examination — To note consistency, colour, visible blood, mucous.

(ii) Chemical examination — to detect pH, lactose, starch, total fat excretion and other tests of malabsorption.

(iii) Microscopic examination in saline and iodine mount (direct and concentration) — to detect cyst and trophozoites of protozoa, ova, larva and adult worm of helminths.

(iv) Microscopy of stained preparation —

(a) Ziehl-Neelsen method and modified Z. N. method (after formol ether concentration) — to detect acid fact bacillus and oocysts of protozoa (coccidia).

(b) Heidenhain's iron-haematoxyline method (after fixation of film in Schaudinn's fluid) — to detect protozoal cysts.

(v) Culture —

(a) Bacteriological — to detect bacterial pathogen of intestine.

(b) Harada-Mori culture — to detect larva of hook-worm and species identification.

(vi) P.C.R. — to detect coccidian parasites (e.g. *Cryptosporidium*), viruses causing diarrhoea (e.g. *Astrovirus*).

(vii) RNA-PAGE — to detect molecular marker of Rota virus.

This chapter is devoted to discuss the microscopic examination of stool for parasitic infestation of gut.

METHOD OF MICROSCOPIC EXAMINATION FOR PARASITES IN STOOL

A. Sample

(i) Freshly voided stool in a stool collection container is preferable, especially for trophozoites of *E. histolytica* and *G. lamblia* and helminthic larva.

(ii) NIH swab for ova of *E. vermicularis*.

(iii) Sigmoidoscopic specimen of large gut ulcer areas — for trophozoites of *E. histolytica*.

B. Transport : Stool should be examined as quickly as possible. If there is delay, it is preserved with Polyvinyl Alcohol (PVA). Stool : PVA ratio should be 1 : 10. Otherwise one part stool sample in 3 parts 10% formaldehyde in normal saline solution may be used.

C. Direct saline (0.85%) and iodine (1 : 1 mixture of 0.5% Lugol's iodine and 50% Acetic acid solutions) mount preparation :

- Label a clean dry glass slide with the specimen number.
- Wear protective latex gloves.
- Place one large drop each of normal saline and iodine on the centre of either end of the slide.
- Using a wooden or broom-stick applicator, lift as small portion of stool from several part of the sample. Take care not to miss the mucous and visible bloody areas.
- Make an uniform emulsion of the stool on the slide with the normal saline drop. The emulsion should not be too thick or too thin.
- Using the same applicator, make a similar emulsion with lugol's iodine.
- Discard the applicator in freshly prepared 1% sodium hypochlorite solution.
- Place cover slips on emulsions on slide, taking care not to form air buble.

Microscopic examination :

Using low power objective (10 ×) scan the mounts thoroughly for helminthic ova and larva. Next scan the mounts with high power objective (40 ×) for protozoa. Characteristic movement of the protozoa, often is of diagnostic importance, is demonstrated in saline mount. Intracellular details (eg. nucleus, nuclear chromatin, chromatoid bar, glycogen vacuole etc.) are better visualised in iodine mount.

D. Concentration methods

Indication : Scanty parasite in stool and difficulty in demonstration by direct wet mount.

Methods :

1. **Floating method** :
   (a) Saturated sodium chloride solution floatation.
   (b) Zinc sulphate centrifugal floatation.
2. **Sedimentation method** :
   (c) Formol ether sedimentation technique.

(a) Saturated NaCl solution floatation method—

- In a small container place about 10 g. of stool.
- Using an applicator and with gradual addition of saturated sodium chloride solution (sp. gravity 1.2) make an emulsion. Continue the procedure till the container is full almost to the brim.
- Coarse materials on top is then removed.
- Add little more saline to form a convex meniscus at top.
- Place carefully a glass slide (size large enough to cover the open end of the container) in contact with convex meniscus of saline.
- Wait for 15 minutes.
- Carefully lift the slide and invert. Place a cover slip over the preparation side.
- Examine under microscope, first directly, and then, if required, with addition of lugol's iodine.

The method is useful for demonstration of fertilised eggs of *Ascaris lumbricoides*, *Enterobius vermicularis*, hookworm, *Trichuris trichiura*. Unfertilised egg of *Ascaris*, ova of *Cestodes* and *Trematodes*, protozoal cysts cannot be demonstrated by this technique, as these are sedimented.

(b) Zinc sulphate centrifugal floatation —

- In a 15-20 ml capacity centrifuge tube mix 10 gm of stool with distilled water to form a suspension.
- Filter the faecal suspension through two layers of gauze in a funnel into another centrifuge tube.
- Spin at 1800 r.p.m. for 5 minutes. Discard the supernatant, and resuspend the deposit in freshly added distilled water. Repeat centrifugation continue the procedure of washing repeatedly till the supernatant is clear.
- Then add Zn SO_4 solution (sp. gr. 1.180) to resuspend the deposit. Centrifuge at 1800 r.p.m. for 3 minutes.
- Place few loopful of surface fluid from meniscus on a glass slide. To one add one drop of lugol's iodine. Place cover slips and examine microscopically.

The method is useful to detect egg of hookworm, fertilized egg of *Ascaris*, *Trichuris*, tapeworm and *protozoan cysts*. It fails to demonstrate unfertilised Ascaris eggs, nematode larvae, eggs of most trematodes and large tapeworms (eg. Taenia).

(c) Formol ether sedimentation technique —

- Mix $^1/_2$ t.s.f. stool in normal saline thoroughly. The suspension is filtered through 2 layers of gauze in a funnel, into a 15 ml centrifuged tube (screw capped).
- Discard the supernatant after centrifugation at 1800 r.p.m. for 5 minutes.
- Resuspend the deposit in 10 ml of 10% formalin and allow to stand for 5 minutes.
- Then add 3 ml ether and close the screw cap. Shake the content vigorously.
- Next centrifuge at 1500 r.p.m. for 10 minutes.
- Sediment is to be used for preparation of wet mounts and smears for staining by modified Z.N. method or Trichrome stain.

The method is useful for demonstration of all varieties of parasitic elements in faeces. This is a must for detection of oocysts of coccidian protozoa (eg. *Cryptosporidium*, *Cyclospora*, *Isospora* and *Microspora*) in diarrhoeic stool of AIDs cases.

MICROSCOPIC MORPHOLOGY OF HELMINTHIC EGGS IN STOOL IN WET MOUNT

Ascaris lumbricoides

Three type of morphology is found in stool — (a) fertilised egg, (b) unfertilised egg, (c) degenerated egg (in older sample without preservative).

Fertilised Egg (Fig. 8.1)

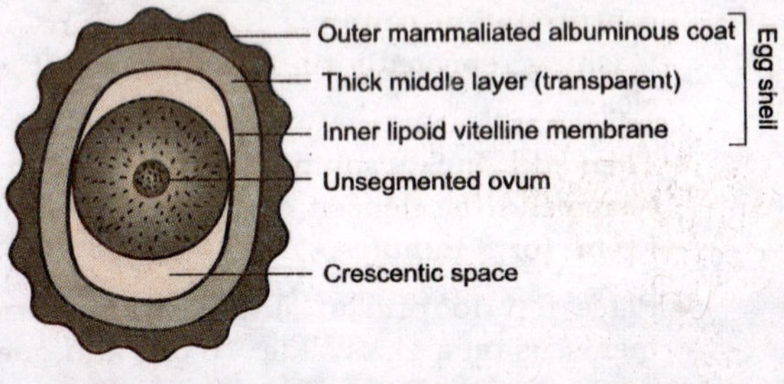

Fig. 8.1 : Eggs of *Ascaris lumbricoides (fertilised)*

Shape — Round or oval.

Size — Length 60-75 µm × breadth 40-50 µm.

Colour — Bile stained (brown or yellowish brown).

Saturated salt solution — Egg floats.

Features :

- Large unsegmented ovum at innermost part.
- Coarse yolk granules obscures the nucleus.
- Inner vitelline membrane surrounds the ovum. Often difficult to see.
- Ovum with vitelline membrane is surrounded by thick translucent shell.
- Two crescentic space in between ovum and vitelline membrane at two poles.
- Outer coat — a bile stained thick albuminous coat showing rugosity or mammillations. Sometimes, this coat is found missing, when it is called decorticated egg.

Unfertilised Egg (Fig. 8.2)

Shape — Elongated, narrow and more elliptical.

Size — Length–about 80 µm × breadth about 55 µm.

Colour — Bile stained.

Salt floatation — Heaviest of all helminthic eggs, does not float.

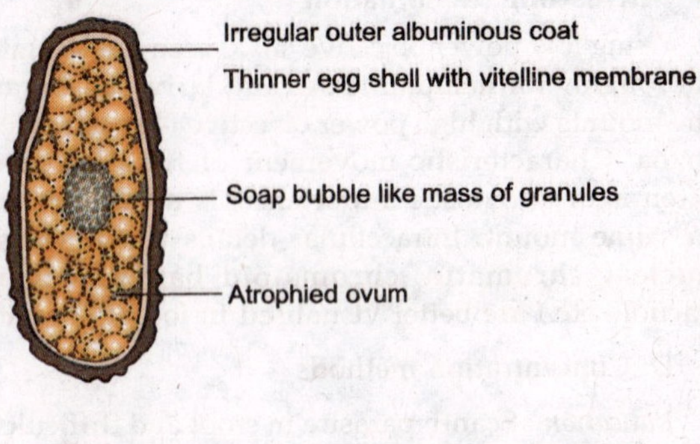

Fig. 8.2 : Eggs of *Ascaris lumbricoides (unfertilised)*

Features :

- Irregular outer albuminous coat
- Thinner egg shell with vitelline membrane
- Ovum atrophied
- Soap bubble like mass of granules

Degenerated Egg

Similar to fertilised egg, but mammillation is absent (decorticated), ovum not visible, yolk is coarser.

It is to be noted that both fertilised and unfertilised ora may be found in the same sample.

Trichuris trichiura (Fig. 8.3)

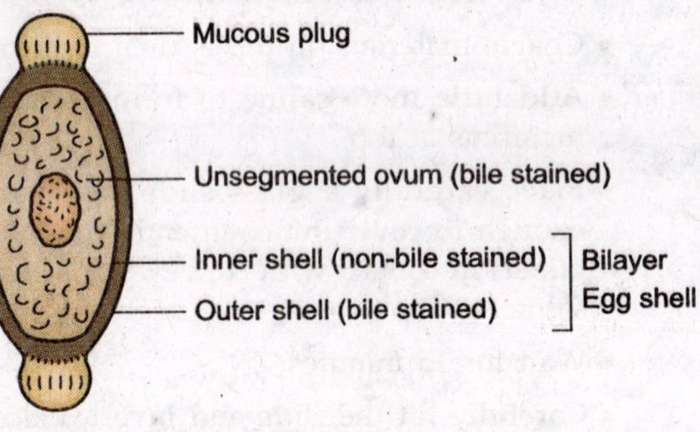

Fig. 8.3 : Egg of *Trichuris trichiura*

Shape — Barrel like with protuberant mucous plug at each pole.

Size — Length–about 50 µm × breadth about 25 µm.

Colour — Dark brown to yellow brown due to bile staining.

Floatation — Floats in saturated solution of common salt.

Features :

- Unsegmented bile stained granular mass is the ovum, encased in egg shell.
- Smooth egg shell is bilayered. Outer one is bile stained and inner one is transluscent.

[Differential diagnosis : *Capillaria philippinensis* egg looks similar to *Trichuris trichiura* egg. Former is distinguished by smaller size (45 × 21 μm), peanut shape, bipolar flattened mucous plugs and pitted egg shell].

Enterobius vermicularis (Fig. 8.4)

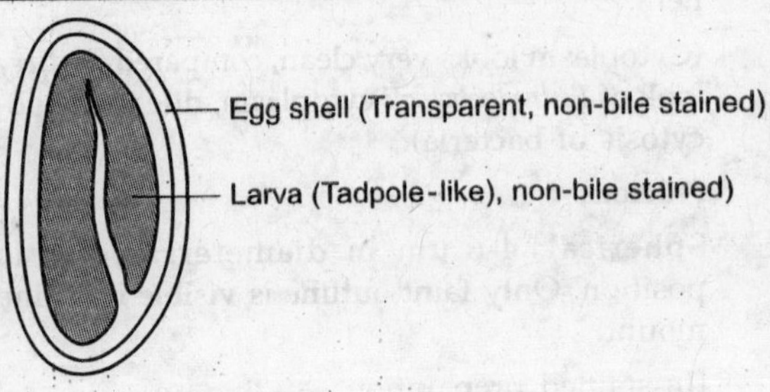

Fig. 8.4 : Egg of *Enterobius vermicularis*

Shape — Asymmetric. Ventral side flattened and dorsal side convex — giving planoconvex appearance.

Size — Length 50-60 μm × breadth about 30 μm.

Colour — Colourless, transparent, non-bile stained.

Floatation — Floats in saturated common salt solution.

Features :

- Coiled larva inside the egg shell.
- Egg shell is transparent and double layered.

(Instead of stool, the egg is better demonstrated in morning perianal NIH swab).

Hookworm (Fig. 8.5)

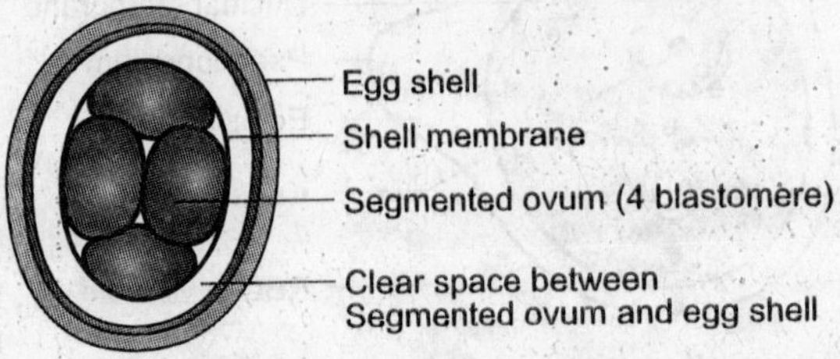

Fig. 8.5 : Egg of hookworm

Shape — Oval or elliptical in shape.

Size — Length 65 μm × breadth 40 μm.

Colour — Colourless. All layers are non-bile stained.

Floatation — Floats in saturated solution of common salt.

Features :

- Ovum is segmented in 4 blastomeres.
- Ovum is immediately surrounded by hyaline shell membrane.
- Egg shell is transparent.
- Clear space between egg shell and ovum.

Hymenolepis nana (Fig. 8.6)

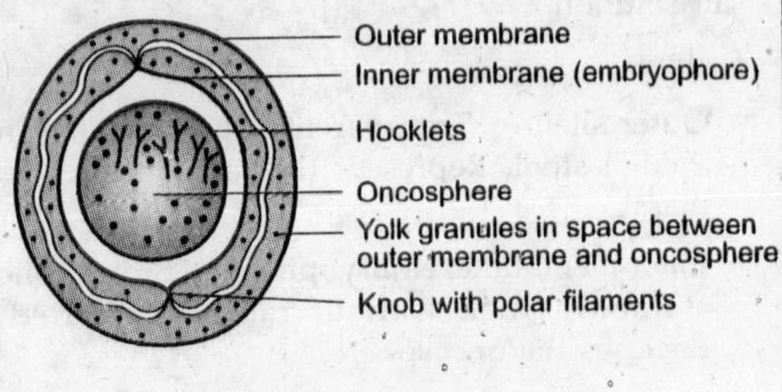

Fig. 8.6 : Egg of *Hymenolepis nana*

Shape — Spherical or oval.

Size — Diameter 35-45 μm.

Colour — Colourless. No element is bile stained.

Floatation — Floats in saturated common salt solution.

Features :

- Two distinct membranes encloses an oncosphere.
  Outer membrane is thin and colourless.
  Inner membrane, embryophore, encloses the oncosphere and shows two polar knobs, from which polar filaments (6-8) originates.
- Oncosphere is colourless and shows 3 pair of hook lets.
- Space between outer membrane and embryophore is filled with yolk granules and polar filaments.

[Differentiating points from H. diminuta : H. diminuta egg is larger, outer shell is yellowish and is devoid of polar filaments]

Taenia Spp. (Fig. 8.7)

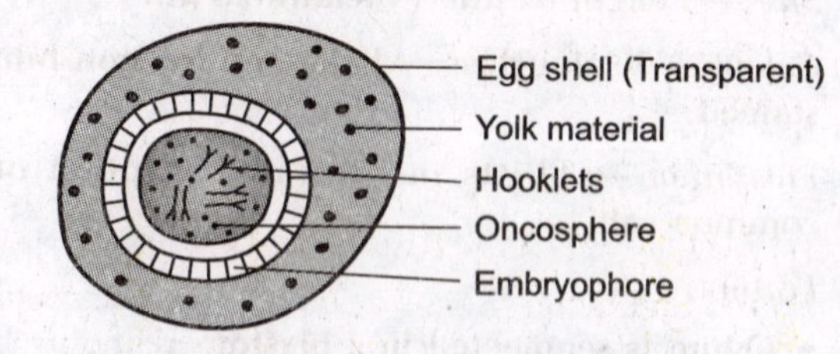

Fig. 8.7 : Egg of Taenia spp.

Shape — Spherical.

Size — Diameter 31-43 µm.

Colour — Brown (bile stained).

Floatation — Do not float in saturated common salt solution.

Features :

- Outer shell — Transparent. Often missing in voided stool. Represent the remnant of yolk mass.
- Inner membrane, embryophore — Brown (bile stained), thick walled, radially striated. Encloses the oncosphere.
- Oncosphere — 14-20 µm in diameter, shows 3 pairs of hooklets.

[By morphology *T. solium* and *T. saginata* eggs cannot be differentiated; both looks same. For species identification examination of proglottides (segments) or scolex (head) is necessary].

MICROSCOPIC MORPHOLOGY OF PROTOZOA CYSTS IN WET MOUNT EXAMINATION OF STOOL

Entamoeba histolytica

A. Trophozoite (Fig. 8.8B)

For demonstration of E. histolytica trophozoite, saline mount of mucous part of freshly voided stool is to be examined. It is desirable to use a warmer stage of microscope when temperature is below 30°C.

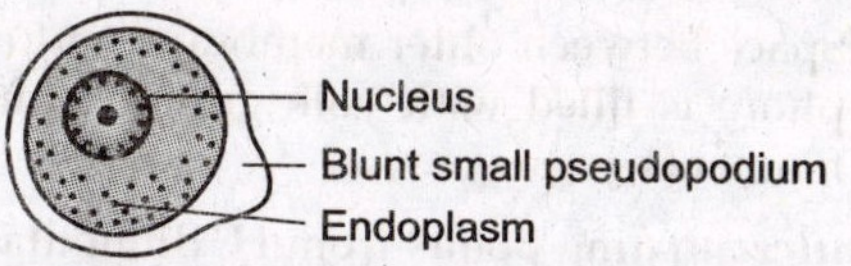

Fig. 8.8A : Pre-cyst of *Entamoeba histolytica*

Features —

- Slow gliding movements.
- Pseudopodia is thrown from one end only, with a jerky movement resembling ejection under high pressure. This is followed by flowing of the entire endoplasm.
- Shape — No fixed shape.
- Size — Range 18-40 µm. Average 20-30 µm.
- Cytoplasm —

Outer ectoplasm— Clear translucent.

Inner endoplasm — Granular. RBC is found here.

(Cytoplasm looks very clean, compared to dirty look of *Entamoeba coli* cytoplasm, due to phagocytosis of bacteria).

- Nucleus

Spherical. 4-6 µm in diameter. Eccentric position. Only faint outline is visible in saline mount.

[In stained preparation —

- Karyosome — Dot-like, central position, surrounded by a clear halo.
- Nuclear membrane — delicate, lined by regularly arranged fine chromatin granule.
- Linin network — of fine thread, arranged radially].

B. Pre-cystic stage (Fig. 8.8A)

Size — Smaller — 10-20 µm.

Shape — Round or ovoid with a small blunt pseudopodium.

Nucleus — Same as trophozoite.

Endoplasm — No RBC.

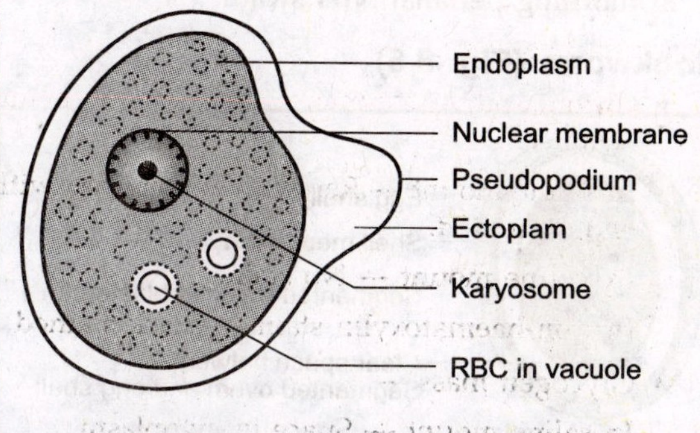

Fig. 8.8 B: Trophozoite of *Entamoeba histolytica*

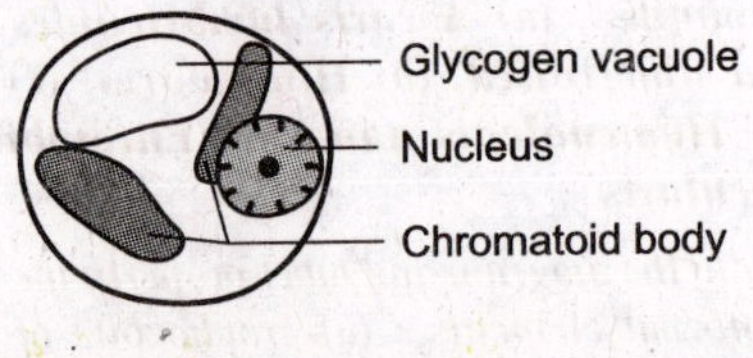

Fig. 8.9 : Uninucleate cyst

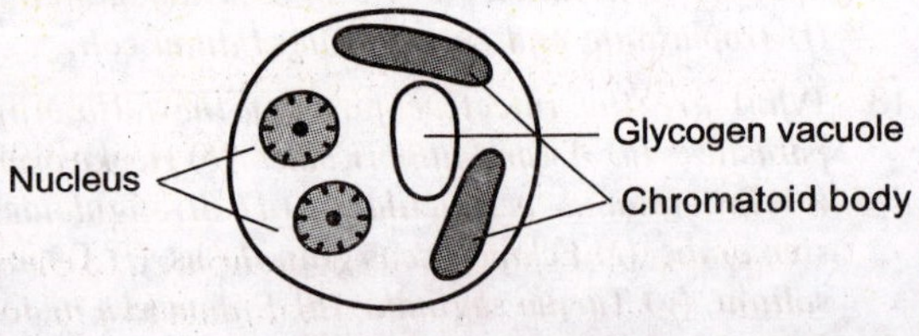

Fig. 8.10 : Binucleate cyst

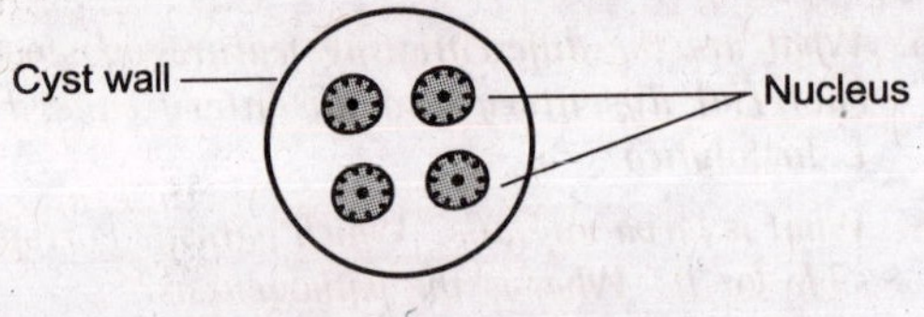

Fig. 8.11 : Tetranucleated cyst of *Entamoeba histolytica*

C. Cyst (Figs. 8.9, 8.10, 8.11)

Size — 'Small race' — 6-9 µm; 'Large race' 12-15 µm.

Shape — Rounded.

Cyst wall — Refractile membrane.

Nucleus — According to stages of development, it might be uninucleate, binucleate or quadrinucleate mature cyst. Nucleus is stained by iodine and bears similar characters as the trophozoite or precyst.

Cytoplasm —

(a) Early stage :

- Chromatoid or chromatoidial bars — 1 to 4 in number.

  In saline mount — Refractile oblong bar with ends rounded.

  In iodine mount — No stain.

  In iron-haematoxylin stain — Black stained.

- Glycogen mass —

  In saline mount — Space in cytoplasm

  In iodine mount — Stains brown.

[Maturity of the cyst is associated with —

- Nucleus number changes from one to four,
- Chromatoid bars and glycogen vacuole disappears].

Giardia intestinalis

A. Trophozoite (Fig. 8.12)

Found and better demonstrated in saline mounts of freshly voided diarrhoeic stool or after purgative.

Size — Length 14 µm × Breadth 7 µm.

Shape —Flat view — Tennis or badminton racket like.

Side on view — Longitudinally split pear like.

Dorsal surface — Convex.

Ventral surface — Concave.

Anterior end — Broader and rounded.

Posterior end — Tapered.

Symmetry — Bilaterally symmetrical. All the organs are paired.

Features —

- Axostyle — Two central supporting rod, running longitudinally.
- Sucking disc — Found on ventral surface at anterior end.
- Nuclei — Two.
- Flagella — Four pair.

Movement : Looks like a falling leaf in saline mount of freshly voided diarrhoeic stool.

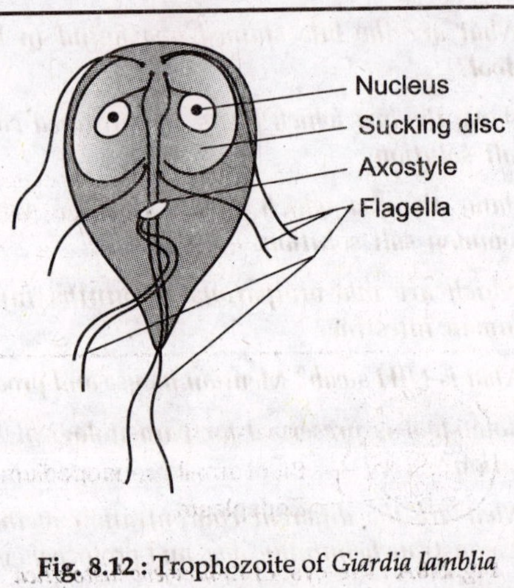

Fig. 8.12 : Trophozoite of *Giardia lamblia*

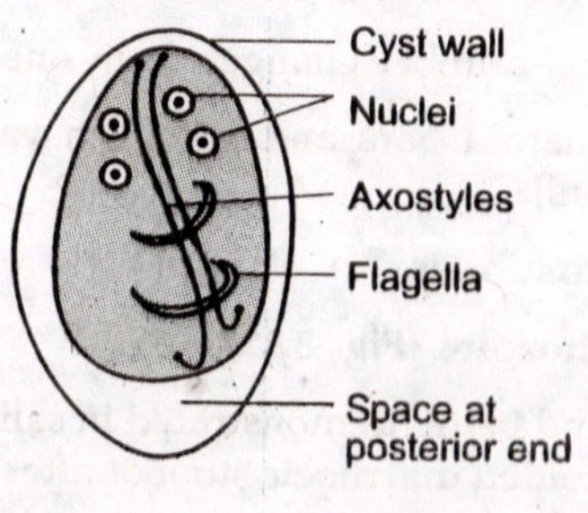

Fig. 8.13 : Cyst of *Giardia lamblia*

B. Cyst (Fig. 8.13)

Better demonstrated in iodine mount. Iodine stains the internal structures.

Size — **Length 12 μm × Breadth 7 μm.**

Shape — **Oval or elliptical.**

Cyst wall — **Refractile.**

Nucleus — **Four in number, forming a cluster at one end.**

Axostyle — **Set diagonally.**

Rudimentary flagella — **arranged in pair across the axostyle.**

Space between cell wall and cell membrane — **It is pronounced at the posterior end.**

QUESTIONS RELATED TO STOOL EXAMINATION

1. *Enumerate the nematodes infesting human gut.*
2. *Name the cestodes infesting human.*
3. *Name the larva found in human stool.*
4. *What are the bile stained ova found in human stool?*
5. *Name the ova which floats on saturated common salt solution.*
6. *Name the ova which do not float on saturated common salt solution.*
7. *Which are ovo-viviparous helminths infesting human intestine?*
8. *What is NIH swab? Mention its use and procedure.*
9. *How stool is preserved for parasitological examination?*
10. *What are the different concentration methods to demonstrate helminthic ova, and protozoal cyst and oocyst?*
11. *Draw diagram and label the eggs of following helminths : (a)* ***Ascaris lumbricoides*** *fertilised and unfertilised, (b)* ***Hookworm****, (c)* ***Taenia****, (d)* ***Hymenolepis nana****, (e)* ***Enterobious vermicularis****.*
12. *Draw the diagram and label properly the following protozoal elements : (a) trophozoite of E. histolytica, (b) cysts of different stages of E. histolytica, (c) cysts of Entamoeba coli, (d) trophozoite of Giardia lamblia, (e) cysts of Giardia lamblia, (f) trophozoite and cyst of Balantidium coli.*
13. *What are the infective form of the following parasites : (a) Ascaris lumbricoides, (b) Hookworm, (c) Enterobious vermicularis, (d) Strongyloides stercoralis, (e) Echinococcus granulosus, (f) Taenia solium, (g) Taenia saginata, (h) Entamoeba histolytica?*
14. *How will you distinguish between cysts of E. histolytica and E. coli?*
15. *What are the differentiating features of stool of bacterial dysentery and dysentery caused by E. histolytica.*
16. *What is larva migrans? Which parasite is responsible for it? What is the pathogenesis?*
17. *What is the causative parasite for Löeffler's pneumonia?*
18. *What are the principal clinical presenting features and pathogenic mechanisms of the following parasitic infestations : (a) Ascaris lumbricoides, (b) Hookworm, (c) Trichuris trichiura, (d) Enterobious vermicularis, (e) Entamoeba histolytica, (f) Giardia lamblia, (g) Taenia solium, (h) E. granulosus?*
19. *What are the skin penetrating larvae of helminths infesting man?*
20. *How will you identify the human pathogenic species of following parasites : (a) Hookworm, (b) Taenia, (c) Trichomonas, (d) Entamoeba.*
21. *What is free living amoebae and what are the diseases produced by them?*
22. *Name the helminths and protozoa affecting C.N.S.*
23. *Name the opportunistic coccidian protozoa infesting human intestine. What are the clinical presenting features? How will you demonstrate the protozoa in stool. Draw microscopical picture of all of these protozoan elements found in stool.*
24. *How will you confirm the infestations of following parasites : (a) extra-intestinal amoebiasis, (b) Toxoplasma, (c) Taenia solium, (d) Meningitis by free living amoebae, (e) Echinococcus?*

Immunoassays (Serological Tests)

9

When an antigen combines with its specific antibody in presence of an electrolyte (NaCl) in an optimum concentration at an optimal pH and temperature (37°C), the antigen and antibody complex forms an insoluble precipitate.

Important tests for antigen-antibody reactions include *precipitation, agglutination, complement fixation, neutralisation*, and labelled assays (immunofluorescence, enzyme immunoassay, radioimmunoassay) (Table 9.1). These reactions are greatly improved by the availability of highly specific monoclonal antibodies.

Antibody titre

The term titre is used to denote the highest dilution of the serum at which antibody activity is demonstrable, which is usually expressed as the reciprocal of the dilution of the serum, e.g. 64, when antibody was detected at a final serum dilution of 1 in 64. The antigens and antibodies taking part in the reaction are also measured by their mass weight, e.g. mg nitrogen.

Tests for antigen-antibody reaction

1. Precipitation reaction (Table 9.2)

When a soluble antigen reacts with its specific antibody at an optimum proportion, pH and temp, Ag-Ab complex forms an insoluble precipitate, e.g.

(a) **Simple precipitation tests**: Ring test, slide test, slide flocculation test (VDRL), tube flocculation (Kahn) test.

(b) **Immunodiffusion**: Single diffusion in one dimension, double diffusion in one dimension, double diffusion in two dimensions, counter-immunoelectrophoresis.

2. Agglutination

It is an antigen-antibody reaction in which an antibody (usually patient's serum and soluble)

Table 9.1 : Antigen-Antibody reactions

Receptor	Immunoglobulin			Modified tests
	IgG	IgM	IgA	
Precipitation	S	W	V	Immunoelectrophoresis, Immunoprecipitation
Agglutination	W	S	M	Latex agglutination, Indirect haemagglutination, Coagglutination, Antiglobulin (Coombs' test).
Complement fixation	S	W	N	Conglutination.
Neutralisation	S	W	N	Plaque assay, Measurement of lethal dose (LD).
Immunofluorescence	S	W	N	Indirect immunofluorescence, Immunofluorimetric assay.
Enzyme immunoassay	S	W	N	Enzyme-linked immunosorbent assay.
Radioimmunoassay	S	W	N	Immunoradiometric assay.

S = Strong, W = Weak, V = Variable, N = Negative, M = Moderate.

Table 9.2 : Precipitation tests

Test	Procedure	Diffusion	Uses
Simple precipitation (Precipitation in liquid medium)			
1. Ring test (Fig. 9.1)	Ag solution layered over a column of whole serum (Ab) in a narrow test tube	A ring of ppt. forms at junction of two	Ascoli's thermoprecipitin test, streptococcal grouping
2. Slide test	A drop each of Ag solution and serum placed on a slide, mixed by shaking	Floccules formed	VDRL
3. Tube flocculation	Serial dilutions of Ag made in test tube to which fixed amount of serum added	Amount of Ag that flocculates the serum is called Lf dose	Kahn test
Immunodiffusion (Precipitation in gel)			
1. Oudin [Fig. 9.2(i)]	Serum (Ab) incorporated in agar gel in a test tube and Ag solution layered over it	Antigen diffuses downward forming line of ppt	Single diffusion in one dimension
2. Oakley Fulthorpe variation of Oudin [Fig. 9.2(ii)]	Ab incorporated in gel, above which is placed a column of agar and Ag is layered on surface of plain agar	Ag and Ab move towards each other through plain agar and forms a band of ppt	Double diffusion in one dimension — used in Elek test
3. Radial (Fig. 9.3)	Ab incorporated in agar gel in Petri dish or slide, Ag kept in well cut out gel	Ag diffuses, concentric bands of precipitin form around the well	Single diffusion in two dimensions — used in complement components detection and their assay
4. Ouchterlony (Fig. 9.4)	Agar gel poured on a slide, wells are cut using a template. Ab placed in central well and Ags in surrounding wells	When adjacent Ags are identical, lines of ppt fuse; if unrelated, lines of ppt cross each other	Double diffusion in two dimensions — used in detection of Ags and their relatedness
5. Immunoelectrophoresis (Fig. 9.5)	(i) Ag placed in a well in agar gel in a slide. Electric current passed. Ags get separated. (ii) A trough is then cut in agar and filled with Ab.	By diffusion lines of ppt formed with each separated Ag	Detection of myeloma band
Counter immunoelectrophoresis (Fig. 9.6)			
	Simultaneous electrophoresis of Ag and Ab in gel is done in opposite direction	Ppt occurs at a point between the two	

combines with a particulate antigen in presence of an electrolyte and at an optimal temperature and pH resulting in visible clumping (aggregation of the particles, such as agglutination of bacteria, erythrocytes, latex particles etc.), e.g.

(a) **Slide and tile agglutination test**: Detection of isolated bacteria by slide agglutination test.

(b) **Tube agglutination test**: Widal test.

(c) **Heterophile agglutination test**: Weil-Felix

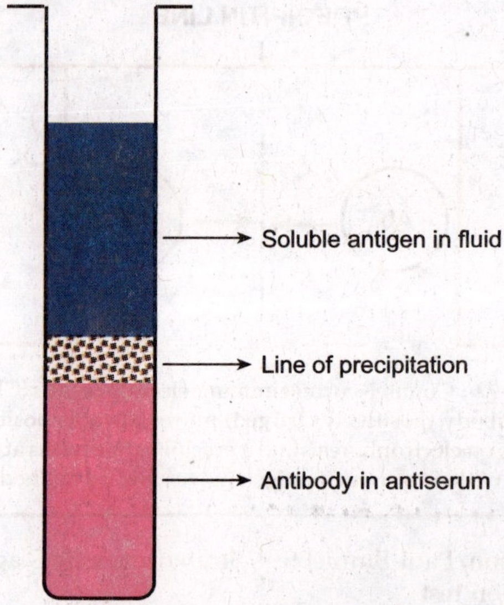

Fig. 9.1 : Tube precipitin test

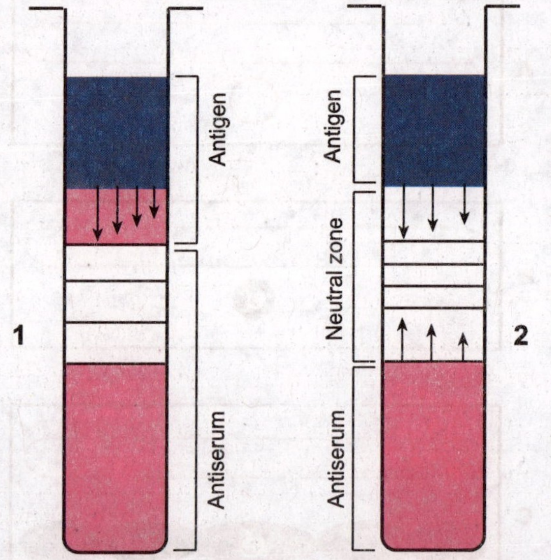

Fig. 9.2 : Gel diffusion precipition reactions — (1) Single diffusion in one dimension; (2) Double diffusion in one dimension. Arrows show direction of diffusion. Broad line = precipitation hands

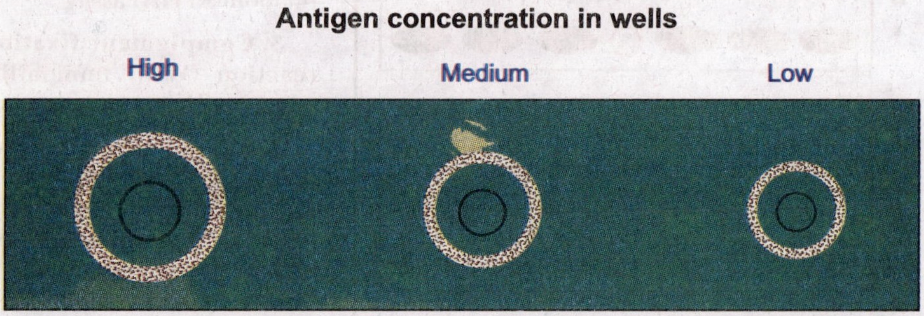

Fig. 9.3 : Single radial diffusion. Unknown Ag in well and specific antibody in the agar

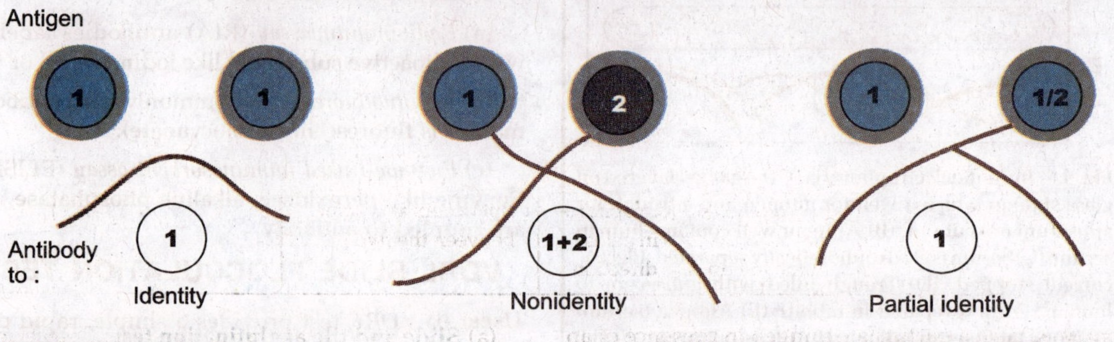

Fig. 9.4 : Commonly observed pattern of precipitation band in double diffusion test (Ouchterlony immunodouble diffusion) : (1) Line of confluence with two antigens that cannot be distinguished by the antiserum used (reaction of identity), (1 + 2) Crossing-over of lines obtained with two serologically different antigens (reaction of nonidentity), (1) "Spur" formation by partially related antigens at the junction of precipitin bands (reaction of partial identity).

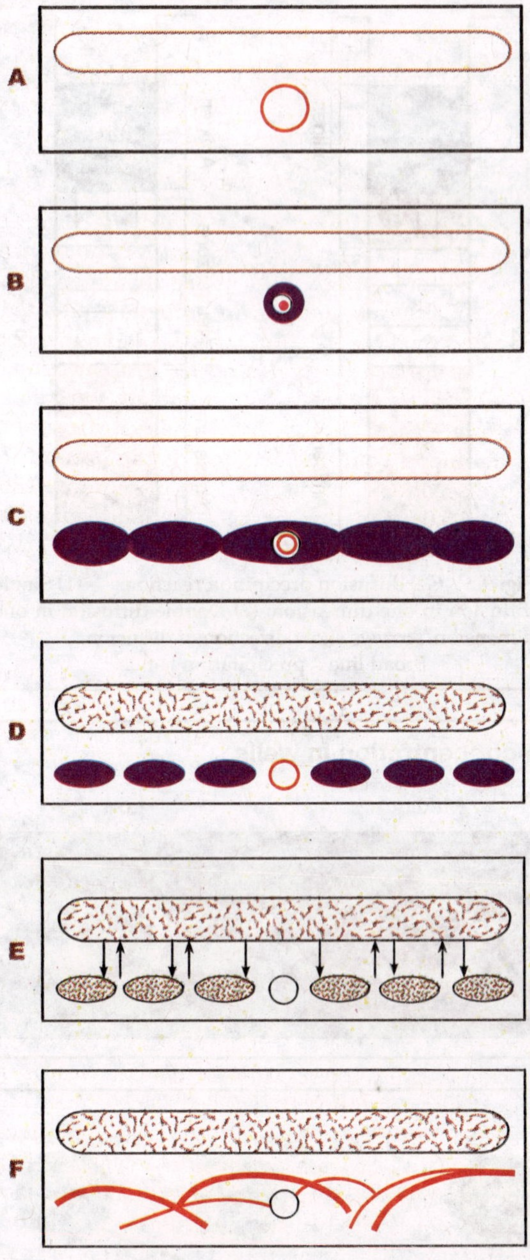

Fig. 9.5: Immunoelectrophoresis: (A) Agar gel layered on glass slide in which a well for antigen and a trough for antiserum are cut out. (B) Antigen well contains human serum. (C) Serum is electrophoretically separated. Electric current stopped. (D) Trough filled with antiserum to human serum (prepared in rabbit). (E) Antigen (serum) antibody (anti-serum) allowed to diffuse into agar. (F) The two components diffuse to each other and form precipitate bands. Precipitin bands form for individual serum protein. The band can be shown more clearly by staining with a protein stain.

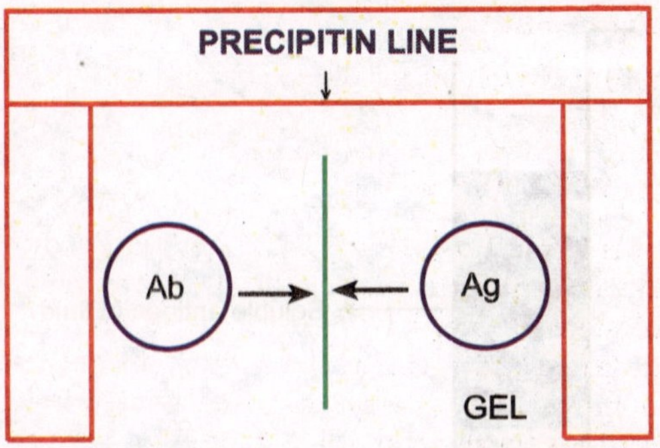

Fig. 9.6: Counter-current immunoelectrophoresis (CIE). Antibody (positively charged) moves towards positive pole on electrophoresis and a precipitin line forms at the site of their meeting (antigen moves toward antibody).

reaction, Paul-Bunnel test, Streptococcus MG agglutination test.

(d) **Antiglobulin test**: Coombs' test.

(e) **Microtitration agglutination**: Indirect passive haemagglutination test, haemagglutination inhibition (HI) antibody test, reverse passive haemagglutination (RPHA) assay.

3. Complement fixation test: Wassermann reaction (WR), immobilisation test, immune adherence test, cytolytic or cytocidal reaction.

4. Neutralisation test: When an antibody (antitoxin) combines with specific antigen (toxin), the biological effects of the toxin (antigen) are neutralised e.g. Neutralisation test (guinea pig inoculation) and neutralisation *in vivo* (agar gel precipitation test), both tests are done for detection of diphtheria toxin.

5. **Labelled Immunoassay**:

(a) *Radioimmunoassay* (RIA) antibodies labelled with radioactive substances like iodine — ^{125}I or ^{131}I.

(b) *Immunofluorescence* (commonly used antibody marker is fluorescein isothiocyanate).

(c) *Enzyme-linked immunosorbent assay* (ELISA): Enzyme like peroxidase, alkaline phosphatase, etc. are coupled to antibody.

VDRL SLIDE FLOCCULATION TEST

Uses: (i) VDRL test provides a simple, rapid convenient and economical, procedure for serologic testing for diagnosis of syphilis.

(ii) It has high sensitivity. Test is non-specific. It can be used for rapid and exact quantitative titration of reactive serum samples for screening and monitoring treatment.

(iii) It is well-suited for mass surveys.

Reagents

1. ***VDRL Antigen***

It is an alcoholic solution and contains cardiolipin 0.03 per cent, purified lecithin 0.21 per cent, and cholesterol 0.9 per cent. The antigen is serologically standardised by comparison with an antigen of known reactivity. The antigen is dispensed in 0.5 ml quantities (with a sufficient excess for convenient withdrawal of the required amount) in sealed glass ampoules which should be stored in a cool dark place.

2. ***Buffered saline solution***

The buffered saline has the following composition :

Formaldehyde	....	0.5 ml
Na_2HPO_4	....	3.037 gm
KH_2PO_4	....	0.170 gm
NaCl	....	10.0 gm
Distilled water	....	1000 ml

and has a pH of 6.0 ± 0.1.

3. ***VDRL slide***

Glass slides (2 × 3") with 12 paraffin rings or cavities of approximately 14 mm inside diameter are used. Similar slides with permanently fixed ceramic rings (5 rings) (Fig. 9.7) should be more convenient but are somewhat expensive.

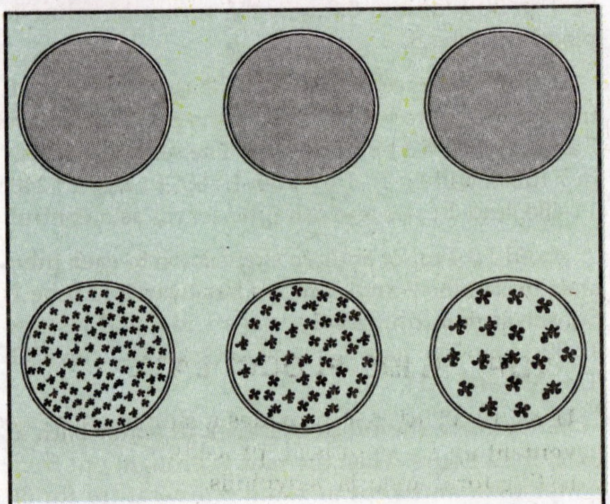

Fig. 9.7 : VDRL slide flocculation test result

Procedure

1. ***Preparation of Serum***

Serum is inactivated for 30 minutes at 56°C. Sera to be tested more than 4 hours after being heated; should be reheated at 56°C for 10 minutes.

2. ***Preparation of Antigen Emulsion***

0.4 ml of buffered saline is pipetted into the bottom of a 1 oz. reagent bottle with flat or concave inner bottom surface. Add 0.5 ml of antigen, drawn from an ampoule into a 1.0 ml pipette graduated to tip, directly on to the saline while rotating the bottle on a flat surface. Antigen is added drop by drop but rapidly so that it takes approximately 6 seconds to complete the delivery. Blow the last drop of the antigen and continue rotation of the bottle for 10 more seconds. Then add 4.1 ml of buffered saline from a 5.0 ml pipette. Stopper the bottle and shake it vigorously for approximately 10 seconds. Temperature of buffered saline solution and antigen should be preferably between 23°C to 29°C during the preparation of antigen emulsion.

Maturation of the antigen increases the sensitiveness and this is almost complete **in 15 to 30 minutes**. The antigen emulsion may then be used during the whole day. Under conditions of high temperature and low humidity, the antigen emulsion is stored in a refrigerator but should be restored to room temperature before the test. Antigen emulsion should be shaken gently every time before use. This quantity (5.0 ml) is sufficient for 250 serum tests.

The preparation of antigen emulsion should first be examined by testing known reactive and nonreactive sera. This is done by adding one drop of antigen emulsion to 0.05 ml of each serum and completing the test as described under Quantitative Serum Test. These tests should present typically reactive and non-reactive results, respectively and the number and distribution of antigen particles per microscopic field in the negative sera should be optimum. An unsatisfactory antigen emulsion should be discarded.

Qualitative Serum Test

A volume of 0.05 ml heat inactivated (56°C for 1 hour) serum is pipetted into one ring of a VDRL glass slide. The serum should spread.

Now add one drop (1/60 ml) antigen emulsion on to the serum by a syringe dropping 1/60 ml antigen per drop. Rotate the slide for 4 minutes.

(If rotated by hand on a flat surface this movement should roughly circumscribe a 5 cm diameter circle 120 times per minute).

Reading and reporting the results

The tests are read immediately after rotation under a microscope with low power objectives at 100 × magnification. The antigen particles are seen as small fusiform needles which remain more or less evenly dispersed in a non-reactive serum and aggregate into clumps in reactive sera.

No clumps or very slight	—	Non-reactive (N)
Small clumps	—	Weakly reactive (W)
Medium and large clumps	—	Reactive (R)

Zone reactions are recognised by the irregular clumping. Clumps are not compact and very small. Large clumps may be seen in the same field. In such cases, the results are reported on the basis of quantitative reaction done on the same serum.

Quantitative Serum Test

Quantitative test is performed on all reactive serum samples and on all samples showing weakly reactive or "rough" in the qualitative test. Successive two fold dilutions of the serum are made in 0.9 per cent saline and each dilution is treated as an individual serum and tested as described under Qualitative Serum Tests. The results are reported in terms of the highest dilution which gives a frank reactive reaction.

Reporting results of the Quantitative Tests

The results are reported in terms of the highest dilution of the serum that produces a definite reaction (not weakly reactive). Some examples are shown below (Fig. 9.8) :

Serum dilution							
1/1	1/2	1/4	1/8	1/16	1/32	1/64	Report
R	W	N	N	N	N	N	R 1 dil
R	R	W	N	N	N	N	R 2 dils
R	R	R	W	N	N	N	R 4 dils
W	W	R	R	W	N	N	R 8 dils
N	W	R	R	R	N	N	R 16 dils
W	N	N	N	N	N	N	W 0 dil
W	W	N	N	N	N	N	N R

Fig. 9.8 : Reporting results of the quantitative VDRL tests

VDRL Antigen can also be used for the VDRL Tube Flocculation test and for testing spinal fluids.

WIDAL TEST

Principle

It is used for detection of antibodies produced by the host against determinants on the surface of a bacterial agent in response to infection with *Salmonella typhi* and *S. paratyphi*. Patient's serum show agglutinating antibodies that cause agglutination of the bacterial antigens. The patient's serum is tested by agglutination for its titres of antibodies against H and O suspensions of *S. typhi* and *S. paratyphi*.

Materials required

1. Small test tubes (Kalin tube). Dreyer tubes may be used for testing H-agglutination.

2. Antigen suspensions, prepared from suitable stock cultures in the laboratory, but generally commercially prepared suspensions are used.

3. 0.85% NaCl.

4. Water bath.

Procedure

Patients serum is tested in a series of dilutions against each of the different antigen suspensions :

1. Eight tubes are taken for each series — seven for serum dilutions and the eighth for non-serum control (C).

2. Add 0.4 ml saline in tubes 1 to 7. Dilute patient's serum 1 in 15 in saline and add 0.4 ml of this to tubes 1 and 2. Dilution of serum in tube 2 will be 1 in 30 (volume 0.8 ml). No serum or saline is placed in tube 8.

3. Mix the contents of tube 2 thoroughly and transfer 0.4 ml to tube 3. Repeat the process till tube 7 and discard 0.4 ml in the end. The serum dilutions in 7 tubes will be 1 : 15, 1 : 30, 1 : 60, 1 : 120, 1 : 240, 1 : 480, and 1 : 960 and 8th tube serves as a control.

4. Add 0.4 ml of antigen suspension to each tube, start from tube 7 and working backwards to tube 1. So, the serum dilutions in tubes 1 to 6 will be now 1 : 30-1:960. The four different antigens used are TO, TH, AO and AH.

5. Incubate the tubes in a rack in water bath at 37°C for 2 hours. Then the rack is brought out from water bath and kept at room temperature for 30 minutes. H-agglutination is noted at this point. Then the rack is again kept in water bath at 37°C for

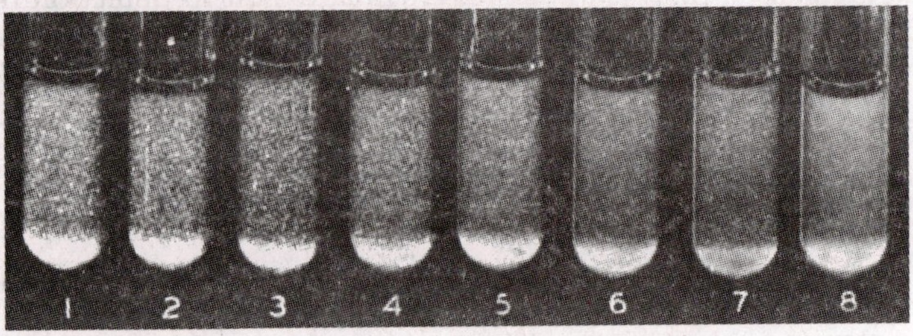

Fig. 9.9 : Macroscopic agglutination (Widal) test — flagellar agglutination of *Salmonella* (Tubes 2 to 8). The control tube (8) 'C' contains only bacterial suspension but no antiserum. Successive serum dilution in tube 2 to 8 are 1 : 15, 1 : 30, 1 : 60, 1 : 120, 1 : 240, 1 : 480, and 1 : 960

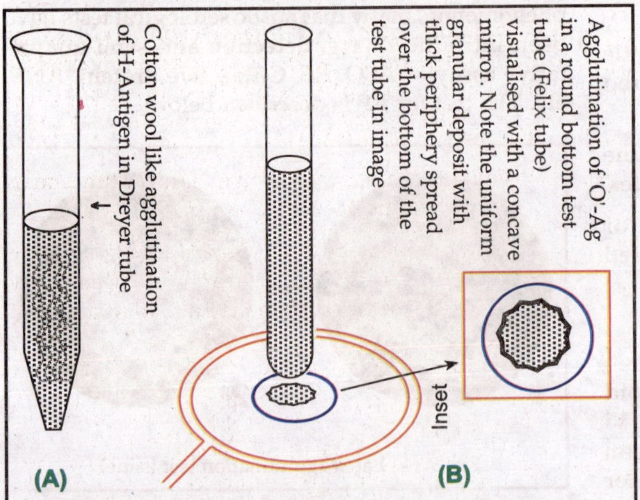

Fig. 9.10 : Widal tube test showing bacterial agglutination

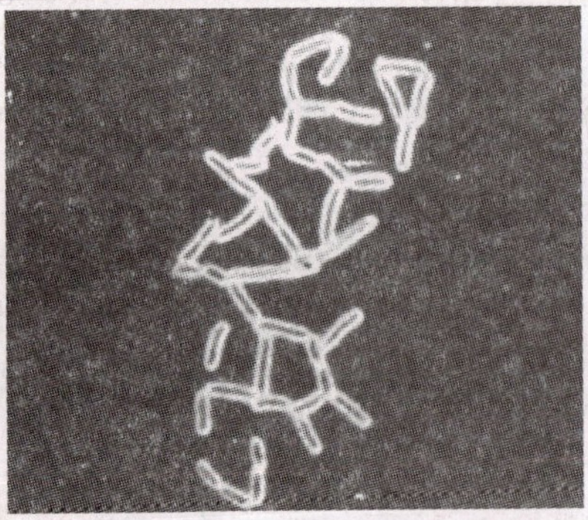

Fig. 9.12 : Somatic ('O') agglutination of *Salmonella* by O antiserum (examination of deposit by coverslip preparation) shown a polar attachment of bacterial cells

another 2 hours, followed by preservation in refrigerator for overnight period before O-agglutination is noted.

Results

1. H-agglutination, appears as large flakes is read by viewing the tubes under good light against a dark background with the aid of a magnifying lens (Figs. 9.9 to 9.11). O-agglutination form fine granular deposit, best viewed with a concave mirror (Figs. 9.12 and 9.13). If necessary, the tubes can be gently rotated, to swirl up granules from the deposit.

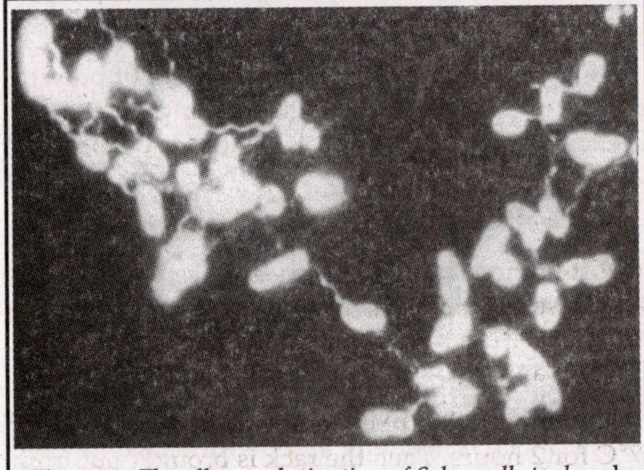

Fig. 9.11 : Flagellar agglutination of *Salmonella typhosa* by H antiserum : clumps of cells formed by intertwining of thickened flagellar structures (Electron microscopy)

2. The titre of the serum is the highest dilution of serum giving visible agglutination.

Remarks

1. A progressive rise in titre between first and second week after onset of fever is highly significant. A positive or a negative result in a single test is not significant.

2. Since the antibodies are detected only after seven to ten days of illness, test should be done later.

3. The serum of some uninfected subjects causes agglutination at dilutions of about 1 in 60. So titres are considered significant when agglutination occurs in serum dilution above 100.

4. H-agglutinins tend to persist longer than O-agglutinins. Persons immunised with TAB vaccine

may show high titres of antibodies to all the antigens and so only a marked rise in titre is considered significant.

5. Early administration of antibiotic cause arrest of titre.

RAPID SLIDE TEST

Commercial kits are available for the purpose :

1. Place 0.01 ml serum on each of five squares on a glass plate.

2. Add 0.03 ml of antigen (1 drop) from a bottle of antigen suspension. Antigen is thoroughly mixed before use.

3. Mix well by a stick (toothpick). Then lift the plate and slowly tilt back and forth for 2-3 minutes.

Reading : Result is read in a viewing box or against a flat black background. Test with diluted serum is done to find out titre.

Vi AGGLUTINATION (Fig. 9.13)

Antibodies to Vi-antigen appear during typhoid fever but disappear after recovery from disease. Vi antibodies are detected in current or recent infection but soon disappear. Vi antibodies persist in carrier state. Antibody to Vi antigen (1 : 10 or above) is present in serum of most carriers (Fig. 9.13) :

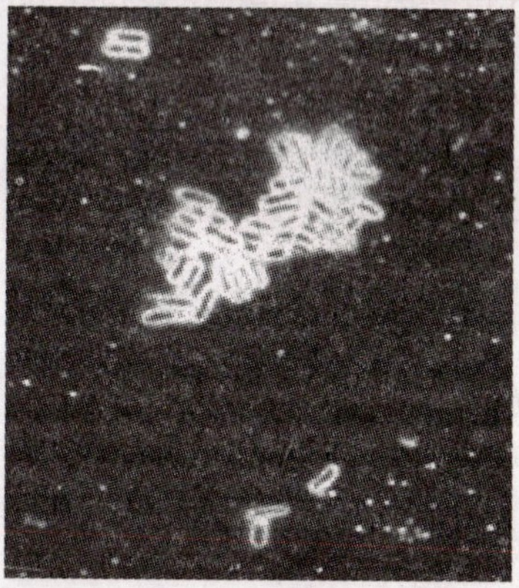

Fig. 9.13 : Vi agglutination of *Salmonella typhi* by Vi antiserum — side-to-side attachment of cells has produced a dense mass of agglutinated cells

Convalescent carriers and some individuals with subclinical infection (*healthy carriers*) of typhoid fever continue to excrete organisms in faeces, less commonly in the urine for about 2 months to a year. Incidence of chronic carriers is lower in paratyphoid than typhoid fever. In addition to detection of antibody to Vi antigen in patient's serum repeated stool cultures may be required to detect the bacilli. Aspirated bile and duodenal drainage cultures are helpful.

LATEX AGGLUTINATION TEST (Fig. 9.14)

Latex or polystyrene particles coated with Ag or Ab react with specific corresponding Ab or Ag to produce clumping of the particles. Based on this phenomenon, many diagnostic serological tests have been introduced : e.g. detection and semi-quantitative assay of ASO, RF, C-Reactive protein, ANF, etc. The test for RF is described below.

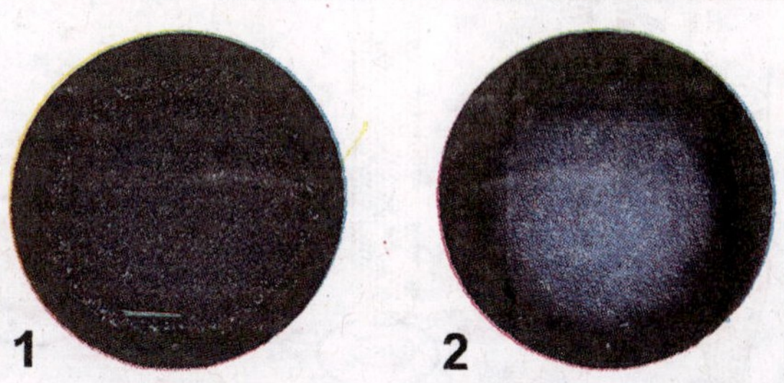

Fig. 9.14 : Latex agglutination test (slide)

Principle

RF slide test for detection of rheumatoid factors is based on the principle of agglutination. The test specimen is mixed with RF latex reagent and allowed to react. If RF (anti-human IgM) is present within detectable levels then a visible agglutination is observed. If RF is absent below detectable levels, then no agglutination is observed.

Reagent required

1. RF reagent : A uniform suspension of polystyrene latex particles coated with suitably modified Fc fraction of IgG. The reagent is standardised to detect 10 IU/ml of RF or more.

2. Positive control serum, reactive with the RF reagent.

3. Negative control serum, non-reactive with the RF reagent.

Each batch of reagents undergoes rigorous quality control at various stages of manufacture for its specificity, sensitivity and performance.

Reagent contains **0.1% Sodium azide** as preservative. Avoid contact with skin and mucosa. On disposal, flush with large quantities of water.

The reagent can be damaged due to microbial contamination or on exposure to extreme temperature. It is recommended that the performance of the reagent be verified with the positive and negative controls provided with the kit. Shake the RF latex reagent well before use to disperse the latex particles uniformly and improve test readability.

Specimen

Only serum should be used for testing. Should a delay in testing occur, store the sample at 2-8°C. Samples can be stored for up to a week. Do not use haemolysed serum.

Material required

1. RF latex reagent, Positive control, Negative control.

2. Glass slide with six reaction circles. Samples dispensing pipettes, Mixing sticks, Rubber teat.

3. Stopwatch, Test tubes, a high intensity direct light source, isotonic saline.

Procedure

Bring reagent and samples to room temperature before use.

(a) **Qualitative Method**

1. Pipette one drop of serum onto the glass slide using the disposable pipette.

2. Add one drop of RF latex reagent to the drop of serum on the slide. Do not let the dropper tip touch the liquid on the slide.

3. Using a mixing stick, mix the serum and the RF latex reagent uniformly over the entire circle.

4. Immediately start a stopwatch. Rock the slide gently, back and forth, observing for agglutination macroscopically at **2 minutes**.

(b) **Semi-quantitative Method**

1. Using isotonic saline prepare serial dilutions of the serum sample positive in the qualitative method 1 : 2, 1 : 4, 1 : 8, 1 : 16, 1 : 32, 1 : 64 and so on.

2. Pipette each dilution of the serum sample onto separate reaction circles.

3. Add one drop of RF latex reagent to each drop of the diluted serum sample on the slide. Do not let the dropper tip touch the liquid on the slide.

4. Using a mixing stick, mix the sample and the latex reagent uniformly over the entire circle.

5. Immediately start a stopwatch. Rock the slide gently, back and forth, observing for agglutination macroscopically at **2 minutes** (Fig. 9.14).

Interpretation

Qualitative method : Agglutination is a positive test result and indicates the presence of rheumatoid factors in the test specimen. No agglutination is a negative test result and indicates the absence of rheumatoid factors in the test specimen.

Semi-quantitative method : Agglutination in the highest serum dilution corresponds to the approximate amount of rheumatoid factors in IU/ml present in the tests specimen.

To calculate the RF in IU/ml, use the following formula :

RF (IU/ml) = S × D

where, S = Sensitivity of the reagent, **i.e. 10 IU ml**

D = Highest dilution of serum showing agglutination.

Notes :

1. Markedly lipemic, haemolysed and contaminated serum samples could produce non-specific results.

2. Use of plasma rather than serum can lead to false-positive results.

3. Do not read results beyond two minutes.

4. Rheumatoid factors are not exclusively found in rheumatoid arthritis but sometimes in syphilis, systemic lupus erythematosus, hepatitis, hypergammaglobulinaemia also.

5. It is recommended that results of the test should be correlated with clinical findings to arrive at the final diagnosis.

6. The RF reagent is free from prozone effect at RF levels between 10 IU/ml to 2300 IU/ml of RF concentration.

7. RF reagent is sensitive to the presence of IgM RF with heterogeneous specificity.

Summary

Autoantibodies are sometimes produced by the human body against self-antigens. The precise role that this aberrant immunity plays in the pathogenesis of certain rheumatoid diseases is unknown. The presence of these autoantibodies serve as credible marker of the disease.

In rheumatoid arthritis, diagnostically useful autoantibodies termed as "Rheumatoid factors" (RF) can be detected which are immunoglobulins of the class IgM, IgG, IgA and IgE. Practically, IgM class RF with specificity to human IgG (Fc) is the most useful prognostic marker of RA. The clinical significance of RF determinations consists in differentiation between rheumatoid arthritis, in which RF of modified IgM class have been demonstrated in the serum of approximately 80% of the cases examined and rheumatic fever, in which RF are almost always absent. The agglutination test is most frequently used because of its greater sensitivity and simplicity.

INDIRECT HAEMAGGLUTINATION ASSAY (IHA)

Principle

When a particulate antigen is mixed with its antibody in the presence of electrolytes at a suitable temperature and pH, the particles are clumped or agglutinated. Agglutination occurs optimally when antigens and antibodies react in equivalent proportions.

This test measures as little as 1-10 µg/ml of antibody. RBCs are used in the test as they are extremely convenient passive carriers of antigen and give a visible reaction and many antigens can be coated on complex surface of RBC. RBCs used can be of Human group "O" as it does not contain antigen and of Sheep (or RBCs of Horse, Monkey, Turkey Guinea-pig, etc. can be used).

Reagents

1. *Phosphate buffer* solution (PBS) (pH 7.4) – 0.15 M
2. *Alsever's solution* :

Sodium citrate	: 0.08 g
Dextrose	: 2.05 g
Sodium chloride	: 0.42 g
Distilled water	: 100 ml

Adjust pH to 6.1 with 10% citric acid (autoclave at 10 pounds for 15 minutes).

3. *Tannic acid (TA)*

Dissolve 1 mg in 20 ml of normal saline and store at 4°C. (1 : 20,000 dilution).

4. Rabbit Serum Saline (RSS)

1% Rabbit serum in PBS.

Preparation of sensitised RBC's

1. To collect sheep blood in Alsever's solution.
2. To wash the RBCs thrice in PBS by centrifugation at 1,000 rpm.
3. The RBCs are packed at 2500 rpm by washing with PBS (pH 7.2) for 5-10 minutes.
4. Make 2.5% suspension of RBCs in PBS (pH 7.2) (make upto 2 ml.).
5. Add equal volume of Tannic acid.
6. Incubate at 37°C for 15 min. in a water bath.
7. Wash the RBCs thrice with PBS.
8. For sensitisation of RBCs add 1.5 ml of tanned cells to 1.5 ml of antigen [diluted in PBS (pH 6.4)] (Antigen is titrated first against positive serum of known titre by chequer board and finally minimum antigen concentration which gives agglutination with known positive serum at same dilution is used).
9. Incubate at 37°C for 30 minutes in water bath.
10. Centrifuge at 1,000 rpm for 10 minutes.
11. Wash with 1% Rabbit Serum Saline (RSS).

Procedure (Figs. 9.15, 9.16)

1. The test sera is inactivated at 56°C for 30 minutes.
2. 1 per cent RSS is used for serial dilutions of serum samples.
3. Make 4-fold dilutions of all serum samples in perspex plates with the help of microdiluters starting from 1 : 8 to 1 : 2,048 (take 50 µl of diluted serum).

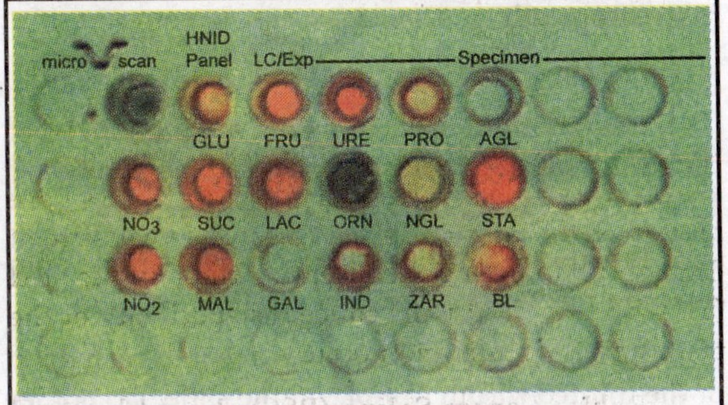

Fig. 9.15: Microtitration plate: Results of indirect haemagglutination tests are shown

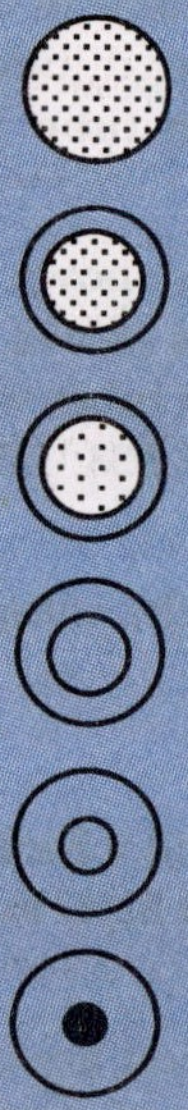

POSITIVE (4+) Uniform mat of cells covering the entire well base, may be with folded margin

POSITIVE (3+) Uniform mat of cells partially covering the well base

POSITIVE (2+) Uniform mat of cells margined by a ring of cells

WEAK POSITIVE (1+) Smaller mat encircled by a smaller ring of cells

INDETERMINATE (1+) Button cells with a clear centre

NEGATIVE (•) Compact button in the well

Fig. 9.16 : Interpretation of haemagglutination test results

4. Two controls, i.e. tanned RBCs control and antigen control should always be put with every test.

5. Add 0.025 ml (one drop of a microdiluter) of sensitised RBC's in each well (except in antigen control well). Mix by shaking.

6. Incubate for 1 hour at 37°C and then overnight at 4°C.

7. Agglutination, characterised by uniform mat of cells covering the entire bottom of the well, suggests positive reaction and button (of RBCs) suggest negative reaction (Fig. 9.16). So the titre of antibody will be the highest dilution of antibody which will give agglutination reaction.

Remarks

1. Tanning of RBCs is important, as it exposes the surface receptors and also reduces the electrostatic charges. RBCs are negatively charged and so are always repelling each other. To cause enhancement of agglutination, if the concentration of tannic acid (TA) is too high, it will reduce the specificity of the test as autoagglutination occurs.

2. Rabbit Serum Saline (RSS) should be used because it prevents autoagglutination of tanned cells and acts as a stabiliser by balancing out the agglutinating effect of TA resulting in greater sensitivity of the test. Rabbit serum should also be inactivated at 56°C for 30 minutes.

3. Plates are thoroughly washed and cleaned and serum should be free of contamination.

4. Sometimes the test shows false-positive results, because of the presence of artifacts in plates or insufficient stability of RBCs or because of autoagglutination of cells by excessive tanning or by using excess of antigen. So all these should be standardised properly and time given for each step should be adhered to — to avoid false-positivity.

5. False-negative results do occur when the concentration of antigen is low, or by undertanning RBCs. So proper precautions should be taken.

6. Cold centrifuge should preferably be used for all steps as the test is very sensitive to high temperatures.

7. Instead of normal saline (as it can resist the changes in pH) PBS is used as the test is very sensitive to changes in pH.

8. Preferably fresh RBCs should be used, as preserved cells are less sensitive than (preservative formalin) fresh ones.

9. Alternatives for tannic acid are Bis-diazotised benzidine and chromium chloride.

ANTI-STREPTOLYSIN O (ASO) TEST
(TUBE DILUTION METHOD)

Principle

It is a neutralisation test used to measure the ability of a patient's serum to neutralise the erythrocyte lysing capability of streptolysin O, an extracellular enzyme produced by ***Streptococcus pyogenes*** during infection.

Materials

1. *Antigen* : Streptolysin O — available commercially, is reconstituted before use.
2. *ASO buffer* : Phosphate buffered saline (pH 6.4).
3. *RBC suspension* : 5% suspension of RBCs in ASO buffer : Human blood group 'O' or rabbit erythrocytes.
4. *Water bath.*

Procedure

1. *Serum dilution* (Table 9.1)

Serum is at first diluted in 3 master dilution tubes as follows :

Master dilution tube I (1 : 10) : A volume of 0.2 ml. serum is added to 1.8 ml ASO buffer.

Master dilution tube II (1 : 100) : A volume of 0.05 ml of serum is diluted in 4.95 ml ASO buffer.

Master dilution tube III (1 : 500) : A volume of 0.5 ml of 1 : 100 dilution serum from master dilution tube II is tranferred master dilution tube III containing 4.5 ml of ASO buffer.

Now place the diluted sera in tubes as shown in Fig. 9.15. Then add buffer to the tubes as shown in Table 9.3. The dilution in different serum tubes will be 12, 50, 100, 125, 166, 250, 333, 500, 625, 833, 1250, 2,500.

2. *Addition of antigen* : Add 0.5 ml of the antigen to all the tubes.

Incubate at 37°C for 15 minutes.

3. *RBC suspension* : After incubation add 0.5 ml of washed 5% RBCs, shake and incubate at 37°C for 1 hour.

4. *Control* : Controls used with this test are cell control, antigen control and a standard serum control.

Results

1. Reading can be taken as such but centrifugation of tubes makes reading easier.

2. The titre of ASO is the highest serum dilution causing no haemolysis. Significant titre is considered to be 250 or more.

Table 9.3 : Anti-streptolysin O (ASO) test by tube dilution method

Tube No.	1	2	3	4	5	6	7	8	9	10	11	12	Cell control	Lysin control	Serum control
1 : 10 serum dilution	0.8	0.2	—	—	—	—	—	—	—	—	—	—	—	—	1.0
1 : 100 serum dilution	—	—	1.0	0.8	0.6	0.4	0.3	—					—	—	1.0
1 : 500 serum dilution	—	—	—	—	—	—	—	1.0	0.8	0.6	0.4	0.2	—	—	1.0
Buffer	0.2	0.8	0	0.2	0.4	0.6	0.7	0	0.2	0.4	0.6	0.8	1.5	1.0	1.0
Antigen (Streptolysin O)	0.5	0.5	0.5	0.5	0.5	0.5	0.5	0.5	0.5	0.5	0.5	0.5	0	0.5	—
	Shake gently. Incubate 15 minutes at 37°C.														
5% cell suspension	0.5	0.5	0.5	0.5	0.5	0.5	0.5	0.5	0.5	0.5	0.5	0.5	0.5	0.5	0.5
Value of tube in Todd units	12	50	100	125	166	250	333	500	625	833	1250	2500	—	—	—
	Shake gently. Incubate 45 minutes at 37°C. Refrigerate overnight or centrifuge tube one minute at 1,500 r.p.m. and read														

Remarks

1. Serum is to be inactivated at 56°C for 30 minutes before use.

2. A rise in ASO is detectable after 1 week of infection and very high titres are observed between third and fifth week.

3. False-positive results are observed due to increased levels of B lipoproteins in serum or contamination of serum by *S. aureus* or Pseudomonas species or by oxidation of ASO.

ROSE-WALLER TEST
(Differential Sheep Cell Agglutination Test)

Principle

It is an agglutination (antiglobulin) test using sheep RBCs sensitised with a subagglutinating dose of rabbit anti-sheep erythrocyte serum IgG. Rheumatoid factor, 19 S IgM, will combine with the fixed 7S IgG and produce agglutination.

Materials required

1. *Sheep RBCs.*

2. *Anti-sheep RBC serum* (A-SRBC) : The titre of antiserum which fails to agglutinate the SRBCs should be determined.

3. *Sensitised RBCs* : 2% RBC suspension is added to an equal volume of diluted antiserum with constant stirring. This can be used within few minutes.

Procedure

1. A serial two-fold dilutions of patients serum (0.2 ml) is made in saline in ten test tubes, such as 1 : 4, 1 : 8, 1 : 16, 1 : 32 and 1 : 64. The last tube is kept as control for SRBC suspension.

2. A volume of 0.2 ml of **sensitised RBCs** is added to all tubes and incubate at 37°C for one hour and then at 4°C for 2 hours.

3. Known positive and negative serum is included as control.

4. One row of ten tubes is taken as **control** in which unsensitised SRBCs are added to diluted patient's serum for **detection of heterophile antibodies.**

Findings

1. If the cells are agglutinated then that serum dilution is taken as the positive. The highest dilution of serum showing definite haemagglutination is taken as the end point.

2. The serum titre is determined by taking the ratio between the dilution agglutinating unsensitised and the sensitised RBCs. It is expressed as the reciprocal of the highest dilution of patient's serum showing agglutination.

3. A significant titre is 1 : 16 or above.

Remarks

1. The serum is to be inactivated.

2. Controls with unsensitised SRBC should always be included and there should be no agglutination in these tubes.

3. Ratio's of 1 : 8 considered as doubtful and less than that is not significant.

4. Latex particles coated with human gammaglobulin can be used instead of sheep RBCs.

5. For determining the dilution of the antiserum to be used for sensitisation of RBCs different dilutions tested should be from 1/100 to 1/6,400 and from 1 : 140 to 1/8,960 by making two fold dilutions.

ELISA TEST

Principle and uses : See Textbook of Microbiology by Dr. P. Chakraborty.

The ELISA (*enzyme-linked immunosorbent assay*) is so named as the test technique involved use of an enzyme system and an immunosorbent. The absorbing material may be particulate e.g. cellulose or agarose or a solid matrix, e.g. microwells, membranes etc.

(A) Plate format test

Materials required :

1. Microtie plate or tray.
2. Wash buffer (PBS with triton).
3. Sample diluent (PBS with bovine albumin).
4. Conjugate, substrate and stop solution (Table 9.4).
5. Strongly reactive control.
6. Non-reactive control.

- **Coat the wells of a PVC microtitre plate with Ag**
  - (i) Fill the wells with Ag at a conc of 1-10 μg/ml in carbonate/bicarbonate buffer (pH 7.4).
  - (ii) Cover the plate with an adhesive plastic and incubate at 4°C.
  - (iii) Remove the coating solution containing unbound Ag and wash the wall twice with 200 μl PBS Triton.

Table 9.4 : Common conjugate, corresponding substrate, stop solution and wavelength of filter for reading

Conjugate	Substrate	Buffer	Stop	Colour of end products	Filter
Alkaline phosphatase (pNPP)	p-nitrophenyl phosphate pH 9.5	pNPP – 1 mg/ml in 10 mM diethanolamine + 0.5 mM $MgCl_2$,	1 M NaOH	Y (nitrophenol)	405 nm
Horseradish peroxidase	H_2O_2 (0.003–0.015 %)	(1) 3, 3'5, 5'-Tetramethylbenzidine, i.e. TMB : 0.1 mg/ml in 0.05-0.1 M phosphate-citrate buffer, pH 5	1 M H_2SO_4		450 nm
		(2) 2, 2'–Azino-di-(3-ethyl-benthiazoline-6-Sulphonic acid), i.e. ABTS : 0.4 mg/ml in 0.05 M phosphate-citrate buffer pH 4	–Do–	Green	416 nm
		(3) O-phenylenediamine HCl, i.e. OPD : 0.5 mg/ml in 0.05-0.1M phosphate-citrate buffer, pH 5	–Do–		492 nm

- **Blocking and adding samples**
  - (i) Remaining protein-binding sites in the coated wells is blocked by adding 200 µl blocking buffer, 5% non-fat dry milk/PBS, per well.
  - (ii) The plate is covered with adhesive plastic and incubated for 2 hours at room temperature or, overnight at 4°C.
  - (iii) Wash wells with 200 µl PBS-Triton twice as above.
  - (iv) 100 µl of appropriately diluted samples are added to the previously demarked wells. Standards in duplicates or triplicates and blanks are concurrently tested for calculating accurate quantitative result. After addition of samples, blank solution and controls, the plates are incubated at 37°C for 60-90 minutes.
  - (v) The wells are washed twice with 200 µl PBS with triton.
- **Addition of 2nd step antibody (conjugate)**
  - (i) 2nd step antibody (i.e. antibody against the antibody to be detected in the sample) conjugated with Alkaline phosphatase or Horseradish peroxidase is to be appropriately diluted according to its titration result done beforehand.
  - (ii) 100 µl of the 2nd step antibody conjugate is added to the reaction wells, where 1st Ab present in serum is already fixed. Incubation is done for 1 hour.
  - (iii) Repeat washing as above.
- **Addition of substrate**
  - (i) Prepare substrate solution. Substrate depends on the enzyme conjugated with the 2nd antibody. Add 50 µl of the substrate solution in each well. Keep the plate at room temperature in dark for 60 minutes.
  - (ii) Add appropriate stop solution in 50 µl quantity.

Reading

The colour developed is measured (optical density) using appropriate filter.

Result

Qualitative : Cut off value is calculated from the OD of blank and controls. A test result above the cut-off value is taken as reactive.

Quantitative : Graph is prepared using OD values corresponding to controls. By plotting the OD value of test on the graph, quantitative estimation could be done.

Modifications

Above basic protocol may be modified according to the need :

(i) *To detect Ag*, coating of wells is done with corresponding monoclonal antibody.

(ii) To increase the sensitivity of *Ab detection*, sandwich method (Ag is captured between two layers of antibodies) is adopted where 2nd Ab used is a non-conjugated one, and a 3rd Ab used is within conjugated with enzyme and raised against the 2nd Ab in a different animal.

(iii) *In competitive ELISA*, used to detect an Ag, the coating is done with monoclonal Ab. The test sample and measured amount of Ab mixture is added in 1st reaction. Ab in sample competes with the bound Ab for binding the epitopic sites of the Ag. After first wash unbound Ag and free Ab is washed out. The rest of the steps are similar to sandwich ELISA protocol. Here decrease in OD compared to control one (without free Ab in the 1st reaction) is proportional to the concentration of Ag.

(B) ELISA PROTOCOL FOR MEMBRANE FORMAT

Liquid with Ab and Ag may flow through or move laterally in a membrane like nylon, nitrocellulose or other membranes. ELISA test may be performed using these membranes as solid phase on which Ag or Ab is immobilised in a spot or line according to the need. An absorbent material is placed below these membrane. The two membranes together forms the card on which the test is performed. Known Ag or Ab, according to the need, is impregnated on non-absorbent nylon or nitrocellulose membrane. The absorbent membrane below serves to pull the reactants through the membrane and help to separate non-reactant components from Ag-Ab complex bound on the membrane.

Different tests

1. Immunocomb test.
2. Flow through test — e.g. spot test.
3. Lateral flow test — e.g. immunochromatographic strip test.

1. IMMUNOCOMB TEST

This is basically an indirect solid-phase enzyme immunoassay (EIA). The solid phase is a card with a number of projections (teeth), mimicing a comb (Fig. 9.17A).

Each tooth is impregnated on two spots :

Upper spot – by human IgG or IgM, as required, for internal control.

Lower spot – by purified Ag.

Procedure

Initially, patient's serum (treated and suitably diluted) is allowed to react with the Ag spot by immersing the tooth in the well of row 'A' of a developing plate (Fig. 9.17B) containing the test serum. If specific Ab is present, it binds with the Ag. Unbound components are then washed in row 'B'. In row 'C', captured Ab of test serum at lower spot and human IgG or IgM on the upper spot (internal control), will react with alkaline phosphatase (AP) labelled anti-human IgM antibody. In the next two rows, unbound components are removed by washing. In 'E' row, the bound alkaline phosphatase will react with chromogenic components. The results are visible as grey spots on the surface of the teeth of the card.

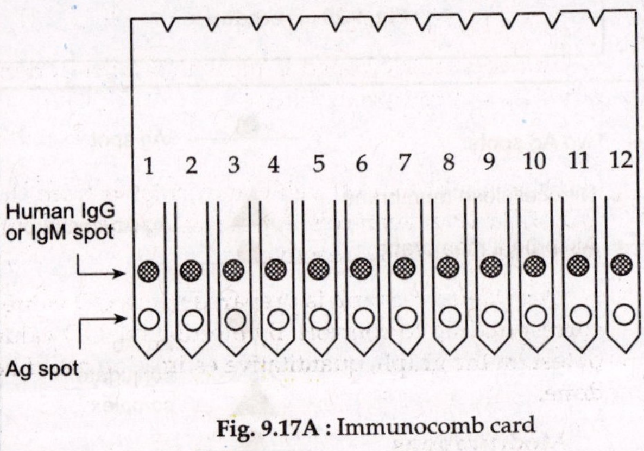

Fig. 9.17A : Immunocomb card

Note : Reaction and washing steps are done in the rows of walls of a developing plate

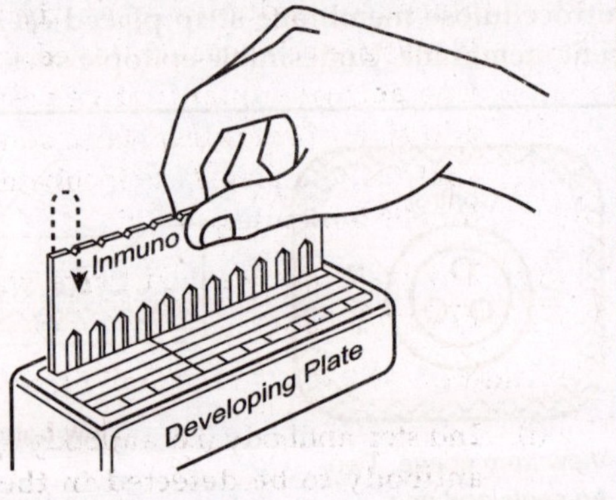

Fig. 9.17B : Developing plate containing rows of wells containing diluted serum, reagents and washing solutions. Combs are immersed in the well for stepwise ELISA reactions and washing.

Interpretation (Fig. 9.18) :

1. Positive — two spots develop on the card tooth.
2. Negative— the upper spot is developed only.

All specimens must produce an upper spot as internal control for validation of test.

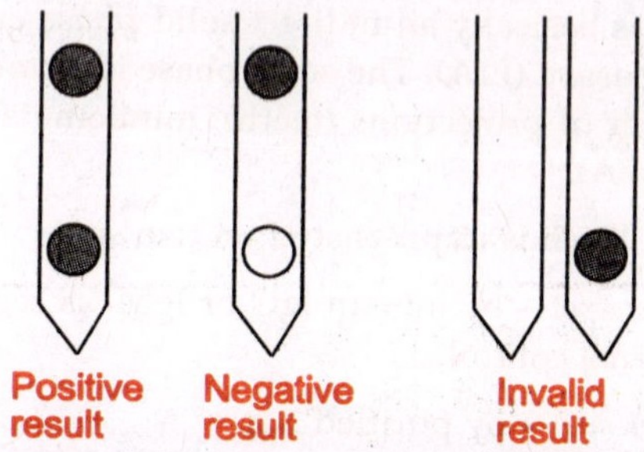

Fig. 9.18 : Interpretation

2. SPOT TEST (Membrane flow through test)

The flow through characteristic of nylon, nitrocellulose and other membranes, on which Ag or Ab is impregnated, is employed in Spot-ELISA test. This enhances the speed, sensitivity and simplicity of ELISA reaction process. Absorbent material below helps to pull the liquid reactants through the membrane and thus separates non-reactant components from Ag-Ab complexes (Fig. 9.19). This simplifies the washing steps.

Procedure

According to the need Ag (e.g. synthetic peptide Ag of HIV-1 or HIV-2) is impregnated on a nylon or nitrocellulose membrane strip placed on an absorbent membrane. Undesirable epitopic sites of Ag are blocked by blocking solution (Hammersten Casein in 0.05%. Tween 20 in P.B.S.). Such test strips are readily available for many common sero-diagnostic tests, e.g. HIV.Tri-Dot detecting HIV-1 and HIV-2 Ab in patient's serum (Fig. 9.19).

Test serum suitably diluted is dropped in adequate quantity on the reaction strip and allowed to incubate at room temperature for 10 minutes. This will allow formation of Ag-Ab complex on Ag/Ab spots, if the patient's serum contains desired Ab/Ag, respectively. Any unbound material flows through towards underlying absorbent material. As in conventional ELISA, a wash step is followed using droping a wash buffer over the spots. Next, a conjugate (Antihuman IgG conjugated with colloidal gold is added. This will cause development of colour spots over the Ag spots if the serum contains corresponding Ab. Control spot containing human IgG will react with the conjugate to form colour spot declaring validity of the test (Figs. 9.20 and 9.21).

The procedure may detect Ag (e.g. P-24 Ag of HIV) if the corresponding monoclonal Ab is spotted on membrane and a second Ab is used to sandwich the Ag between two antibodies.

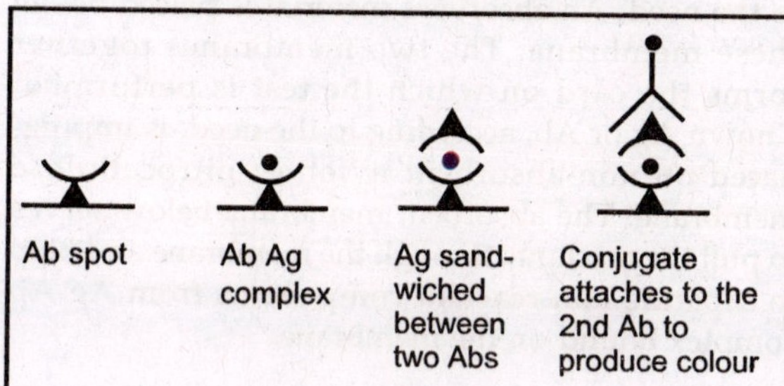

Fig. 9.20 : Procedures

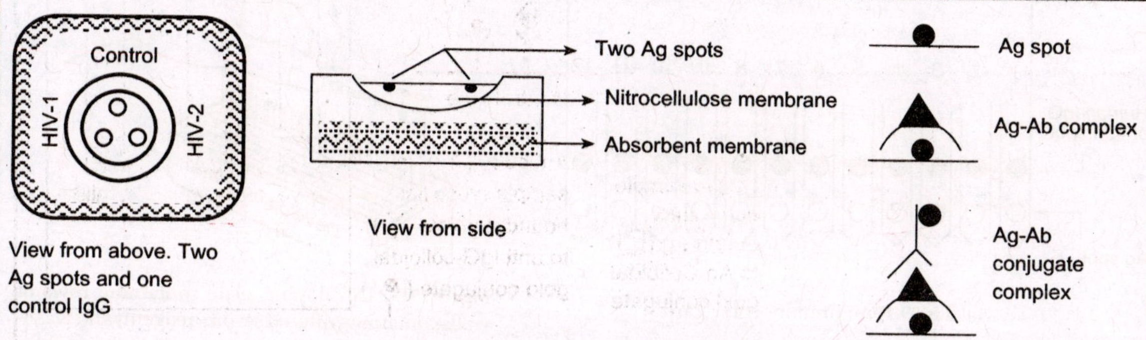

Fig. 9.19 : Spot ELISA Test Card)

Interpretation (Fig. 9.21)

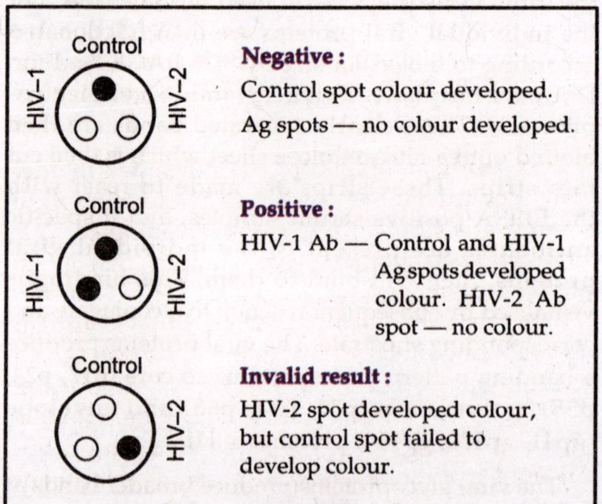

Fig. 9.21

3. Lateral flow membrane test (Fig. 9.22)

This is an immunochromatographic test (rapid) for qualitative detection of Ag (e.g. Ag of P. falciparam) or Ab (eg. HIV-1 or HIV-2-Ab) in serum, plasma or whole blood. The strip consists of a nylon or nitrocellulose membrane, supported on an absorbent membrane. The first one is impregnated by human IgG (control line) and Ag or Ab in test line.

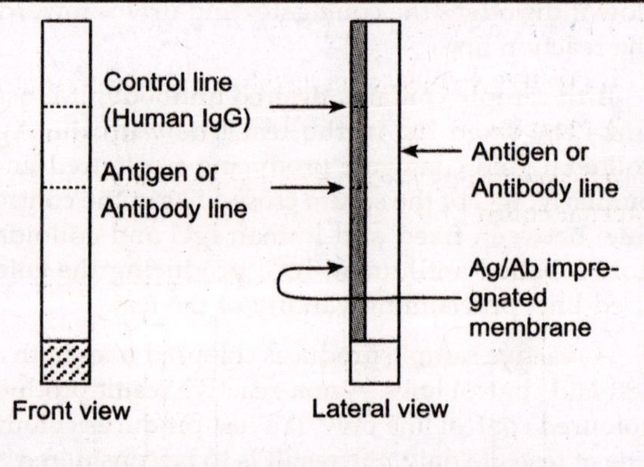

Fig. 9.22 : Lateral flow test strip

Principle and Procedure

(a) Ab detection (Fig. 9.23)

For Ab detection, corresponding purified Ag is impregnated in test line. In the control line 'human anti IgG-Ab' is fixed for establishment of validity of the test. In the absorbent pad, colloidal gold conjugated to Ag and anti-human-IgG is loosely absorbed.

When sample is added to the absorbent pad (which is often arranged to dip in small well containing diluted sample), it moves up by capillary action towards the test and control lines. During this

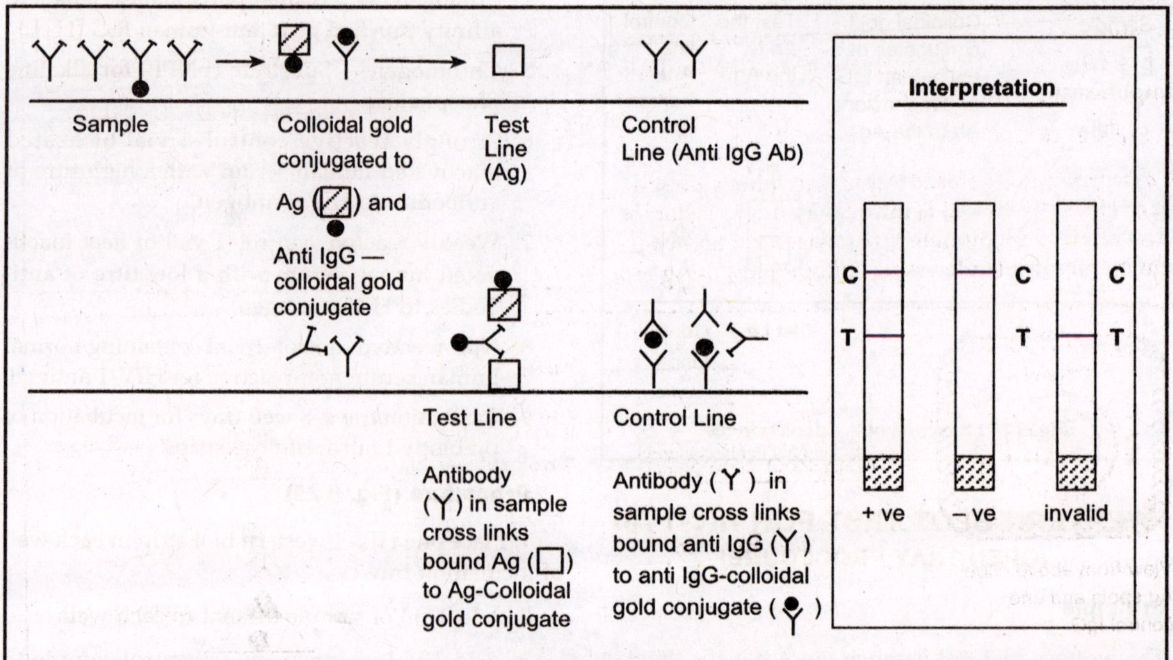

Fig. 9.23 : Ab detection

flow it dislodges the conjugates and drives towards the reaction lines.

If th sample contains desired antibody, it cross-links the fixed Ag in the test line with the Ag-colloidal gold conjugate producing a coloured line. Similarly, IgG of the serum cross-links at the control line, between fixed anti-human IgG and colloidal gold labelled antihuman-IgG, producing the coloured line, proclaiming validity of the test.

A reactive sample produces coloured lines both at test and control lines. A non-reactive result produce coloured control line only. If a test produces colours line at test site only, the result is to be considered as invalid.

(b) **Ag detection** — Lateral flow membrane ELISA may be employed for detection of Ag also (eg. Ag of *P. falciparum*). The test is similar. The differences are —

(i) at test line, monoclonal antibody against the Ag to be detected is fixed.

(ii) in the absorbent pad, colloidal gold conjugated with monoclonal Ab to the Ag and antihuman globulin is added. Reaction is depicted in Fig. 9.24.

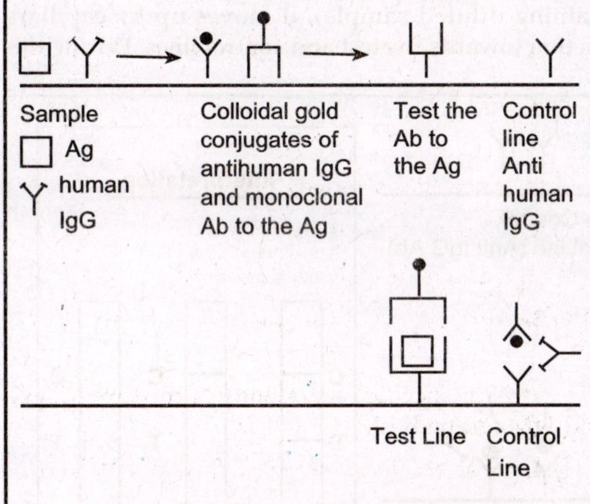

Fig. 9.24 : Reaction of Ag detection test

WESTERN BLOT TEST FOR HIV-1 Ab (OPEN TRAY PROCEDURE)

Principle

The western blot test is much more specific than an ELISA, as it detects antibodies to specific proteins of HIV-1. The western blot assay begins with the same virus preparation used in the ELISA, but the individual viral proteins are then fractionated according to molecular size by SDS-PAGE (Sodium Dodecyl Sulphate–Polyacrylamide gel electrophoresis). These clearly separated bands are then blotted onto a nitrocellulose sheet which is then cut into strips. These strips are made to react with the ELISA positive serum samples, and if specific antibodies are present to the individual viral proteins, they will bind to them. This binding is visualised by subsequent reaction to a conjugate and corresponding substrate. The viral proteins produce a banding pattern corresponding to core (p17, p24, p55), polymerase (p31, p51, p66) and envelope (gp41, gp120, gp160) proteins of HIV-1.

The viral glycoproteins produce broader bands at 41, 120 and 160 KD.

A serum or a plasma sample that is positive in both the ELISA and the western blot is presumed to have come from a person exposed to HIV-1.

Materials required

1. HIV-1 western blot strips : Preblotted strips with resolved HIV-1 specific viral proteins.
2. Wash buffer (PBS with Triton).
3. Sample diluent (PBS with bovine albumin).
4. Conjugate — Alkaline phosphatase labelled, affinity purified goat anti-human IgG (H+L).
5. Chromogen — Substrate (pNPP) for alkaline phosphatase.
6. Strongly reactive control–1 vial of heated inactivated human serum with a high titre of antibodies to HIV-1 antigen.
7. Weakly reactive control–1 vial of heat inactivated human serum with a low titre of antibodies to HIV-1 antigen.
8. Non-reactive control–1 vial containing normal human serum non-reactive for HIV-1 antigen.
9. Incubation trays–8 well trays for incubation of preblotted nitrocellulose strips.

Procedure (Fig. 9.25)

1. Place one HIV-1 western blot strip in each well of incubation tray.
2. Add 1 ml of sample diluent to each well.
3. Add 10 μl of specimen or control sample to each well.

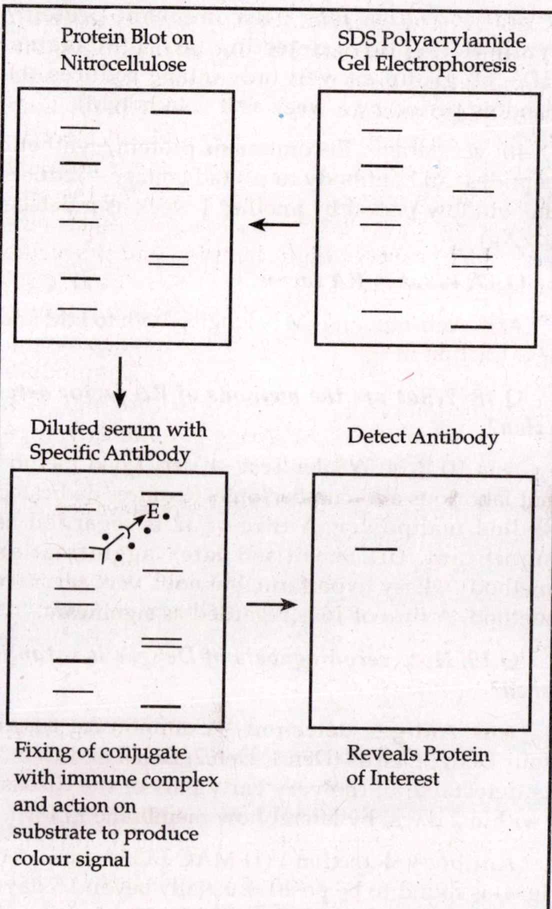

Fig. 9.25. Scheme of events in Western Blot test

4. Incubate the tray on a rocker or rotatory platform with gentle shaking for 30 minutes.

5. Aspirate the mixture from the wells into a tray containing disinfectant.

6. Wash for three minutes with gentle shaking with 1 ml/well of wash buffer. Repeat the washing three times.

7. Add 1 ml of conjugate solution and incubate with gentle shaking for 30 minutes at room temperature.

8. Aspirate the conjugate and do washing three times with wash buffer.

9. Add 1 ml of chromogen solution and incubate with gentle shaking for 10 minutes at room temperature.

10. Aspirate the chromogen and wash the strips two times with water.

11. Air dry the strips (for 30 minutes) completely before reading.

Interpretation of results

Non-reactive control :

No HIV-1 specific bands should be observed.

Weakly reactive control :

Bands must be present at p24 and gp120/gp160 — other bands may or may not be present.

Strongly reactive control :

Bands must be present at p17, p24, p31, gp41, gp51, p66 and gp120/gp160. Other bands may or may not be present.

Remarks

1. Non-reactive and weakly reactive controls must be run in each assay regardless of the number of samples to be tested. The non-reactive and weakly reactive controls are used to establish criteria for reactivity of bands.

2. In the first run of a kit, the strongly reactive control must be assayed.

QUESTIONS RELATED TO SEROLOGICAL TESTS

Q.1. ***What are the different antigen-antibody tests?***

Ans. Already discussed.

Q.2. ***What is VDRL test?***

Ans. It is a slide flocculation test.

Q.3. ***What type of antibody is detected by VDRL test?***

Ans. Non-specific reagin body (a mixture of IgG and IgM antibodies).

Q.4. ***What are the other modifications of VDRL test ?***

Ans. Rapid plasma reagin (RPR) and Toluidine red unheated serum test (TRUST).

Q.5. ***Name other non-specific tests for diagnosis of syphilis.***

Ans. CFT (Wassermann reaction).

Q.6. ***What are the specific or treponemal tests for detection of syphilis?***

Ans. FTA-ABS,TPI, TPHA.

Q.7. ***Name the biologically false-positive reactions with non-treponemal antigen.***

Ans. Measles, malaria, leprosy, autoimmune disease, pregnancy.

Q.8. ***What are the titres of reagin antibody in untreated syphilis?***

Ans. A 1 : 8 or greater rise of reagin titre in acute infection, and a titre of 1 : 32 or higher, are seen in secondary syphilis by VDRL test.

Q.9. ***How do you interpret Widal tests?***

Ans. Already discussed in Chapter 7.

Q.10. ***Name a haemagglutination test frequently done for serodiagnosis.***

Ans. TPHA (Treponema pallidum haemagglutination test).

Q.11. ***What is the significant titre in TPHA test?***

Ans. A titre ≥ 80 is regarded as significant.

Q.12. ***How long the high titre of TPHA is maintained after treatment?***

Ans. Many years.

Q.13. ***Which serological test for syphilis is used for monitoring treatment efficacy in syphilis?***

Ans. VDRL test/RPR test, as the titre quickly comes down to base level after successful treatment.

Q.14. ***Arrange the following tests for detection of Ag according to sensitivity :***

Haemagglutination, complement fixation, RIA, ELISA, chemiluminescence test.

Ans. Chemiluminescence > RIA > ELISA > CFT > Haemagglutination.

Q.15. ***Name some of the modification of agglutination tests.***

Ans. Sensitised Latex particle agglutination test, Passive haemagglutination test, Reverse Passive Haemagglutination test, Haemagglutination Inhibition test, Staphylococcus co-agglutination test.

Q.16. ***What are the different Ags used for detection of HIV-Ab?***

Ans. *1st generation* : Viral lysate (detects IgG, high rate of false-positivity).

2nd generation : Recombinant protein/synthetic peptides (detects IgG, specificity better than 1st generation Ag).

3rd generation plus : Recombinant protein/synthetic peptides detecting IgG, IgM against HIV-'O' group as well (advantage reduces the window period by a week as it detects IgM).

4th generation : Recombinant protein/synthetic peptides/and antibody to p24 (advantage – reduces the window period by another 1 week as it detects p24 Ag).

Q.17. ***What is RA factor?***

Ans. Anti-human IgM belonging both to IgM and IgG fraction of Ig.

Q.18. ***What are the methods of RA factor detection?***

Ans. (i) Rose Waaler Test — Very good method but laborious and cumbersome. Requires dedicated skilled manpower. A titre of 32 is regarded as significant. (ii) Sensitised latex agglutination method — Easy to perform, but not a very sensitive method. A titre of 16 is regarded as significant.

Q.19. ***How serodiagnosis of Dengue is established?***

Ans. **Antigen detection**— Common Ag for all four Dengue virus (Den 1, Den 2, Den 4 and Den 3) is detectable in the very early part of the disease (within 2 days) by lateral flow membrane ELISA.

Antibody detection : (1) MAC ELISA (to detect IgM) is found to be positive usually beyond 5 days. If the patient had a previous attack of other serotype of Dengue virus (usually Den 1), IgM is very quick to appear within 2 days. Usually by 5 days 80% cases show reactive sera. By 10 days usually 100% cases are found to be seroreactive. MAC-ELISA is useful for clinical laboratories.

(2) Neutralisation Test (NT) — The test is useful for serotype detection of current epidemic. So useful for research purpose.

(3) HI Test — Good test for Lab. diagnosis, if rising tire (4 fold) could be shown.

Both MAC ELISA & HI Test suffer from cross reactivity, due to antigenic sharing of Dengue virus with other flavi viruses, eg. J.E, West Nile, Yellow Fever viruses.

Q.20. ***How serodiagnosis of chikungunya is established ?***

Ans. Tests for serodiagnosis of chikunguniya are MAC-ELISA and HI Test. Patients become seroreactive by MAC-ELISA (IgM capture ELISA) by 4-7 days. Once reactive, the Ab level persists for 6 months at detectable level. HI test become positive after cessation of viraemia. All patients are usually positive by 5-7 days. Demonstration of 4 fold rising titre or falling titre at 1 week apart clinches the diagnosis.

Q.21. *How the serodiagnosis of Japanese Encephalitis is established ?*

Ans. IgM capture ELISA is found to be positive in > 95% cases in CSF after a few days. Sera reactive in HI test a titre of > 20 is suggestive of Japanese Encephalitis, but a rising titre in paired sera is required for confirmation. Tests are done in reference laboratory.

Q.22. *How serodiagnosis of 'West-Nile' fever is established ?*

Ans. HI test result showing a titre of > 20 and a rising titre in paired sera is diagnostic. MAC-ELISA may be done. Tests are available in reference laboratory.

Q.23. *How serodiagnosis of 'Tuberculosis' is established ?*

Ans. Ab detection : Promising Ags for Ab detection by ELISA are Glycolipid Ag and LAM. Several other Ags (P-32, 30 KDa, A60, 45-47 KDa Ag etc.) were given trial, but sensitivity is low. LAM and Glycolipids too show low sensitivity in smear negative cases. Its usefulness lies in showing negative predictive value.

Ag detection : Detection of above mentioned Ags by ELISA in body fluids, supposed to be sterile (CSF, synovial fluid etc.) normally, has a positive predictive value. In an endemic region, like our country with HIV prevalence increasing alarmingly, the test has a low positive predictive value.

SPACE FOR NOTES

Items at Spot Stations/Viva Tables

10

SPOTTINGS

In practical examination spotting stations are arrnaged to test the students familiarity to clinical microbiology laboratory. These are :

(a) Different culture media, commonly used in clinical microbiology with or without growth of corresponding bacteria.

(b) Biochemical test medium with or without reaction.

(c) Lab wares (disposable and non-disposable) commonly used.

(d) Instruments.

(e) Specimens of parasitology.

(f) Entomological specimen visible in naked eye/dissecting microscopic.

(g) Animal model for pathogenicity test.

(h) Microscopic specimens : (i) Saline and iodine mount of stool, (ii) Permanent stained slides of bacteria, fungi, parasites, viruses.

(i) Others.

Students need to visit museum and working labs to gain knowledge about the items. Here are some descriptions of some common medium and growth characteristics.

(A) UNINOCULATED CULTURE MEDIUM

(a) **BASAL MEDIUM**

(1) **Peptone water** (Fig. 10.1) — almost colourless liquid, dispensed in 4" × $^1/_2$" tube, properly cotton plugged. Composition and sterilisation — see chapter 19.

Uses : (i) Basal medium for preparation of nutrient broth and sugar fermentation medium. (ii) Many non-fastidious organism is grown in this medium for preparation of inoculum for antibiogram testing. (iii) It is the medium for indole test.

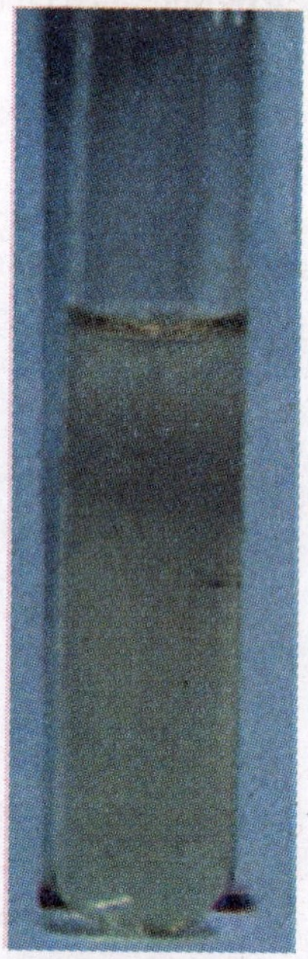

Fig. 10.1 : Peptone water

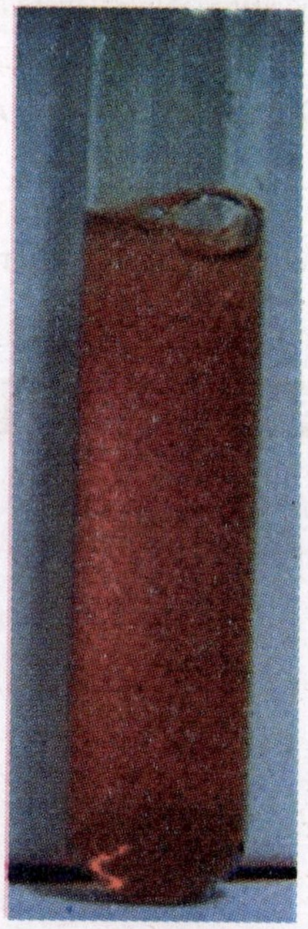

Fig. 10.2 : Nutrient broth

(2) **Nutrient broth** (Fig. 10.2) — faint straw coloured liquid dispensed in 4" × $^1/_2$" tube. Composition and sterilisation — see chapter 19.

Uses : (i) Bacteria is grown in nutrient broth for motility test. (ii) Basal medium for preparation of nutrient agar.

(3) **Nutrient agar** (Fig. 10.3) — Faint straw coloured/colourless solid medium in 45 mm radius petriplates or slants. Its composition and sterilisation — see chapter 19.

Uses : (i) For growth of organism for pigment production, serological test, bacteriocin typing. (ii) To note the colony character. (iii) Basal medium for preparation of blood agar.

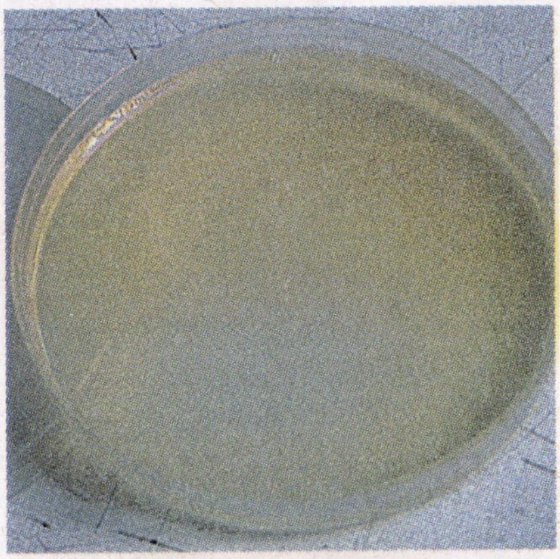

Fig. 10.3 : Nutrient agar

Fig. 10.5 : Chocolate agar

(b) **ENRICHED MEDIUM**

(1) **Blood agar** (Fig. 10.4) — Red, opaque solid medium in 45 mm radius petriplates, slants in test tubes. Composition and sterilisation, see chapter 19.

Uses : (i) Primary culture of throat swab, sputum, pus and other body fluids. (ii) To see haemolytic property of streptococcus. (iii) To perform CAMP test. (iv) To see swarming property of *Proteus* and *C. tetani*.

(2) **Chocolate agar** (Fig. 10.5) — Chocolate coloured opaque solid medium in 45 mm petriplates.

Composition and sterilisation is same as 'Blood agar'. Before medium is poured, it is heated at about 80°C in water bath till blood starts lysing indicated by changing colour from red towards chocolate. Overheating destroys the medium. Lysis of RBC, liberates X-factor in the medium.

Uses : (i) Primary culture of sputum for growth of *H. influenzae*. (ii) Primary culture of urethral and endocervical swab for growth of Neisseria gonorrhoeae. To avoid contaminants vancomycin, colistin and nystatin is added to the medium. (iii) Primary culture of CSF to grow *N. meningitidis* and *H. influenzae*. For the latter 'V' factor disc is placed at the primary inoculum site.

(3) **Löwenstein-Jensen (LJ) medium** (Fig. 10.6) Light green solid medium dispensed in screw cap bottle. Composition and sterilisation, see chapter 19.

Uses : (i) To culture *M. tuberculosis*. (ii) To perform antitubercular drug sensitivity test by absolute concentration method.

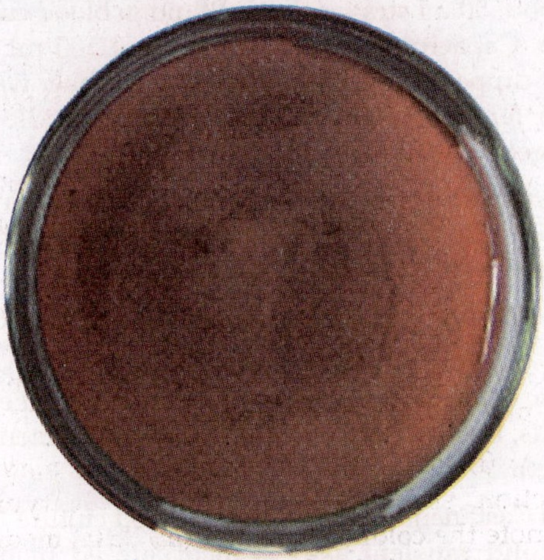

Fig. 10.4 : Blood agar

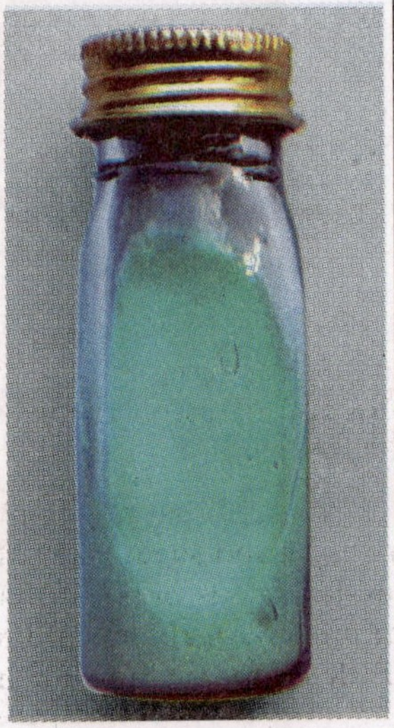

Fig. 10.6 : Löwenstein-Jensen (LJ) medium

Some points to remember :

- Malachite green, imparting green colour to the medium, is inhibitory for growth of contaminants.
- Egg fluid, on inspissation, solidifies the medium. It is the prime nutrient of the medium.

(4) **Dorset egg medium** (Fig. 10.7) — Medium is like a hard boiled egg fluid, dispensed in screw cap bottles (McCartney or Bijou bottle).

Sterilisation : Inspissation.

Uses : (i) Culture of *C. diphtheriae.* (ii) Preservation of bacterial isolates. Culture is done on slope. Once colony appears, 10% Glycerol-saline (sterile) is added to cover the colonies.

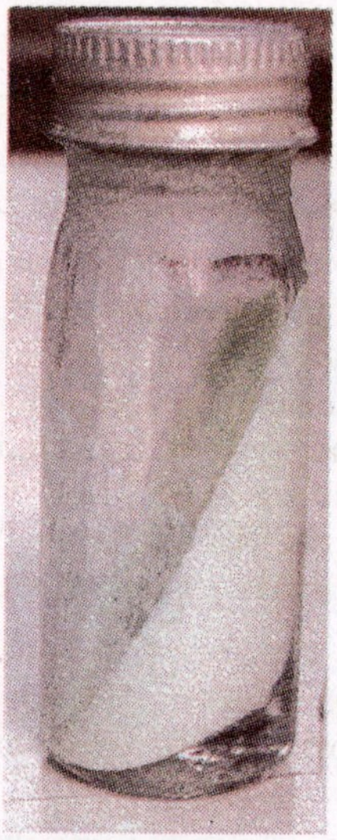

Fig. 10.7 : Dorset egg medium

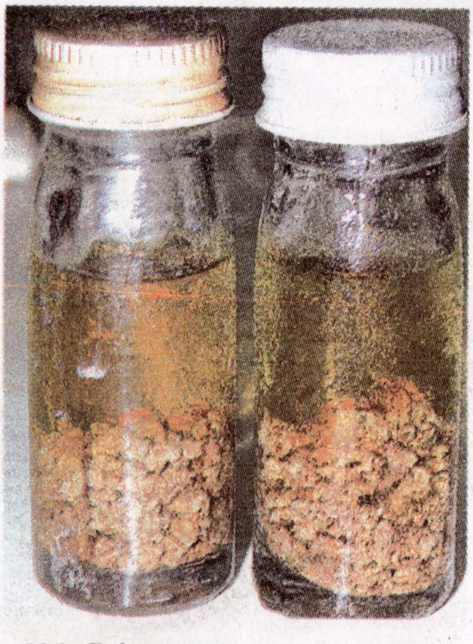

Fig. 10.8 : Robertson cooked meat (RCM) broth

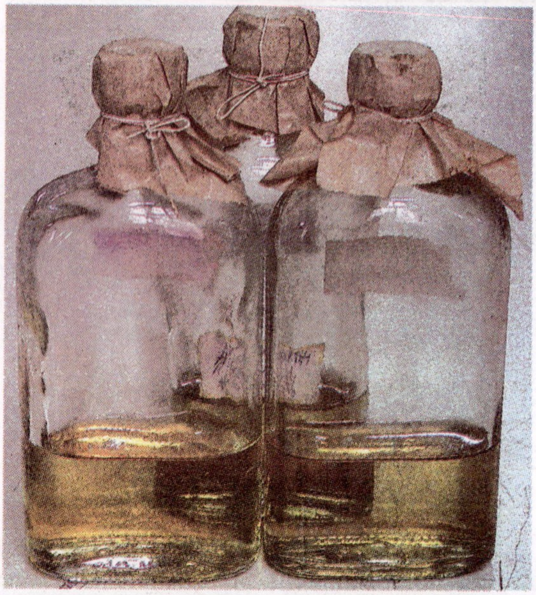

Fig. 10.9 : Blood culture bottle with medium

(5) **Robertson's Cooked Meat (RCM) medium** (Fig. 10.8) —Autoclaved meat particle, covering $^1/_2$ of the container, in nutrient broth. Broth level is about $^1/_2$" above the meat level. In some instances, there is a covering layer of paraffin too. Medium is dispensed in MacCartney's bottle.

Composition : See chapter 19.

Sterilisation : Autoclaving (15 Lb for 20 minutes).

(6) **Blood culture bottle with medium (Fig. 10.9)** — About 50 ml straw coloured fluid in blood culture bottle. Capacity of the bottle is about 100 ml. It is screw capped. Cap is provided with a rubber washer and a fenestration for introduction of needle of a syringe.

Composition : Brain Heart Infusion Broth/Trypticase Soya Broth/Brucella Broth/Hartley's broth/1% Glucose broth/0.5% Bile Broth.

Sterilisation : Autoclaving (15 Lb for 20 minutes).

Use : Blood culture in bacteraemic and septicaemic conditions (e.g. Enteric fever, Bacterial endocarditis, Lobar pneumonia, Meningococcal meningitis etc.).

[In Castaneda medium, liquid blood culture broth and solid nutrient agar is incorporated in blood culture bottle in the form of diphasic medium (Fig. 10.10)].

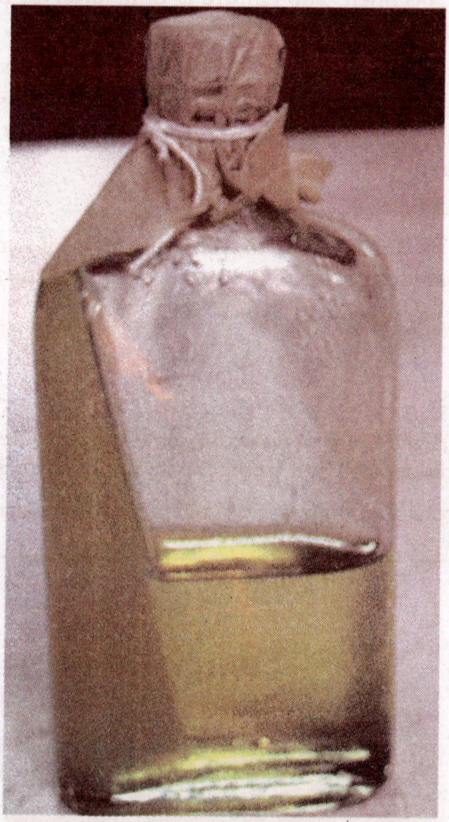

Fig. 10.10 : Castaneda bottle with medium

Advantage : No regular sub-culture is required, as is done in monophasic medium, to note growth of organism. Solid slant provided will show growth of colonies. The inoculated bottle is tilted once daily to facilitate inoculation on solid slant.

7. **Löeffler's serum slope** (Fig. 10.11) — White solid slant dispensed in test tube or screw cap bottles.

Composition : Nutrient broth with serum.

Sterilisation : Inspissation.

Uses : (i) Rapid culture for *C. diphtheriae* for morphology study in 6-8 hours. (ii) With addition of sugar and indicator (phenol red), may be used to study fermentation property of Neisseria.

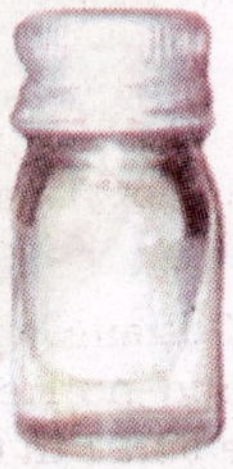

Fig. 10.11 : Loeffler's serum slope

(c) **SELECTIVE AND INDICATOR MEDIUM** :

(1) **MacConkey's agar** (Fig. 10.12) — Red, opaque solid medium in 45 mm radius petriplates, slants in test tubes. Composition and sterilisation, see chapter 19.

Uses : (i) Because of presence of bile salt, it inhibits growth of *Staphylococcus, Micrococcus, Bacillus, E. coli* and *Klebsiella*. So it is used for isolation of salmonella and shigella from stool. (ii) Although it is not an ideal medium, still it is commonly used for urine culture. (iii) It is used to isolate *Enterobacteriaceae, Pseudomonadaceae, A.G.N.Rs, Group D streptococcus* from samples, likely to be contaminated with gram +ve environmental bacteria and skin flora.

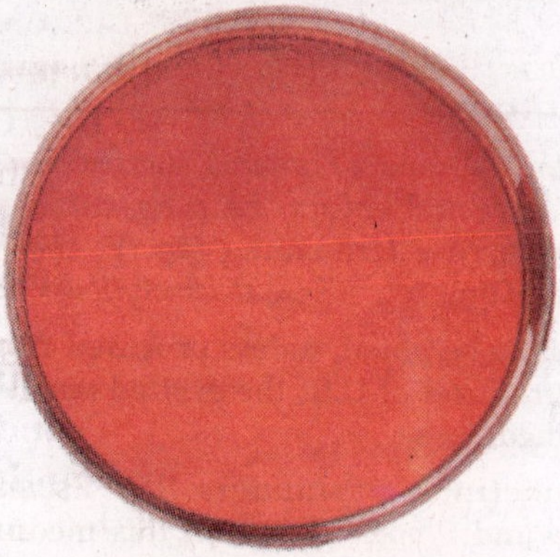

Fig. 10.12 : MacConkey's agar

(2) **T.C.B.S. agar** (Fig. 10.13) — Green solid medium in petri plates.

Composition and sterilisation : See chapter 19.

Use : It is a highly selective medium for *Vibrio*. So it is used to isolated *Vibrio* from stool sample.

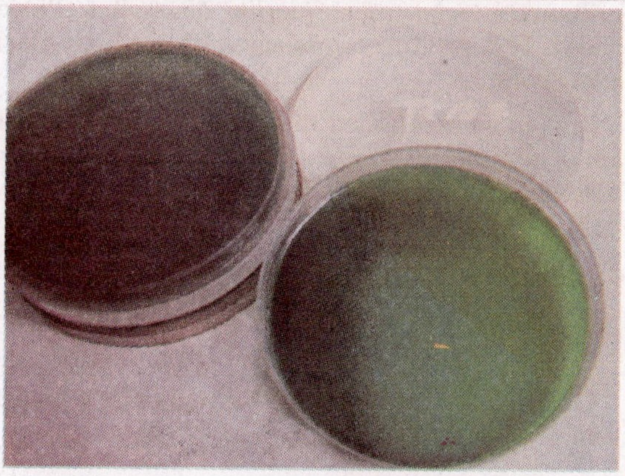

Fig. 10.13 : Thiosulphate Citrate Bile Salt Sucrose (T.C.B.S) agar plate

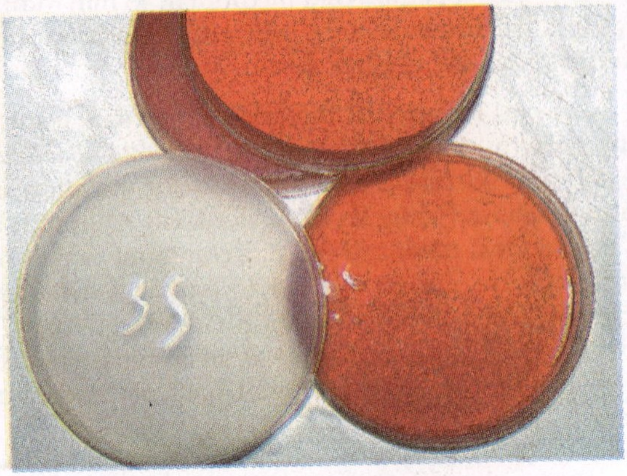

Fig. 10.14 : Salmonella Shigella agar (S.S. agar) plate

Moreover, the media contains sucrose and bromothymol blue indicators, helping differentiation between sucrose fermenting (eg. *V. cholerae*) and non-fermenting (eg, *V. parahaemolyticus*) vibrios.

[• It is to be noted, unless procured from a well known producer of U.S., the desired result may not be obtained.

• Sometimes bystanders like *Pseudomonas*, *Klebsiella* and *Proteus* grows on this medium].

(3) **S.S. Agar** (Fig.10.14) — Pink coloured medium, semitransparent, dispensed in petri plates.

Composition and sterilisation : See chapter 19.

Use : (1) It is a highly selective medium for isolation of *Salmonella, Shigella, Aeromonas* and *Plesiomonas* from stool. (2) It is an indicator medium too and able to differentiate between lactose fermenters (*E. coli, Klebsiella*) from non Lactose Fermenters (*Salmonella, Shigella, Aeromonas, Plesiomonas*). H_2S producers (*Salmonella*) produce black center colonies.

[It is to be mentioned that although inhibitory it cannot completely suppress the growth of *Klebsiella, Citrobacter, Enterobacter, Proteus, Providence and E. coli*].

(d) **ENRICHMENT MEDIUM** :

(1) **Selenite F broth** — Brick coloured liquid medium dispensed in test tubes.

Composition : Follow the manufacturer's instruction.

Sterilisation : Autoclave.

Use : The medium is used for enrichment of the number of *Salmonella, Aeromonas* and *Plesiomonas* in stool specimen. Sub-culture is done after 18 hours of incubation on S.S. Agar.

(2) **Alkaline Peptone water** —10 ml transparent colourless liquid dispensed in 6" × 1/2" test tubes.

Composition: Peptone 0.5%, NaCl 2%, D.W – as required. pH – 8.4.

Sterilisation : Autoclave.

Use : Enrichment of vibrio from stool sample. 1 gm amount of stool is inoculated in 10 ml medium.

(B) INOCULATED CULTURE MEDIUM SHOWING COLONIES

1. **Beta haemolytic Colony on Blood agar** (Fig. 10.15A&B) — Clear zone of haemolysis with definite margin around pin point transparent colonies.

Probable diagnosis : Pyogenic Streptococcus.

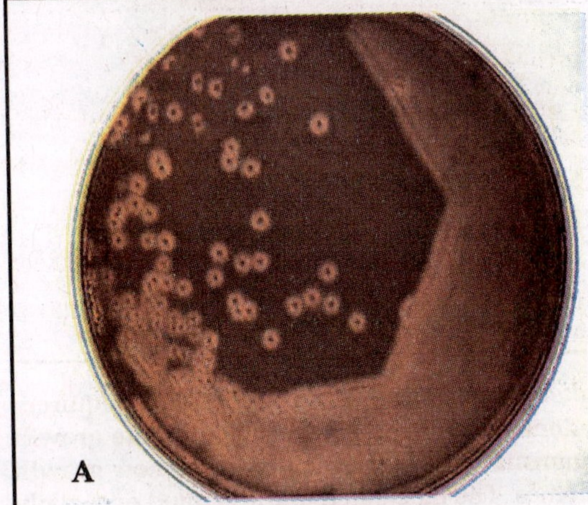

Fig. 10.15A : Beta haemolytic Colony on Blood agar

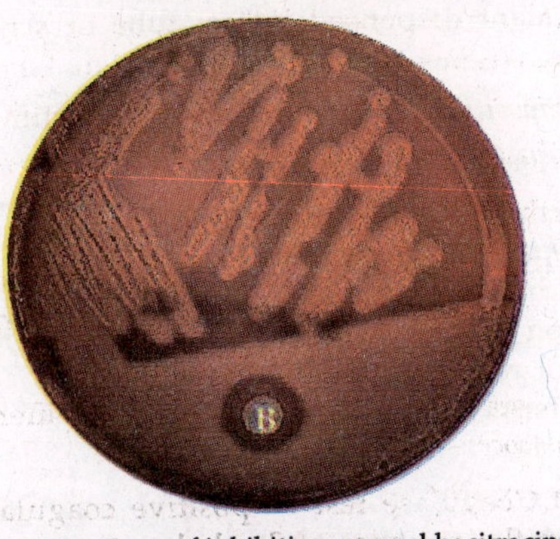

Fig. 10.15B : Zone of inhibition around bacitracin disc by Streptococcus Gr A

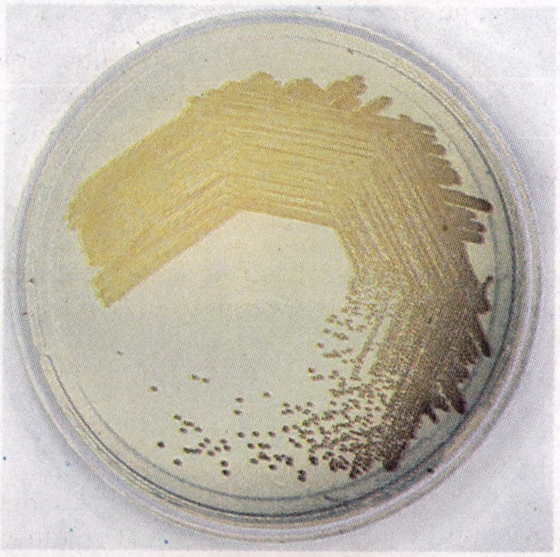

Fig. 10.16 : Colonies of Straphylococcus aureus on Nutrient agar

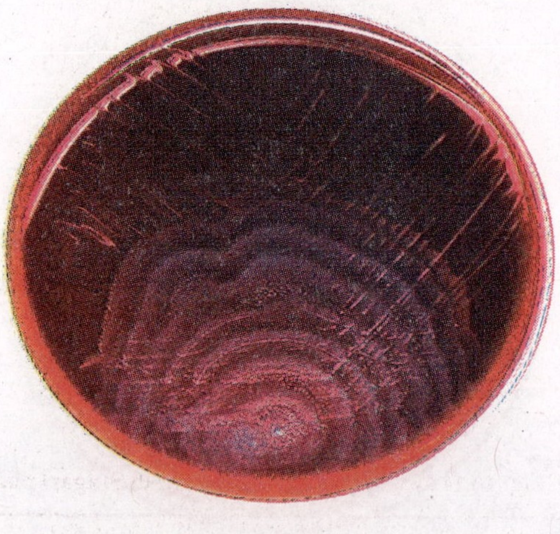

Fig. 10.17 : Swarming proteus ssp on blood agar

Further tests for identification :

(i) Smear examination after gram stain to show gram +ve cocci in long chain, morphologic of *Streptococcus pyogenes.*

(ii) Catalase test — A negative catalase test establish the genus level diagnosis of *Streptococcus.*

(iii) Bacitracin sensitivity test — *S. pyogenes* is sensitive.

(iv) CAMP Test — Positive in *S. agalactiae.*

(v) Carbohydrate Ag extraction followed by sensitised latex agglutination (latex particles coated with Ab against the carbohydrate Ag) test to identify the Lancefield group A, B, C & G.

2. **On Blood agar or Nutrient agar** (Fig. 10.16) — 2-3 mm diameter, dome shaped, smooth surfaced, entire margined, creamy, golden yellow pigmented colonies. Pigment is restricted to the colonies.

Probable diagnosis : *Staphylococcus aureus.*

Further tests for identification :

(i) Gram stained smear examination to show gram positive cocci arranged in grape like irregular cluster.

(ii) Catalase test — positive result differentiate *Staphylococcus* from *Streptococcus.*

(iii) Coagulase test — positive coagulase test confirm the presence of Staphylococcus aureus.

(iv) Phosphatase test — if coagulase test is found negative, phosphatase test clinch the species diagnosis 'aureus'.

(v) Growth on 15% NaCl Agar – confirm genus level diagnosis of *Staphylococcus* when in doubt.

3. **Swarming growth on blood agar or nutrient agar** (Fig. 10.17) — Spreading growth from original colonies in the form of waves covering the plate.

Probable diagnosis : Growth of *Proteus mirabilis* or *Proteus vulgaris.*

Further tests for identification :

(i) Gram stained smear examination — Gram –ve short slender rod, arranged discretely.

(ii) Motility test — Motile bacteria.

(iii) PPA and urease test — Both positive by *Proteus.*

(iv) Indole test — *P. mirabilis* –ve, *P. vulgaris* +ve.

(v) H_2S production — Both *P. mirabilis* and *vulgaris* +ve.

4. **Nutrient agar plate showing irregular margined colonies with greenish pigment diffusing into the medium** (Fig. 10.18).

Probable diagnosis : *Pseudomonas aeruginosa.*

Further tests for diagnosis :

(i) Gram stained smear examination — short slender rods arranged discretely.

(ii) Motility test — Motile

(iii) Oxidase test — Positive.

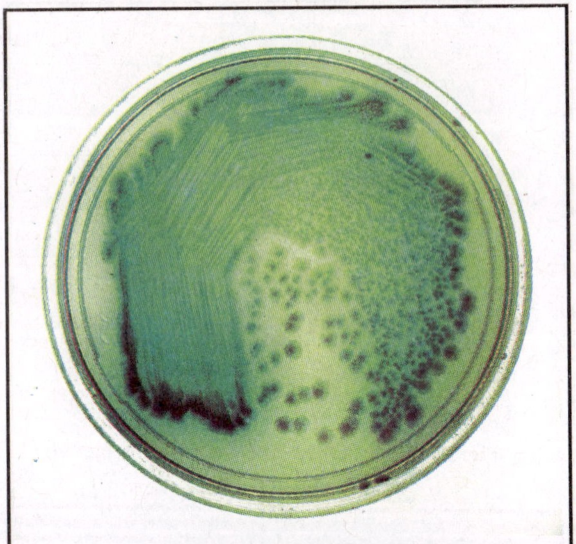

Fig. 10.18 : Nutrient agar plate showing colonies of *Pseudomonas pyocyanea*

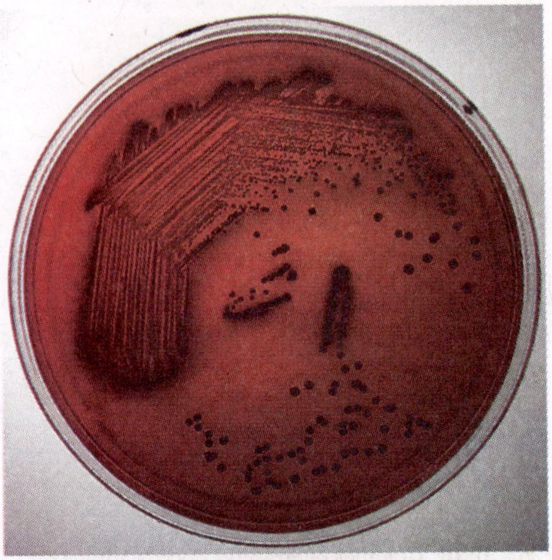

Fig. 10.19 : MacConkey's agar plate with colonies of E. coli

5. **MacConkey's agar plate** showing non-mucoid (Fig.10.19) — Pink lactose fermenting, moderate size, convex, smooth/matt surfaced, entire margined, opaque colonies.

Probable diagnosis : E. coli.

Further tests : (i) Gram stained smear examination — Stout long rods arranged discretely.

(ii) Motility test — Motile rods.

(iii) Indole production +ve, methyl red test +ve, V.P. test –ve, Simmon citrate medium — no growth, H_2S in TSI –ve.

6. **MacConkey's agar plate showing mucoid, pink (LF)** (Fig. 10.20) — large, convex, smooth surfaced, entire margined colonies.

Probable diagnosis : *Klebsiella spp*, or *Enterobacter spp*, or *Hafnia spp*.

Further tests :

	Klebsiella	*Enterobacter*	*Hafnia*
Gram stain	–ve, short plump rod	–ve, short plump rod	–ve, short plump rod
Motility at 37°C	Non-motile	Motile	Non-motile
Motility at 22°C	Non-motile	Non-motile	Motile

Confirmatory test for *Klebsiella pneumoniae* sub-spp *aerogenes* : Indole –ve, M.R. –ve, VP +ve, Simmon's citrate — growth +ve.

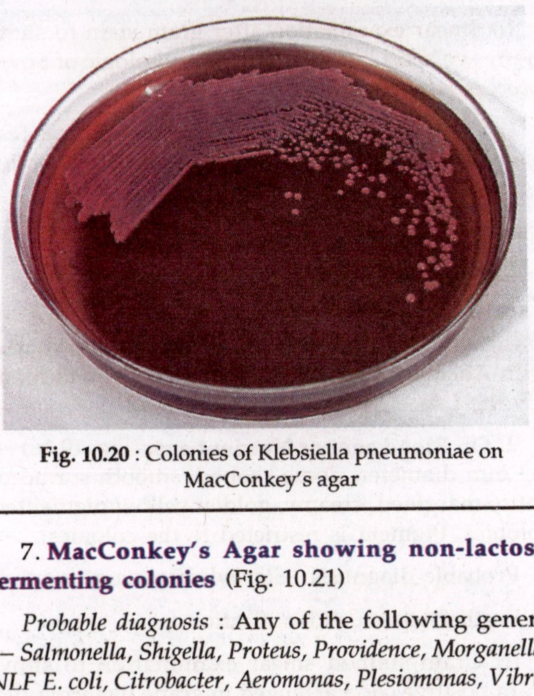

Fig. 10.20 : Colonies of Klebsiella pneumoniae on MacConkey's agar

7. **MacConkey's Agar showing non-lactose fermenting colonies** (Fig. 10.21)

Probable diagnosis : Any of the following genera — *Salmonella, Shigella, Proteus, Providence, Morganella, NLF E. coli, Citrobacter, Aeromonas, Plesiomonas, Vibrio* (if the medium is not NaCl deficient) afermentative, gram negative rods (AGNR), *Pseudomonadaceae.*

Further tests for identification :

Step I : Morphology study by gram stain and motility test. All are gram –ve slender rods. All are motile except *Shigella*.

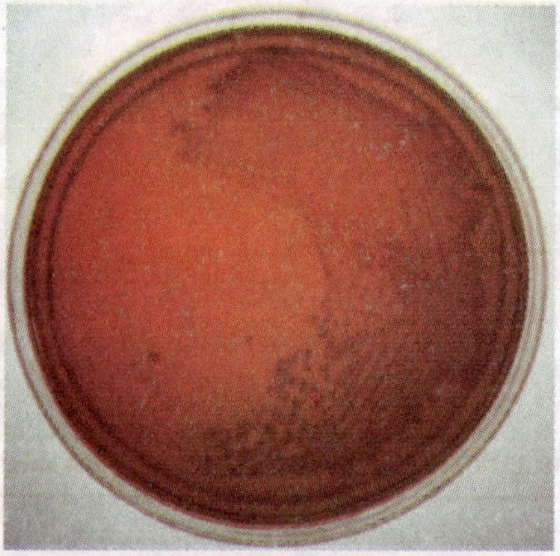

Fig. 10.21 : Non lactose fermenting colonies on MacConkey's agar

Step II :

	Oxidase test	*O.F. test*
Enterobacteriaceae	–	Fermentation +
Vibrionaceae	+	Fermentation +
AGNR *	±	No reaction or Alkali production by *Alcaligenes*.
Pseudomonadaceae	+	Oxidative

* AGNR = Afermentative gram negative rods, eg. *Acinetobacter, Moraxella, Alcaligenes* etc.

Step III : For further tests of individual family/ group see chapter 17.

8. **Nutrient agar plate showing rough surfaced, irregular margined, opaque, non-pigmented colonies** (Fig. 10.22).

Probable diagnosis : *Bacillus spp.*

Further tests for identification :

(i) Gram stained smear examination — Gram +ve stout rods with unstained space for spore. Depending upon the species, arrangement might be in chain, pallisade or discrete.

(ii) Motility test : Motile, except *B. anthracis*.

(iii) Further test for species identification — Position, sizes and shape of spore, gelatin hydrolysis.

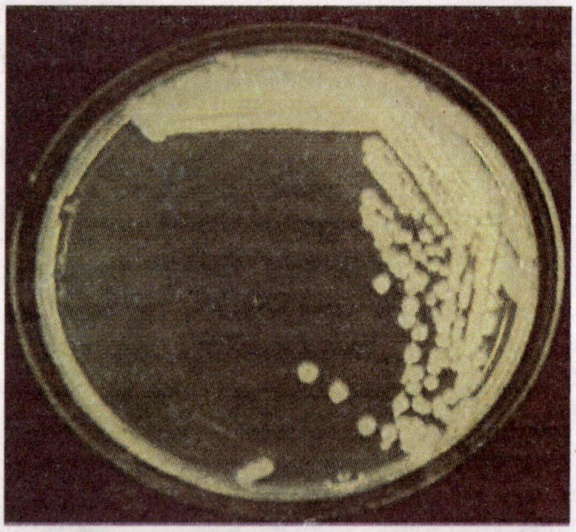

Fig. 10.22 : Nutrient agar plate with colonies of *Bacillus spp.*

Identification of pathogenic species :

(a) *Bacillus anthracis* — Capsule + by 'Polychrome Methylene Blue' stain, Non-motile.

(b) *Bacillus cereus* — Haemolytic colony on Blood Agar. Motility +, Egg yolk reaction +ve.

9. **Löwenstein-Jensen (LJ) medium** showing buff/white/yellow etc. coloured growth (Fig. 10.23A and 23B).

Probable diagnosis : Colonies of Mycobacterium.

Further tests :

(i) **Colony character** — Slow grower/Rapid grower, colour of pigment, whether scotochromogen or photochromogen, rough irregular colony/smooth moist small colonies.

(ii) **Z. N. stained smear examination** — Acid fast bacillus.

(iii) **Biochemical tests** — Niacin test, Aryl sulphatase test, Heat resistant catalase test, Nitratase test.

[Nowadays, conventional tests for identification is being replaced by 'Gene Probe', PCR, G.L.C., Line Probe Assay for quick and more accurate identification.]

10. **S.D.A. medium with growth of dermatophytes** (Fig. 10.24) — Straw coloured slant in 6" × $^3/_4$" test tube with cottony/powdery arial growth and reverse may show leathery growth with brown/red pigmentation.

Further test for identification :

(i) Lactophenol cotton blue mount to show septate branching hyphae with macroconidia. Often microconidia is also seen.

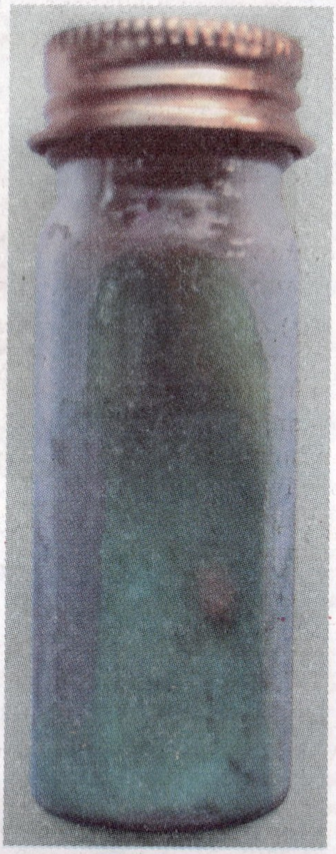

Fig. 10.23A : Colonies of *Mycobacterium Spp* on L J medium

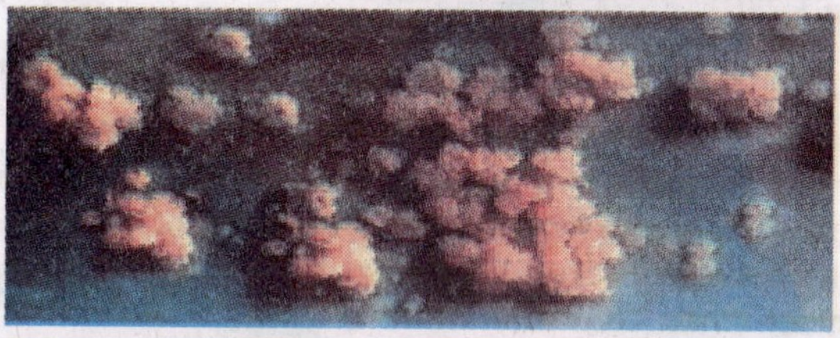

Fig. 10.23B : Rough buff and tough colonies of Mycobacterium tuberculosis

(ii) Slide microculture — followed by lactophenol cotton blue mount to show macroconidial pattern.

11. **S.D.A. medium with growth of C. albicans** (Fig. 10.25) — Straw coloured slant in 6" × 3/4" test tube with big, whitish, creamy, smooth surfaced, regular margined colonies.

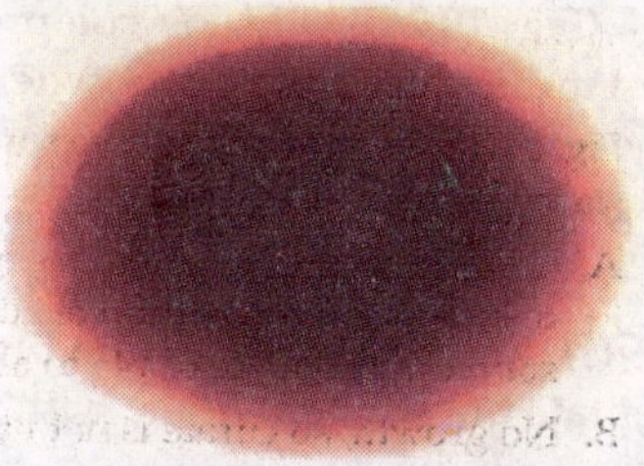

Fig. 10.24 : Colony (*reverse side*) of dermatophyte on S.D.A. medium

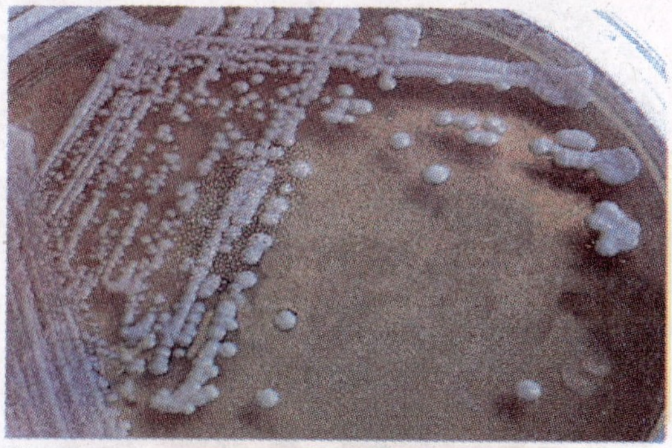

Fig. 10.25 : Candida albicans colonies on SDA medium

Further tests for identification :

(i) Gram stained smear — shows intensely gram +ve budding oval yeast cells.

(ii) Germ tube formation within 2 hours in serum.

(iii) Terminal smooth chlamydospore formation in slide culture in rice meal infusion agar.

(C) MEDIUM FOR BIOCHEMICAL IDENTIFICATION TEST (INOCULATED/UNINOCULATED)

1. **Monosaccharide fermentation** — Monosaccharide fermentation is noted in growth in glucose peptone water with Durham tube to note gas production (Fig. 10.26).

Composition— Peptone water with 1% Glucose with Andrade's indicator, which turns red when pH becomes less than 6.4 due to fermentation of and acid production from glucose.

Sterilisation : Base peptone is sterilised by autoclaving (15 Lb for 20 minutes). Then glucose and Andrade indicator is added, medium is poured in tubes, cotton plugged, followed by free steaming for 1 hour.

Result :

(i) Fermentation with gas production (red medium with gas in Durham tube) — by all enterobacteriaceae (except *Shigella*, *S. typhi*, some species of *Proteus*, *Providence*, *Serratia*, *Klebsiella* and anaerogenic *E. coli*).

(ii) Fermentation without gas production — (red medium and no gas in Durham tube) — by *Vibrio*, *Aeromonas* (except hydrophila) *Plesiomonas*.

(iii) Red at surface only no gas production — indicates oxidative utilisation of glucose. *Example* : Pseudomonas.

(iv) No reaction — *Example* : A.G.N.R.

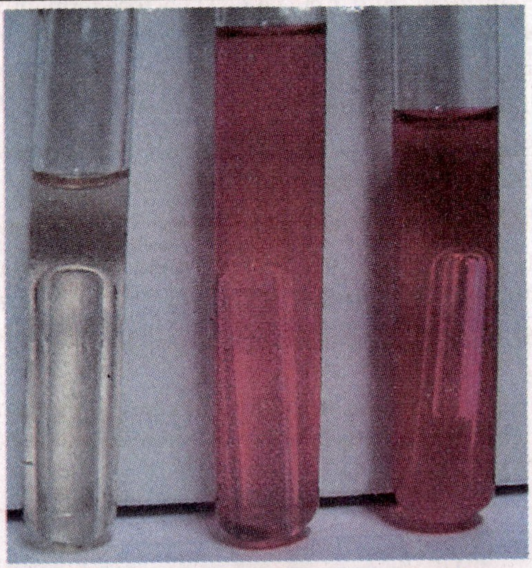

(a) (b) (c)

Fig. 10.26 : Glucose fermentation : (a) No reaction. (b) Fermentation without gas production. (c) Fermentation with gas production in Durham's tube

2. **Disaccharide fermentation** — Feature of the medium and results are very similar to glucose mentioned above. No Durham tube is required here, as we do not note gas production here.

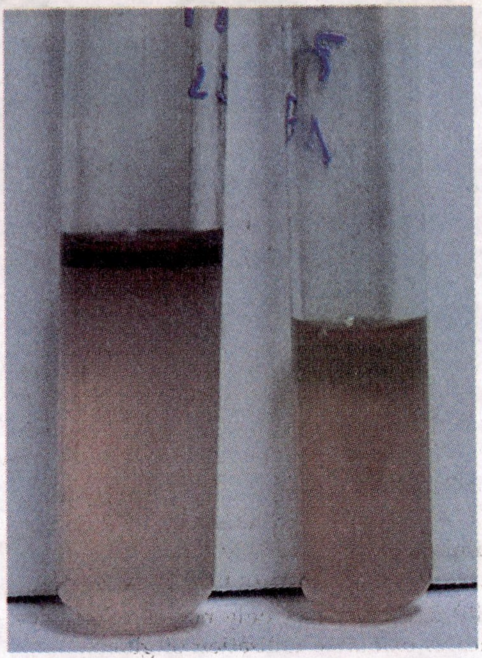

Left tube : –ve result Right tube : +ve result

Fig. 10.27 : Indole production

Commonly used disaccharides fermentation test media are : peptone water with lactose/sucrose/ maltose.

Lactose fermenters : *E coli, K. pneumoniae* (sub spp pneumoniae and *aerogenes*), *Enterobacter, Edwardsiella, Hafnia* (at 22°C).

Sucrose fermenters : *K. pneumoniae* (sub-species pneumoniae and aerogenes), *Enterobacter, Vibrio cholerae*, some serotypes of *E. coli*.

(3) **Test for indole production (Fig. 10.27)** : Some bacteria utilises tryptophan of peptone water medium to produce indole, which could be extracted by amyl alcohol. On addition of p-dimethylaminobenzaldehyde, extracted indole reacts to produce pink ring at surface (Fig. 10.27). +ve reaction : *E. coli, Proteus vulgaris* and others. –ve reaction : *Klebsiella, Enterobacter* and others.

(4) **Test for citrate utilization (Fig. 10.28)** : Some bacteria are able to utilise citrate as sole carbon

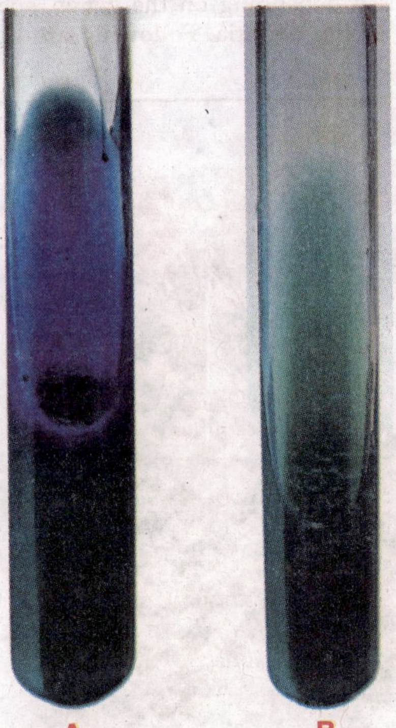

A B

Fig. 10.28 : Test for citrate utilization in Simmon's citrate slant.

A. Growth on slant and change of colour of indicator to blue due to utilisation of citrate as sole carbon source and change of pH to alkaline side.

B. No growth, so citrate is not utilised.

source to produce the required macromolecules for its growth, survival and reproduction. Simmon's citrate medium contain sodium-citrate as sole carbon source. It is a synthetic medium. The test organism is inoculated on the slant. Inoculum should be as small as possible (a few bacteria only). In case of positive result colonies appear with change of pH to alkaline side turning the colour of the indicator from green to blue.

+ve : *Klebsiella aerogenes, Enterobacter, Citrobacter, Providencia rettgeri, S. typhimurium, Pseudomonas etc.*

–ve : E. coli, Shigella, Proteus (other than *spp rettgeri*)

5. **Test for H_2S production (Fig. 10.29)** : H_2S production is tested in Triple Sugar Iron Agar medium. Bacteria to be tested is inoculated using a straight wire. Inoculation is done by stabbing the butt upto the bottom, followed by streaking on surface. On incubation following reactions are encountered depending on the genus, species or serovars of the bacteria. Following are the reactions :

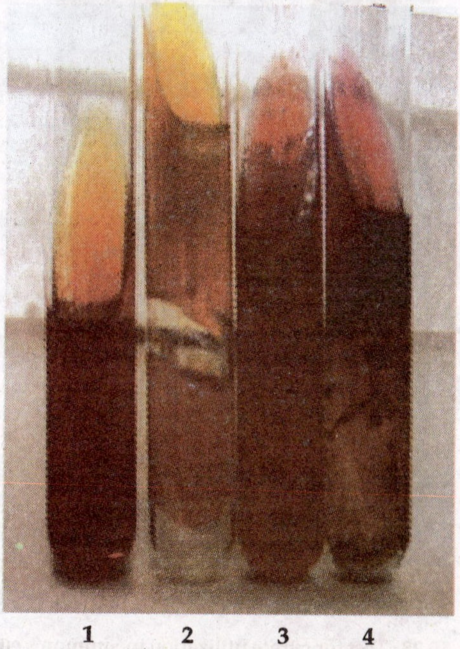

Tube left to right : (1) Uninoculated tube. (2) A/A (acid in butt and slant). (3) K/A (alkaline slant and acid butt). (4) K/A+ (Alkaline slant, acid butt, H_2S produced).

Fig. 10.29 : Test for H_2S production in Triple Sugar Iron agar (TSI)

Slant Acid/Butt Acid (A/A) : Lactose fermenting, H_2S –ve.

Slant Alkaline/Butt Acid (K/A) : Non-lactose fermenting, H_2S –ve.

Slant Alkaline/Butt Acid with black deposit (K/A+) : Non-lactose fermenting, H_2S +ve.

[Acid = Yellow colour, Alkaline = Red colour]

H_2S +ve bacteria : *Proteus, Salmonella* (except *S. paratyphi A*) *Citrobacter freundii.*

6. **Phenyl Pyruvic Acid Deaminase test (PPA) (Fig. 10.30)** :

It is used to test the ability of certain organisms to deaminate phenylalanine to phenylpyruvic acid (PPA).

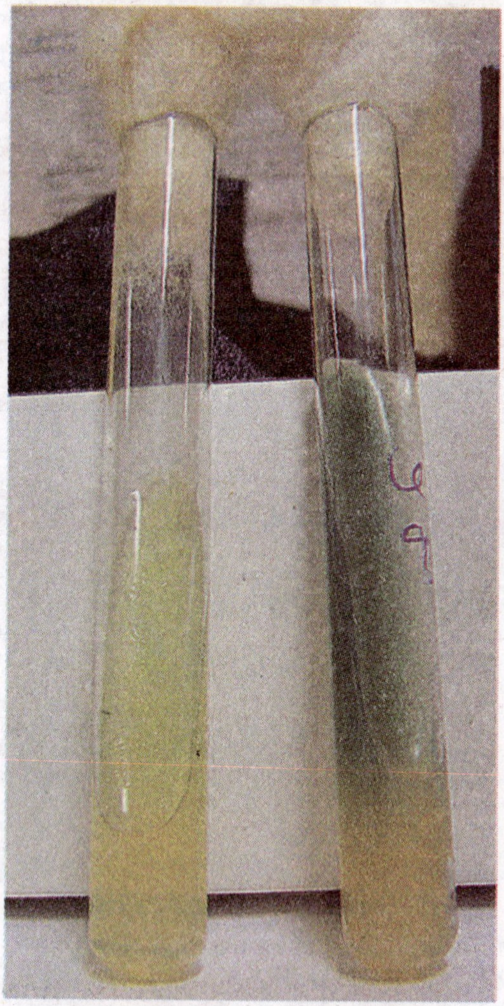

(a) Negative result (b) Positive tesult

Fig. 10.30 : Phenyl Pyruvic Acid Deaminase test (PPA)

Nutrient agar slope containing DL-phenylalanine is inoculated with a fairly heavy inoculum of culture and incubate at 37°C for overnight period. Then a few drops of 10% ferric chloride solution is added.

Result : (i) *Positive PPA test* — Green colour. (ii) *Negative PPA test* — No colour change.

Examples of positive PPA test : *Proteus sp.*, *Morganella sp.* and *Providencia sp.*

D. SLIDES UNDER MICROSCOPE

1. ***Staphylococcus* (Fig. 10.31A & 10.31B)**

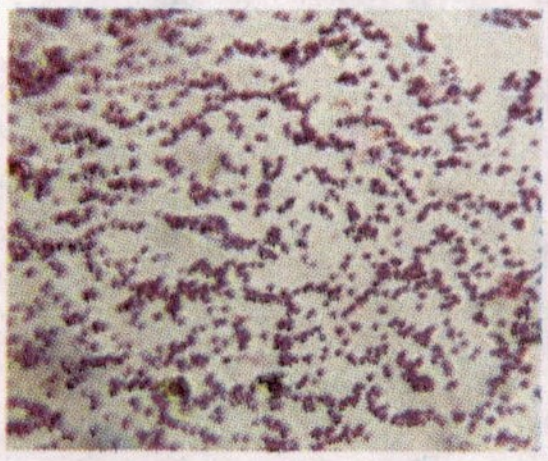

Fig. 10.31A : Gram positive cocci arranged in irregular clusters.

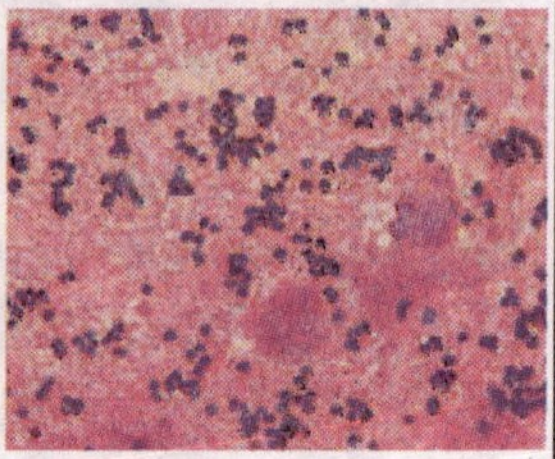

Fig. 10.31B : *Staphylococci in pus*

2. ***Gram negative rods* (Fig. 10.32)**

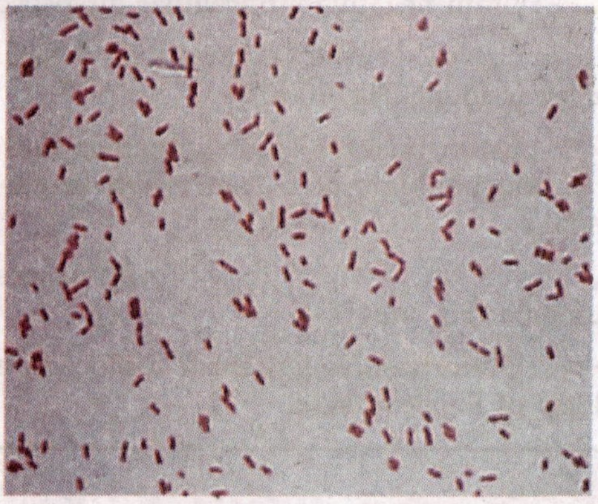

Fig. 10.32 — Note : The individual bacilli are slender, short, sides–parallel, axis-straight. Arrangement discrete. Picture is morphologic of *Salmonella, Shigella, Proteus, Providence, Citrobacter, Pseudomonas* etc.

3. ***Diphtheroid bacillus* (Fig. 10.33)**

4. **Malaria parasites** :

(a) *Ring of P. falciparum* (Fig. 10.34)

Note : No change in RBC. Signet ring, double chromatin and multiple infection.

(b) *Growing trophozoite of P. vivax* (Fig. 10.35)

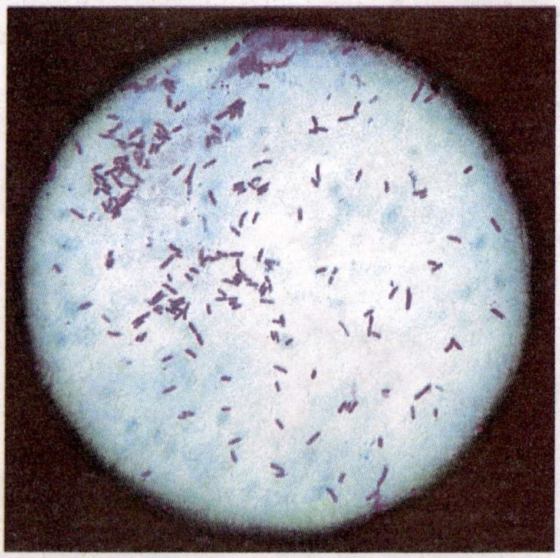

Fig. 10.33 — Note : Gram positive short straight non-spore forming rods arranged in palisade and angular pattern. Individual bacilli shows parallel sides and rounded/ tapering ends.

Note : Infested RBCs are enlarged and altered shape. Cytoplasm of parasite opposite to chromatin is thicker. Irregular cytoplasm is indicative of pseudopodial movement.

(c) *Trophozoites of P. vivax* (Fig. 10.36)

Note : Note RBC is enlarged, irregular, washed out (pale) in appearance and Schuffner's dots. Parasite shows pseudopodial movement, large vacuole, malarial pigment in cytoplasm.

(d) *Female gametocyte of P. vivax* (Fig. 10.37).

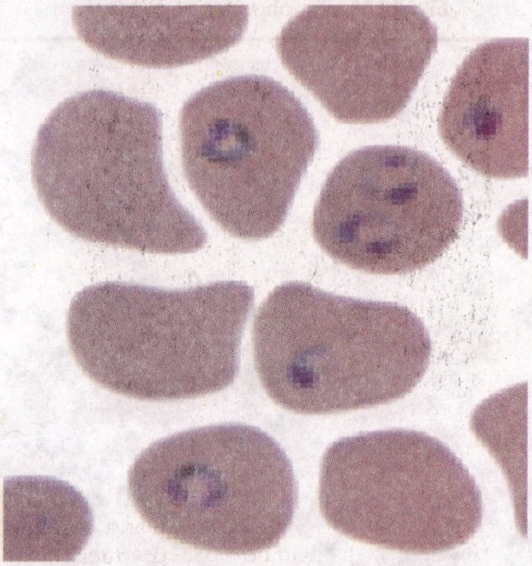

Fig. 10.34 : Ring of *P. falciparum*

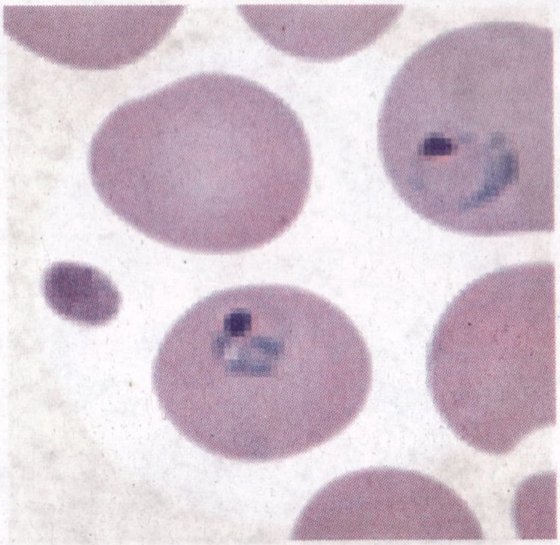

Fig. 10.35 : Growing trophozoite of *P.vivax*

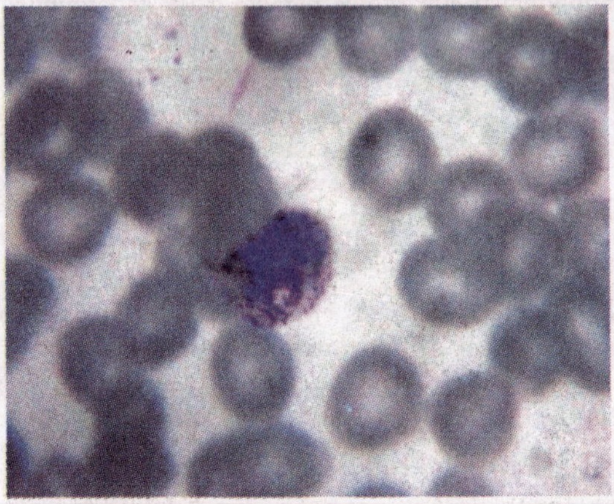

Fig. 10.36 : Trophozites of *P. vivax*

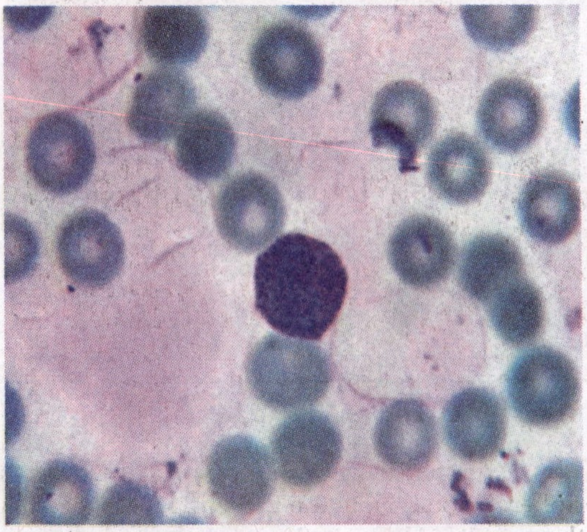

Fig. 10.37 : Female gametocyte of *P. vivax*

Note : Vacuole is absent. Large chromatin at one end.

(e) *Male gametocyte* (Fig. 10.38).

Note : On the right side of the WBC the protozoa inside the RBC, shows diffuse chromatin and no vacuole. (The other parasite is a trophozoite of *P. vivax*).

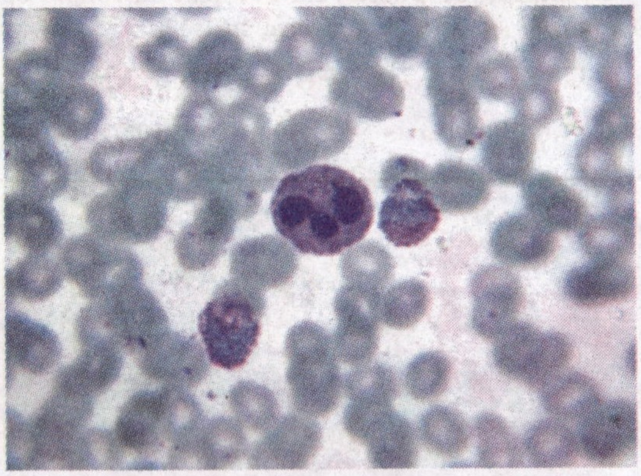

Fig. 10.38 : Female gametocyte of *P.vivax*

5. **Gram stained smear of urethral discharge** (Fig. 10.39)

Note : Gram negative intracellular diplococci.

6. **Gram stained smear of necrotic tissue** in a case of street accident (Fig. 10.40).

Note : Gram positive stout long rods without spores, morphologic of *C. perfringens* in clinical material.

7. **Gram stained smear of sputum** from a case of pneumonia (Fig. 10.41).

Note : Gram positive lanceolate diplococci morphologic of *S. pneumoniae*.

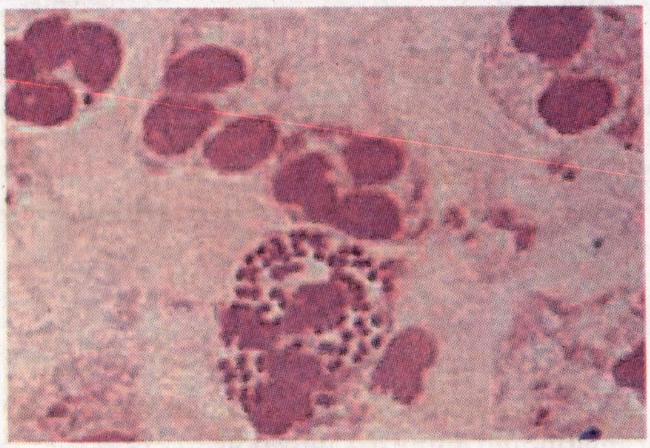

Fig. 10.39 : Gram negative intracellular diplococi

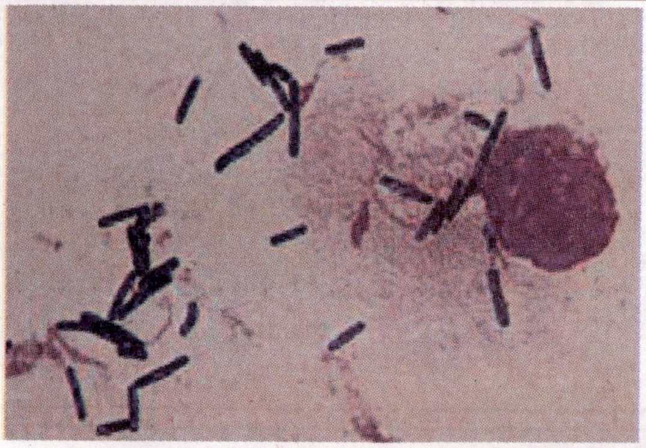

Fig. 10.40

Fig. 10.41

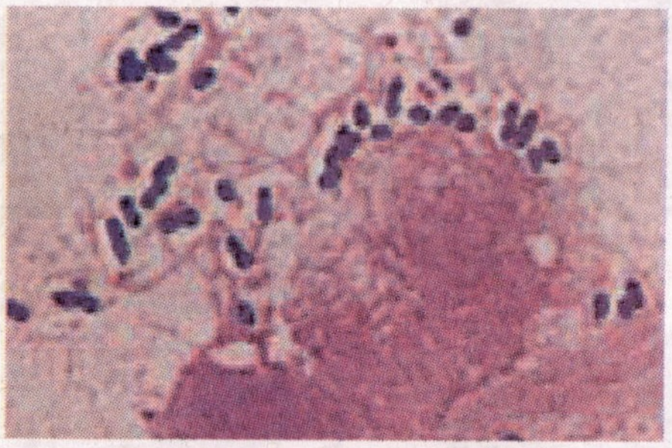

8. **Streptococcus** (Fig. 10.42).

Note : Gram positive cocci in long chains of more than 6 cocci.

9. **Mycobacterium (Z. N. Stained)** (Fig. 10.43)

Note : Bright red acid fast bacillus in a smear of sputum. Other features are 4 degenerated neutrophils (pus cells) and rods taking stain of counterstain (methylene blue). AFB are arranged here in bundle, a characteristic of mycobacterium due to possession of cord factor.

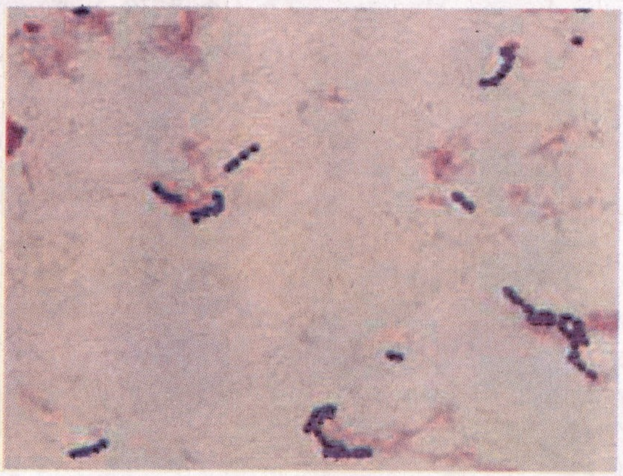

Fig. 10.42 : Streptococcus

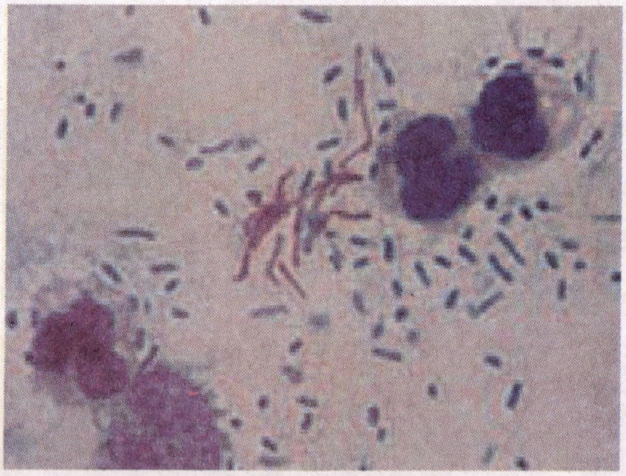

Fig. 10.43 : Mycobacterium (Z. N. stained)

10. Germ tube of candida albicans (after 2 hours incubation in human serum at 22°C) (Fig. 10.44)

Note : Growing tubes from yeast cells, a confirmatory diagnostic test of albican species.

Other confirmatory test — demonstration of terminal smooth chlamydospore in rice meal infusion agar at 22°C).

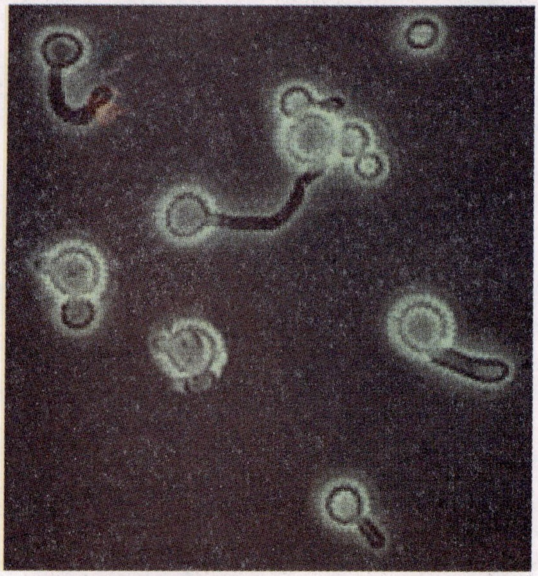

Fig. 10.44 : Germ tube of *Candida albicans*

11. Microfilaria (Fig. 10.45)

Note : Microfilaria of *Wuchereria bancrofti* in peripheral blood. Note the graceful sweeping curve of the parasite. Also note the quadrate cephalic space and nucleus extending upto the tail tip.

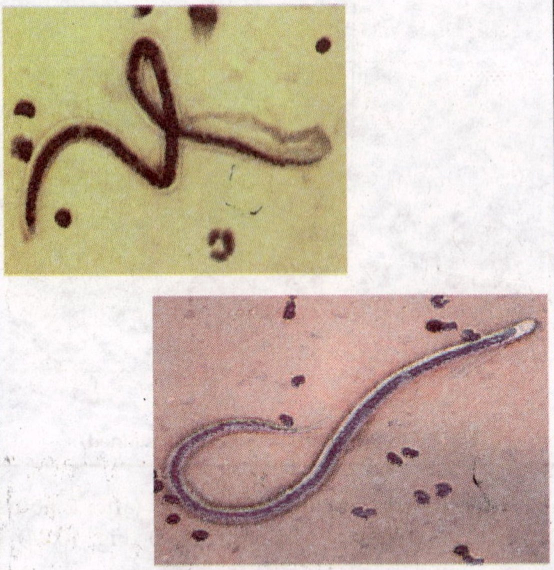

Fig. 10.45 : Microfilaria

12. L.D. body (Leishman stain of bone marrow smear) (Fig. 10.46)

Note : Dots and dashes of L.D. bodies (amastigote form) in mononuclear cells.

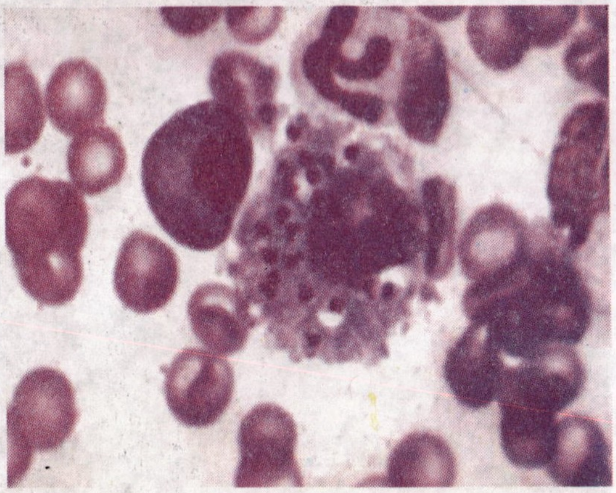

Fig. 10.46 : L. D. body

E. ENTOMOLOGY SPECIMEN

1. *Rat flea* (under low power objective of microscope) — Fig. 10.47.

2. Parasites found on skin of human (Under 10 x objective) — Fig. 10.48

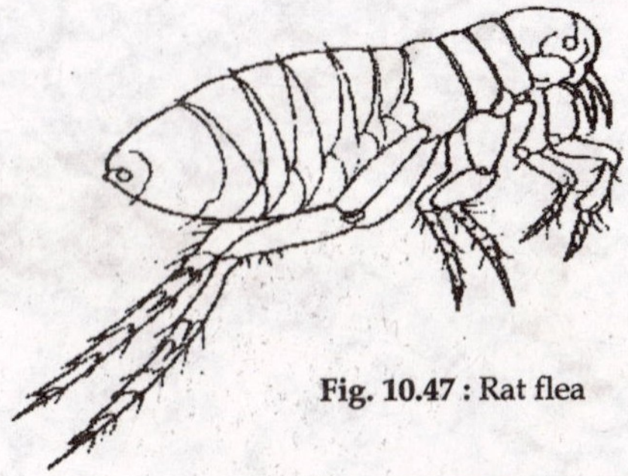

Fig. 10.47 : Rat flea

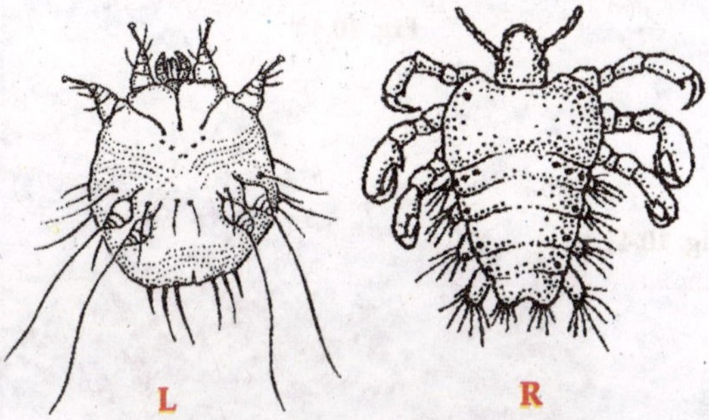

Fig. 10.48 : Parasites found on skin of human
Left : *Sarcoptes scabiei* **Right** : *Phthirus pubis*

3. Female anopheles mosquito — Fig. 10.49B

Note : The posture. Body makes an angle of 45° with the surface. Proboscis is longer than the palpi.

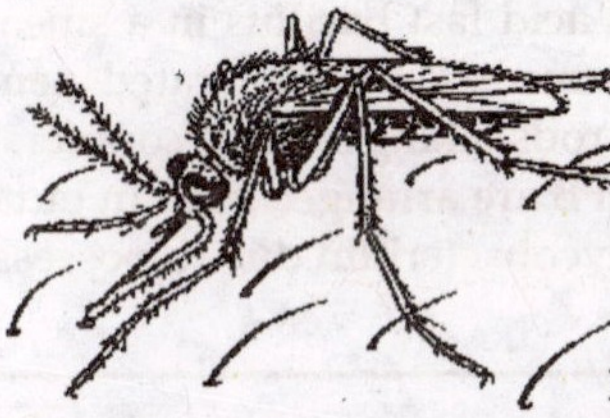

Fig. 10.49A : Culex mosquito, 4 mm

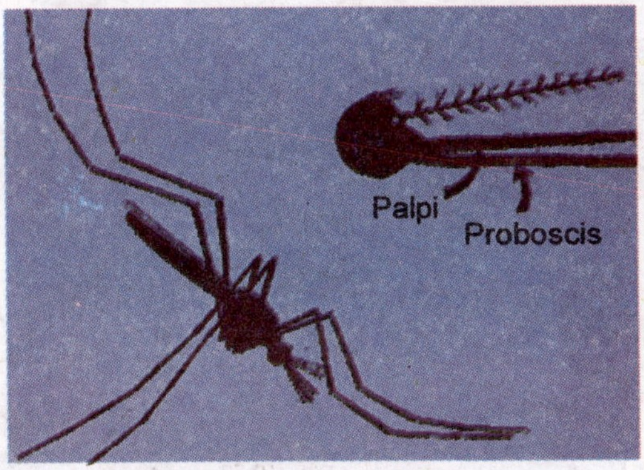

Fig. 10.49B : Female anophele mosquito

4. Aedes mosquito — Fig. 10.50

Note : Sitting posture, short palpi, white bands on abdomen, white spots on wings and legs.

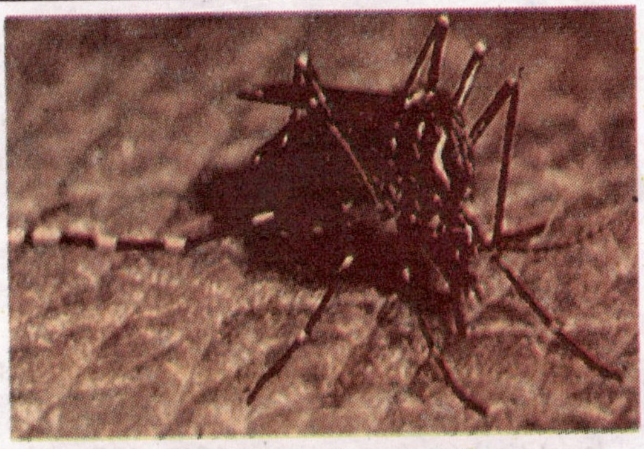

Fig. 10.50 : Aedes mosquito

5. Reduviid bug — Fig. 10.51

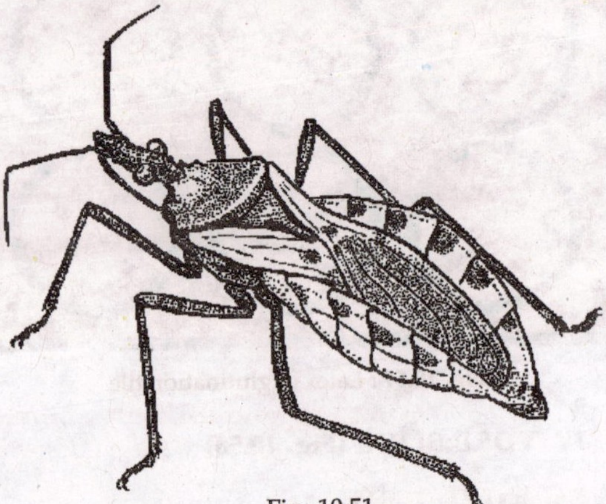

Fig. 10.51

6. Phlebotomus — Fig. 10.52

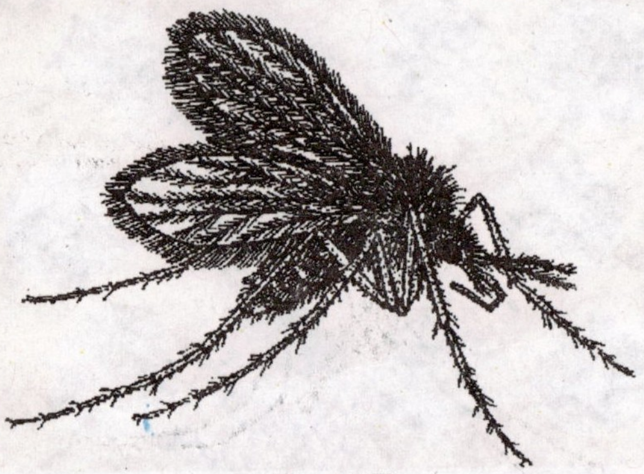

Fig. 10.52

(F) Common Laboratory Equipments

1. Pasteur pipette — Fig. 10.53

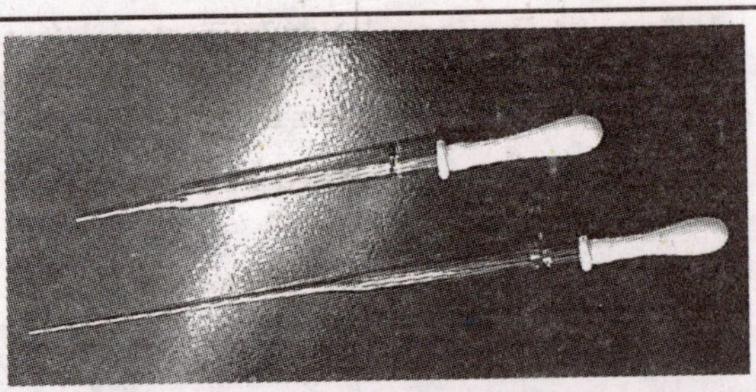

Fig. 10.53

2. Anaerobic jar — Fig. 10.54

Gas pack jars of different sizes

(A)

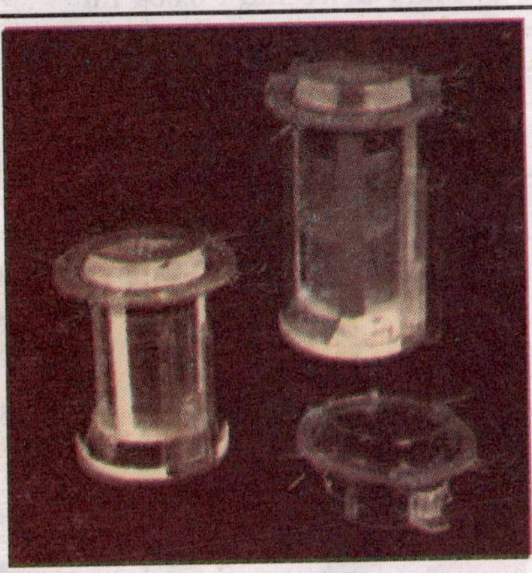

(B)

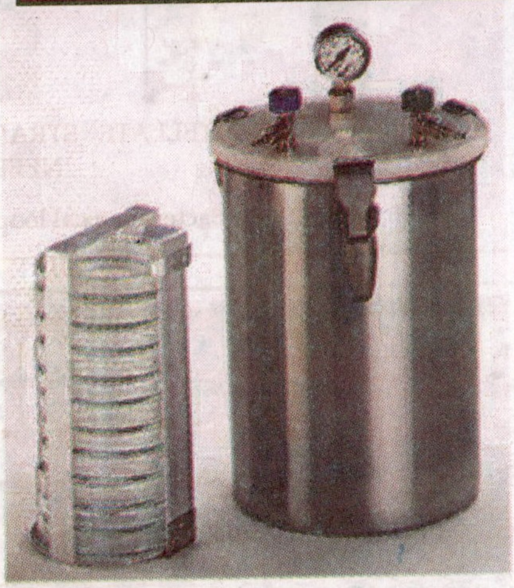

Metal jar with gas inlet, gas outlet and pressure gauge (Fig. 10.54)

(A) : Gas pack jars (with inoculated plates) for chemical generation of H_2 and CO2.

(B) : Inlet and outlet facility for vacuum creation and replacement by N_2 or H_2.

G. MISCELLANEOUS ITEMS

I. BACTERIOLOGICAL LOOP (FIG. 10.55)

1. *Uses* : (i) For inoculation of material from clinical material. (ii) For subculture of bacterial colony from one to other medium.
2. *Sterilisation* : It is sterilised in Bunsen-Burner flame by making it red hot.
3. Specification of loop for urine culture :

   Internal diameter 3 mm.

   External diameter 4 mm.

   Wire thickness 22 G.

   Fluid delivered : 0.004 ml

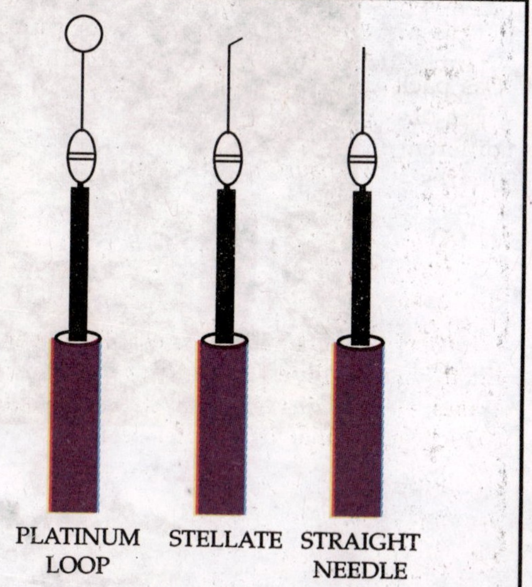

Fig. 10.55 : Bacteriological loop

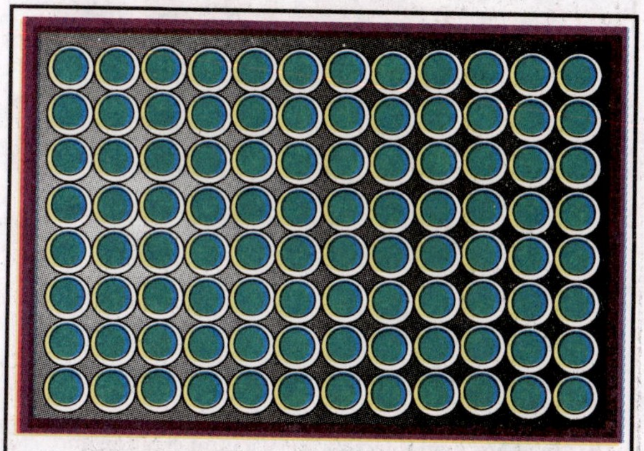

Fig. 10.56 : Microtitre plate

II. MICROTITRE PLATE (FIG. 10.56)

Features

1. *Uses* : For ELISA test.
2. There are 96 (8 × 12) wells.
3. ELISA is used for detection of antigens and antibodies in various micro-organisms, e.g. HIV *antibodies, mycobacterial antibodies* and detection of *hepatitis B markers* in serum.

III. LATEX AGGLUTINATION TILE (Fig. 10.57)

Features

1. *Use* : For performing latex agglutination test.
2. *Uses of latex agglutination tests* : Detection of *hepatitis B surface antigen, ASO, CRP* and *RA factor*.

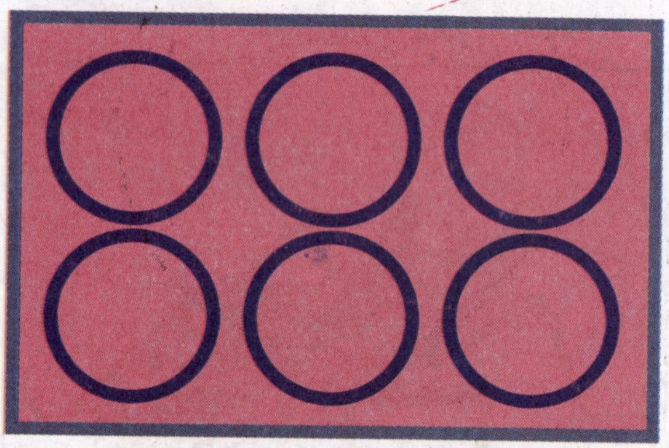

Fig. 10.57 : Latex agglutination tile

IV. VDRL SLIDE (Fig. 10.58)

Salient features

1. *Use* : For VDRL test for serodiagnosis of syphilis.

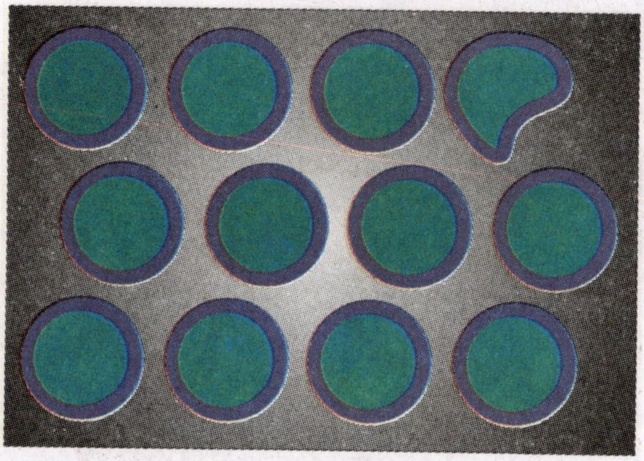

Fig. 10.58 : VDRL slide

2. Causative agent of syphilis : *Treponema pallidum.*
3. VDRL test is a *flocculation test.*
4. *Antigen* : Cardiolipin antigen.

V. CAMP REACTION (Fig. 10.59)

FEATURES

1. *Use* : Detection of group B streptococci.
2. Detection of group B streptococci can also be done by hippurate hydrolysis.
3. Group B streptococci cause neonatal septicaemia and meningitis.

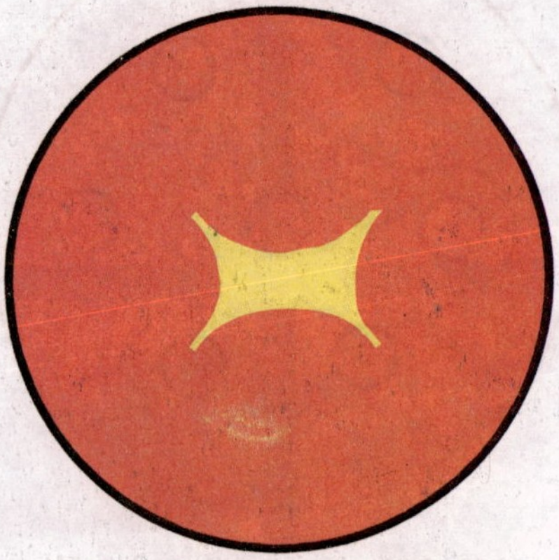

Fig. 10.59 : CAMP reaction

VI. CRAIGIE'S TUBE (Fig. 10.60)

FEATURES

1. It is a wide tube containing 0.2% nutrient agar (soft agar). A short narrow tube open at both ends is kept embedded in the centre of Craigie's tube with one end projecting above the agar.

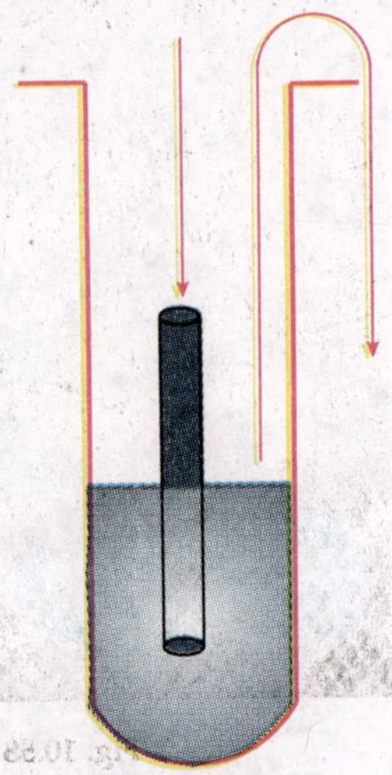

Fig. 10.60 : Craigie's tube

2. Inoculation is made inside inner tube and, after incubation, subculture is taken from surface of agar outside the central tube.
3. *Uses* :
   (i) Demonstration of motility of bacteria.
   (ii) To obtain motile bacteria rich in H antigen, e.g. in *Salmonella typhi.*

VII. MACINTOSH–FILDE'S JAR (see Fig. 10.54, 10.54B)

FEATURES

1. It is a metal or glass jar with gasket to make it air tight.
2. *Principle* : Anaerobiasis is created by (i) placing ignited candle to use up the oxygen or (ii) by gas-out process using vacuum pump and introduction of N_2 or H_2. Palladium beads heated to redness is used inside the jar to absorb remaining O_2.
3. *Use* : For anaerobic culture.

VIII. GAS-PAK JAR FOR ANAEROBIASIS (See Fig. 10.54A)

FEATURES

Principle : By chemical process, H_2 is generated in the jar. Evolved H_2 pushes out the heavier gases, already inside the jar, through a side tube, which act similar to a water seal.

IX. POCKS ON CHORIOALLANTOIC MEMBRANE (Fig. 10.61)

FEATURES

1. Chick egg embryos of 7-12 days old are used.
2. Chorioallantoic membrane (CAM) is inoculated for growing pock forming viruses. Viral replication produces visible lesions (pocks), grey white area in the transparent CAM.

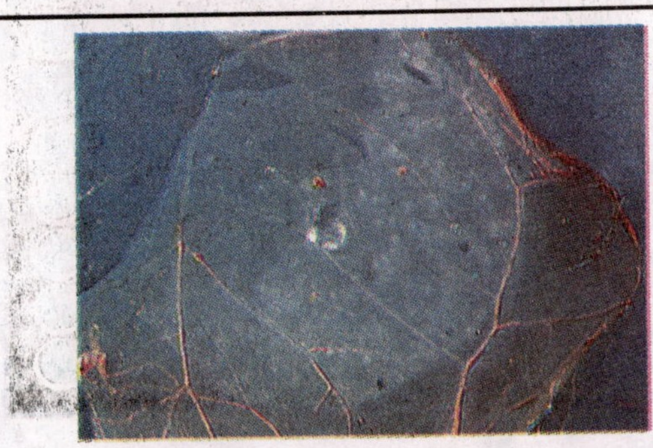

Fig. 10.61 : Pocks on chorioallantoic membrane

3. *Variola, vaccinia*, JE viruses produce pocks on the CAM.

X. STOKE'S METHOD OF ANTIBIOTIC SENSITIVITY TESTING (Fig. 10.62)

1. *Use* : To detect antibiotic sensitivity pattern of bacteria.
2. Müellar-Hinton agar is generally used.
3. Antibiotic discs are applied.
4. Control strain is also inoculated along with test strain.

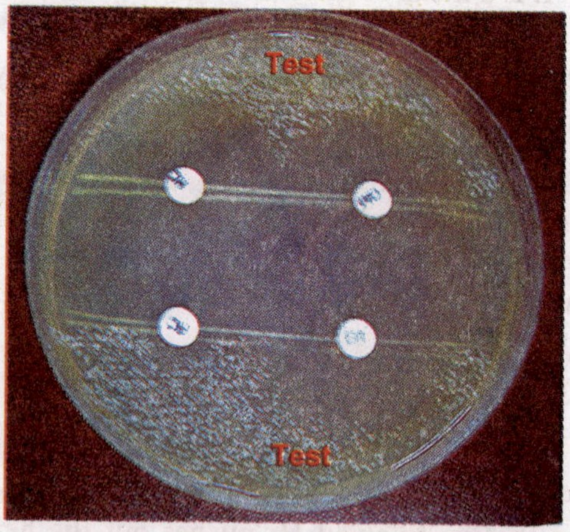

Fig. 10.62 : Stoke's method of antibiotic sensitivity testing

XI. KIRBY-BAUER'S METHOD OF ANTI-BIOTIC SENSITIVITY TESTING (Fig. 10.63)

SALIENT FEATURES

1. *Use* : To detect antibiotic sensitivity pattern of bacteria.
2. Antibiotic discs are used.
3. Control strain is not inoculated.

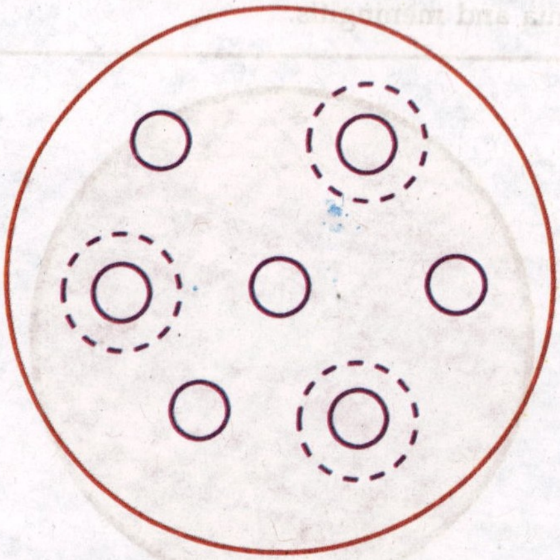

Fig. 10.63 : Kirby-Bauer's method of antibiotic sensitivity testing

Waste Management in health care setting and Universal precautions

11

Nosocomial infection of inpatients and risk of infection in health care delivery workers are very common phenomenon world wide. The vexing problem makes the hospitals an unsafe place. Both patients and HCWs are at risk of acquiring M.R.S.A, V.R.S.A, MDR-TB, MBL producing gram –ve rods, SARS, H_1N_1 virus, HIV, HBV, HCV, NIPAH virus infections to name a few.

To overcome the situation, expert committees suggest to implement 'Hospital Infection Control' measures. The components of HIC are the following:

1. To design the hospital and laboratories in such a way, so that potential infective areas remain separated from rest of the clean areas.
2. To design the isolation rooms, O.T., ICU with maximum containment and air borne infection control measures.
3. Efficient central sterile supply system.
4. Staff education/refresher workshops.
5. Proper waste management.
6. Universal precautions.
7. Antibiotic and disinfectant use policy.
8. Surveillance by 'infection control committee'.
9. Outbreak investigation.

Objective of this chapter is to discuss about proper waste management and universal precaution.

(A) WASTE MANAGEMENT

(I) Classification of hospital waste :

(a) Hazardous (20%)

(i) Infectious (15%) — Non-sharps, sharps, plastics and infectious liquids.

(ii) Non-infectious (5%) — Radioactive materials, glass, pressurized chemical, cytotoxic drugs, incineration waste.

(b) Non-hazardous (80%) — Kitchen waste, fruit peels etc.

(II) Infectious wastes :

These include waste contaminated with blood and body fluids, waste from patients, discarded diagnostic samples, laboratory cultures, stock of infectious agents, waste from laboratory animals, animal carcasses, human body parts (amputed limbs, placenta etc.). On an average 15% of total HW belongs to this category.

(III) Need for proper disposal :

Infectious wastes need proper disposal in right manner for the following reasons :

1. Waste is potentially biohazardous.
2. Pathogens cause disease to HCW and general public.
3. Spread of antibiotic resistance.
4. May lead to poisoning and pollution.
5. My cause injuries. About 10-20 million blood borne infectious take place from sharp.
6. Prevention of access to scavengers.
7. Radioactive accidents.
8. Contamination of drinking water supply.
9. Improper incineration of waste may release potentially toxic gases.

(IV) Components of hospital waste management

(a) Segregation.

(b) Disinfection of selected articles, e.g. used syringe and needle, culture plates etc.

(c) Transport.

(d) Sterilisation, if possible.

(e) Temporary storage (f) Final disposal.

Commonly step 'f' is done by agencies, entrusted for final disposal.

(a) Segregation

This is done at the site of generation in different colour coaded bags kept in bins with lid (to be lifted with foot). Appropriate containers are to be placed at all points of patient care areas. Following is the schedule of colour coading for bio-medical wastes.

1. Non-infectious waste — discarded in black bag. Only non-breakable items are discarded here. If the waste is breakable (e.g. glass), it is first placed in card board box, then discarded in black bag.

2. Sharp — is discarded in puncture proof container, painted blue, bearing biohazard symbol.

3. Infectious plastic items — are to be segregated in red/pink bag. This bag should not be mixed with other items and should not be incinerated in conventional incinerator.

4. Non-plastic infectious wastes — are discarded in yellow bag. Cottons, dressings, anatomical waste, placenta, tissue, experimental animals are included in this category.

(b) Transport

While transporting the observable rules are as follows :

(1) To be done at regular interval.

(2) Avoid spillage by transporting in proper container.

(3) Transportation is to be done by designated trained persons, wearing protective clothing; through the designated areas.

(4) Custom made covered transportation trolleys/trucks are to be used.

(c) Temporary storage

Biomedical wastes after removal from generation areas, are to be placed in temporary storage area. Sharps are left in the wards until the containers are 3/4th full.

(d) Final disposal

- Black bag (non-infectious) — landfill.
- Yellow bag (non-plastic infectious waste) — deep burried.
- Red bag (infected plastic) — treated, shredded and finally go to landfill.
- Blue bag (sharp) — mutilated and landfilled.

(B) UNIVERSAL PRECAUTION

Retrospective data analysis reveals nurses, laboratory workers, physicians, surgical technicians, dialysis technician, respiratory therapist, health aid, embalmer/morgue technician and house keepers are at risk in discharging their professional duties. To avoid contracting the disease in course of their works, 'Universal Precaution' measures are suggested.

(a) Sources of infection

- Blood
- Any fluid containing blood
- Body fluids — e.g. C.S.F., pericardial, amniotic synovial, pleural and peritoneal fluid.
- Semen
- Vaginal fluid
- Aerosols from patients
- Fomites
- Used sharps
- Articles used for procedures etc.

(b) Policy for safer discharge of duties

- Do not harm the patient
- Do not expose provider to unnecessary risk.
- Do not result in waste that is dangerous to others.
- Personal protection.
- Sharp policy.
- Consider all patients are potentially infected and all the areas of hospital contain infectious agents.

(c) Dos and Don't dos of Universal Precautions

1. Personal protection using barriers — e.g. gloves, masks (N-95 for $H_1 N_1$, SARS, Nipah, MDR-TB), apron, eye wear, foot wear.

2. Sharp management :
   - Reduce use.
   - Select devices with protective measures against needle stick injuries.
   - Be careful during use.
   - Don't recap needle after use.
   - Destroy needle, disinfect (if possible), discard in puncture proof blue container with biohazard sign.

3. Hand washing, preferably with alcohol based hand sanitiser, before and after examination of patient or handling clinical sample.
4. Get ready a beaker containing disinfectant (1% sodium hypochlorite) to dispose infected small materials and tackle any infective spillage.
5. Get immunised where applicable (e.g. HBV vaccine).
6. Segregate waste properly.
7. Preserve a sample of serum for assessment of base line titre.
8. Do not take food, drink in work place.
9. Do not move about with open needle in hand.
10. Do not mouth pipette.
11. Do not create aerosol.
12. Do not try to express the last drop of liquid from a pipette.
13. Do not keep unnecessary long hair.
14. Do not allow pregnant staff to perform only in potential infective setting.

SPACE FOR NOTES

Some Important Laboratory Diagnosis of Bacterial Diseases

12

DIPHTHERIA

The genus *corynebacterium* comprises of :

1. Toxin-producing : *C. diphtheriae, C. ulcerans.*
2. Non-pathogenic (commensals) : *C. hofmannii, C. xerosis.* These are also called diphtheroids.

A. BACTERIOLOGICAL STUDIES

For control measures and epidemiological studies laboratory confirmation of diphtheria is necessary. Specific treatment against diphtheria (antitoxin and antibiotic) should be given immediately after clinical diagnosis without waiting for laboratory findings.

Two swabs are taken from the site of lesion (throat, nose or larynx): one for smear examination and other for culture.

1. **Direct smear examination** : Smears stained by *Albert's stain* show beaded slender rods in typical Chinese-letter pattern. The results of microscopic examination of clinical material may not always be reliable. Interpretation of the smear requires technical expertise. Hence smear examination alone is not sufficient for the diagnosis. Specimen should always be cultured.

2. **Culture** : Swab is inoculated on the following culture media —

(a) *Loeffler's serum slope* : Growth appears in 6-8 hours but, if negative, the media will have to be incubated for 24 hours. The microscopic morphology is best seen on Loeffler's medium. Smear from culture stained with Albert stain show typical bacilli.

(b) *Tellurite blood agar medium* and *ordinary blood agar medium* : It is incubated for 36-48 hours. Studies on colonies on tellurite medium is helpful in distinguishing the biotypes of *C. diphtheriae* (Table 12.1). The colonies show characteristic gray-to-black colour on tellurite agar.

Table 12.1 : Differentiating characteristics of *C. diphtheriae* strains

Characteristics strains	gravis strains	intermedius strains	mitis
1. Virulence	Severe	Moderate	Mild
2. Morphology film from Loeffler's medium)	Club-shaped, short rods, few metachromatic granules, uniform staining	Long, poor granulation, barred forms, irregular staining, pleomorphic	Long, curved forms, pleomorphic with classic morphology
3. Colony on tellurite blood agar, 18 hours incubation	1-2 mm size, gray, raised centre, crenated edge with radial striations "daisy head" colonies in 48-72 hours	1 mm size, grayish black, dull granular centre with glistening periphery and a lighter ring near the edge "frog's egg" colony	Size variable, shiny black, circular convex, smooth (poached egg colony)
4. Consistency of colonies	Brittle, not easily picked out or emulsifiable	Intermediate between gravis and mitis	Soft, buttery, easily emulsifiable
5. Haemolysis	Variable	Non-haemolytic	Usually haemolytic
6. Biochemical reaction :			
Glucose	Acid	Acid	Acid
Glycogen	Acid	Negative	Negative
Starch	Acid	Negative	Negative

B. VIRULENCE TEST

All isolates of *C. diphtheriae* should be tested for virulence for toxigenicity which can be done either *in vivo* (animal inoculation) or *in vitro* (Elek's test).

1. **Animal inoculation test** : Guinea pigs and rabbits are susceptible but rat and mice are resistant to the action of toxin.

(a) *Subcutaneous test* : Overnight growth of Loeffler's slope is first mixed with 2 to 5 ml nutrient broth and 0.3 ml from this emulsified growth is injected subcutaneously in thigh in two guinea pigs, one of which has received an intramuscular injection of 500 units of diphtheria antitoxin 18 to 24 hours before the test. The unprotected animal will die within 2 to 3 days. At autopsy, other important findings include : gelatinous, haemorrhagic oedema and often with necrosis at the site of injection; draining lymph nodes–swollen; clear, cloudy or blood-stained pleural and peritoneal fluid; and abdominal viscera–congested. The adrenal gland finding (haemorrhage) is pathognomonic feature. This method is not usually followed because of wastage of animals.

(b) *Intracutaneous test* : Two guinea pigs or rabbits are injected intracutaneously with 0.2 ml emulsion from growth in Loeffler's serum medium, one of which is protected with 500 units of antitoxin the previous day (control animal) and to the other animal 50 units of diphtheria antitoxin is injected intraperitoneally simultaneously with the skin test in order to prevent abrupt death of the animal. The unprotected animal develops local erythematous lesion at the site of injection in 48-72 hours but there is no change in the control animal. By intracutaneous method, 8 to 10 cultures can be tested on a pair of animals and the animals do not die.

2. **In vitro test (Elek's Agar-gel precipitation test)** : This *in vitro* immunodiffusion test, described by Elek (1949), provides a rapid and economic alternative to *in vivo* test. A rectangular strip of filter paper soaked in antitoxin (1,000 units/ml) is placed on the surface of a serum agar plate containing 20% horse serum while the medium is still in fluid form. When the medium solidifies, the testing strain is streaked across the plate at right angles to the filter paper strip and then incubated at 37°C for 24 to 48 hours. Toxin produced by bacterial growth diffuses in agar medium and produces line of precipitation where it meets antitoxin molecules (dispersed from the filter paper) in optimum concentration (Fig. 12.1). Usually the result can be read within 48 hours,

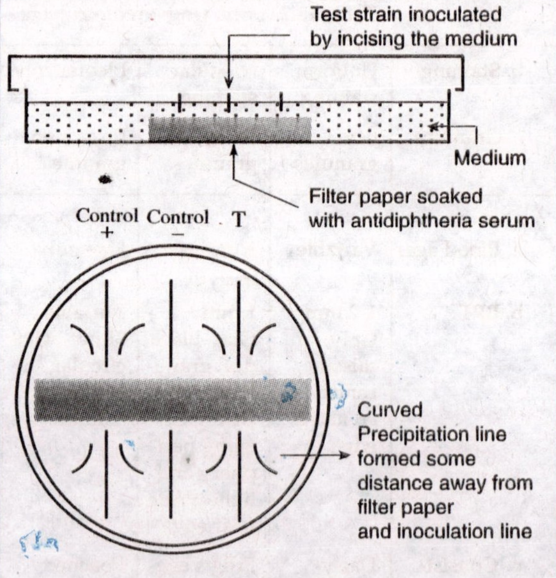

Fig. 12.1 : Elek's test — Toxigenicity test for *C. diphtheriae*

sometimes precipitin lines may take up to 72 hours to develop. This technique is not only very convenient but also economical. The lines of precipitate radiate from the intersection of the strip and the bacterial growth.

3. **Tissue culture test** : This is done by incorporation of test bacteria into an agar overlay of cell culture monolayers. The toxin produced diffuses into the underlying cells causing death of the cells.

The important distinguishing features of *C. diphtheriae* are shown in chapter 3, Table 3.1 (p. 12).

QUESTIONS RELATED TO DIPHTHERIA

Q.1. ***What are the three biotypes of C. diphtheriae and how to distinguish them ?***

Ans. McLeod classified *C. diphtheriae* into three biotypes based on colony characteristics on BPT (see Table 12.2). These three biotypes are :

(a) *Gravis* (b) *Intermedius* (c) *Mitis*

Table 12.2 : Differences between biotypes of *C. diphtheriae*

	gravis	inter-medius	mitis
1. **Morphology**			
a. Length	Short rods	Long forms	Long curved forms

(Table contd. next page)

Table 12.2 contd. from previous page

b. Staining	Uniform staining	Irregular staining	Pleomorphic
c. Granules	Few granules	Poor granules	Prominent granules
2. Culture			
a. Blood agar	Variable	Non-haemolytic	Haemolytic
b. BPT	1-2 mm Gray, raised centre, crenated edge	1 mm Gray-black, dull granular centre with glistening periphery and lighter ring near edge	Variable Shiny-black circular, convex, smooth
c. Consistency of colony	Daisy-head colony Brittle, not easily emulsifiable	Frog's egg colony Intermediate between *gravis* and *mitis*	Poached egg colony Soft buttery, easily emulsifiable
3. Biochemical reaction			
a. Glycogen fermentation	+	–	–
b. Starch fermentation	+	–	–
4. Virulence	Severe	Moderate	Mild
5. Usual complication	Paralytic	Haemorrhagic	Haemorrhagic obstructive

+ = positive, – = negative

Q.2. *Which is the virulence factor? Describe.*

Ans. *Toxin in C. diphtheriae* is responsible for virulence of the organism. It is an exotoxin. The strain universally used for toxin production is the Park-Williams 8. It is a protein having two fragments A and B. Enzymatic activity is present in A, whereas B is responsible for binding and transport of a toxin to cells.

Q.3. *How do you do active immunisation?*

Ans. (i) Diphtheria, Pertussis, Tetanus (DPT) vaccine. (ii) Schedule-3 doses at 4-6 weeks interval by intramuscular route from 6 weeks of age 1st booster at – 1 $^1/_2$ years of age and 2nd booster at 5-6 years. Other vaccine preparations are adsorbed toxoid and formal toxoid.

ENTERIC FEVER

Salmonella typhi causes typhoid fever and *S. paratyphi* A, B and C cause paratyphoid fever.

Enteric fever includes both typhoid and paratyphoid fever. Other important pathogenic salmonellae include enterocolitis group (caused by *S. typhimurium, S. enteritidis, S. dublin* etc.) and septicaemia group (caused by *S. enteritidis*).

Culture and isolation of salmonellae are essential to confirm a diagnosis. Identification of the isolate is based on biochemical characteristics and serology. The optimal specimen for culture varies with presentation.

(a) In a classic case of salmonella gastroenteritis a faecal sample is best. Patient's vomitus and suspected foodstuffs are also useful.

(b) In a suspected case of enteric fever, blood culture or bone marrow aspirate is most likely to yield positive results. Later, with intestinal and renal involvement, culture of faeces and urine is indicated.

The specimens to be tested at different stages of enteric fever and the percentage of positivity are shown in Fig. 7.33 and Table 7.16 (on p. 74). General blood picture in enteric fever may show leucopenia (leucocyte count, 2,000-2,500 cumm) with relative lymphocytosis.

ISOLATION OF THE ORGANISM

1. Culture of blood bone marrow : Specimens of blood or bone marrow in enteric fever; faeces, vomitus or suspected food in gastroenteritis should be collected before starting treatment.

As there is transient bacteraemia, there are small number of organisms in blood. Repeated culture with larger volume (5-10 ml) of blood is necessary. **Blood culture** is positive in 80-90% patients in first week and up to 10 days of fever. The chances of positive culture progressively diminishes with increase in duration of illness (see Fig. 7.33). Blood culture also yields positive result during relapses. **Bone-marrow material** culture is as reliable as blood culture and it yields positive result in 1 to 2 days after commencement of chloramphenicol therapy.

A volume of 5 to 10 ml blood collected aseptically by venepuncture is transferred directly into a blood culture bottle containing 50 to 100 ml 0.5% glucose broth or 0.5% bile broth. Although blood culture in bile broth (selective medium for salmonellae) is most ideal for salmonellae, but, in practice, most laboratories use glucose broth for blood culture because all microorganisms including salmonellae grow in the medium. Larger volume of media helps in dilution of the antibacterial substances present in the blood. **Liquid** (sodium polyanethol sulphonate) may be added in the media which counteracts the bactericidal action of blood.

Alternatively, 5 ml venous blood, collected aseptically, is allowed to clot in a sterile screw-capped universal container. After removing serum, 15 ml. bile salt streptokinase broth streptokinase, 100 units per ml) is added aseptically to each bottle. The streptokinase digests the clot causing its lysis and thereby the bacteria are released from the clot. The separated serum is utilised for **Widal** test. **Clot culture** offers a higher rate of isolation than blood culture as the bactericidal activity of serum is obviated in the technique.

After incubation overnight at 37°C, **subculturing** is done on MacConkey agar or DCA. Subculturing is economically carried out by spreading a loopful of broth over a sector of solid media, one-fourth of an 8.5 cm Petri dish and incubated for 24-48 hours. Colourless colonies (NLF) appear. Cultures may be discarded as negative after 10 days.

As growth may be delayed and also to eliminate the risk of introducing contamination during repeated subcultures, **Castaneda's** method of blood culture may be adopted, which provides both liquid (liver infusion broth) and solid media (3% nutrient agar slope) in one bottle. It is a diphasic medium, broth has an agar slant on one side.

2. **Stool and urine culture** : Culture of faeces and urine are always positive during 3rd and 4th week of enteric fever. Repeated cultures are required for positive result. Stool culture is mainly done for detecting the **carriers**.

3. **Duodenal juice or bile culture** : Bile is cultured to detect ***chronic carriers*** in whom the organisms are present in the biliary tract.

Identification

In MacConkey's agar or DCA, salmonellae grow as non-lactose fermenters which are further studied by *Gram's staining, motility preparation* and *biochemical reactions* in different sugar media. Subculture from the colonies is made in nutrient agar to be utilised for *agglutination test.*

Slide agglutination test : A loopful isolated organism (unknown culture) from the colony in agar is emulsified in a drop of saline on a microscopic slide without spreading the drop. The emulsion must be absolutely smooth and of medium opacity. One small loopful of specific antiserum is added and then mixed by tilting the slide. In the same way, a control of bacterial suspension in normal saline is prepared on other slide and to which no specific serum is added. Clumping of bacteria in test slide occurs within a few minutes if the antigen-antibody reaction is specific. Control saline emulsion of bacteria does not show any change.

Biochemically positive strains (Table 12.3) are first tested with polyvalent O serum, which reacts with salmonella strains in groups A to G, provided agglutination is not blocked by Vi antigen, which can be checked by testing all negative strains using *S. typhi* Vi serum. Positive results with polyvalent O serum indicates a *Salmonella* strain. In the next step, the strain is tested with sera prepared against O antigens of the individual salmonella groups. The following are most useful sera which react with factor 2, Group A; factors 4 and 5, group B; with 6 and 7, group C1; with 8, group C2; with 9, group D; and with 3, 10, 15 and 19, group E.

Table 12.3 : Biochemical reaction patterns of *S. typhi* and *S. paratyphi* (d = delayed)

	S. typhi	*S. paratyphi A*	*S. paratyphi B*	*S. paratyphi C*
Glucose	A	AG	AG	AG
Xylose	d	–	AG	AG
d-tartrate	A	–	–	AG
Mucate	d	–	AG	–

When the strain is positive with individual salmonella O serum and biochemically it is typically *S. typhi*, the strain is tested against *S. typhi* O serum, factor 9. Prompt agglutination indicates that the microorganism belongs to *Salmonella* group D. Its identity is established as *S. typhi* by agglutination with salmonella H specific serum which reacts with flagellar antigen d.

In a non-typhoid salmonella, the strain is tested for agglutination with O and H sera for groups A, B and C. When unusual serotypes are encountered, the same should be referred to the National Salmonella Reference Centre (Central Research Institute Kasauli, for human strain, and Indian Veterinary Research Institute, Izatnagar, for salmonella of animal origin).

Subtyping : Subtyping methods are frequently used for the common serotypes *(S. typhi, S. typhimurium* and *S. enteritidis)* which include phage typing, biotyping, and more recently introduced genotyping methods (plasmid fingerprinting). These techniques are employed in CDC for subtyping within serotypes of *Salmonella.*

SEROLOGICAL TEST

1. **Widal test** : It is an agglutination test which detects presence of *serum agglutinins (H and O)* in patient's serum with typhoid and paratyphoid fever. Salmonella antibody starts appearing in serum at the end of first week (Fig. 7.33) and rises sharply during the 3rd week of enteric fever. It is preferable to test two specimens of sera at an interval of 7 to 10 days to demonstrate a rising antibody titre.

Convalescent sera from salmonella gastroenteritis cases often agglutinate a suspension of the causal serotype which helps in retrospective diagnosis.

Procedure : In Widal test, two types of tubes were originally used : (1) Dreyer's tube (narrow tube with conical bottom) for H agglutination and (ii) Felix tube (short round-bottomed tube) for O agglutination. Nowadays, 3 × 0.5 ml Kahn tubes are used for both types of agglutination.

A serial two-fold dilution of patient's serum in normal saline (1 : 20, 1 : 40 and so on up to 1,280 or more) is prepared in 8 small (3 × 0.5 ml) test tubes for each series; 7 for serum dilutions and 8th for a non-serum control. To the diluted serum and control saline equal volume (0.4 cc) of antigen suspensions (TH, TO, AH and BH) are added and mixed thoroughly by shaking the rack and then the mixtures are incubated at 37°C for 4 hours and read after overnight refrigeration at 4°C. Some workers recommended incubation in a water bath at 37°C overnight.

Observation : Loose and cotton-woolly clumps are formed in *H agglutination* and a disc-like granular deposit in *O agglutination* at the bottom of tube. Control tube shows a compact deposit. The **Maximum dilution** of serum at which agglutination occurs indicate the titre of antibodies. The routinely used antigens are H and O of *S. typhi, H* of *S. paratyphi* A and B. As paratyphoid O antigen cross reacts with typhoid O antigen due to the sharing of factor 12 by them, paratyphoid O antigens are not used.

Preparation of Widal antigen : *H suspension* of bacteria is prepared by adding 0.1% formalin to a 24-hour broth culture or saline suspension of an agar culture. For preparation of *O suspension* of bacteria, the organisms are cultured on phenol agar (1 : 800). Standard smooth strains of the organism are used — *S. typhi* 901, O and H strains are employed for this purpose.

Interpretation of Widal test

1 *Agglutinin* starts appearing in serum by the end of 1st week with sharp rise in 2nd and 3rd week and the titre remains steady till 4th week after which it declines.

2. *Rising titre* : Demonstration of *rising titre* of four-fold or greater of both H and O agglutinins at an interval of 4 to 7 days is the most important diagnostic criterion.

3. In a *single test,* a titre of 100 of O or more and a titre of 200 of H agglutinins signifies presence of active infection, but that has to be interpreted taking into consideration the following factors :

(i) *Local titre* : Due to sub-clinical infection of salmonellosis in endemic area, low titre of agglutinins is present in the serum of normal individuals, which may cause positive reaction. This is known as *local titre.* Local titre is up to 80 in Kolkata and 60 in Siliguri.

(ii) *Immunisation* : In immunisation with TAB vaccine, vaccinated individuals may show high titres of antibody (H antibody titre 160 or more) to each of the salmonellae.

(iii) *Anamnestic reaction* : Persons who had past enteric infection or who have been vaccinated may develop transient fever like *malaria, influenza,* etc.

(iv) *Non-specific antigens* (e.g. *fimbrial antigen)* may produce false-positive result.

(v) *Antibiotic treatment* : When treatment with chloramphenicol is started before the appearance of agglutinins, they are unlikely to appear subsequently; if the antibody is already present, no further rise in titre is expected.

(vi) *Carriers* : Widal tests may be positive in many healthy carriers and some have to be detected by Vi antiserum.

2. **Other serological tests** : ELISA is sensitive method of measuring antibody against the lipopolysaccharide of *Salmonellae,* titre of IgM antibody corresponds fairly well with the Widal O titre.

QUESTIONS RELATED TO ENTERIC FEVER

Q.1. ***What is Vi antigen and its importance?***

Ans. Many strains of *S. typhi* have this antigen —

(a) Felix and Pitt described this antigen and as it was related with virulence, therefore labelled as Vi.

(b) It is a heat-labile surface antigen, like K antigen of coliforms found in many strains *S. typhi*. It covers O antigen and renders the strain inagglutinable with O antisera, hence bacilli inagglutinable with the O antiserum become agglutinable after boiling or heating for 1 hour.

(c) Vi antigen tends to lose on serial subcultures.

(d) It may act by coating bacterial surface and preventing the antibacterial opsonic effect of antibody.

(e) In humans, strains with Vi antigen were found to cause clinical disease more consistently than those lacking the antigen.

(f) It is poorly immunogenic so low titres of antibodies are produced following infection :

- The detection of Vi antibodies is not helpful in diagnosis of cases, hence it is not used in Widal test.
- The total absence of Vi antibodies in a proven case of typhoid fever indicates poor prognosis.
- The antibodies to Vi antigen usually disappear in convalescence and its persistence indicates development of the carrier state.
- It is used for epidemiological typing of *S. typhi* based on specific bacteriophages.

Q.2. ***Name the important strains of salmonellae that are classified serologically — based on Kauffmann-White scheme.***

Ans. The important strains of salmonellae are :

Sero-group	Serotype	O Ag	H phase I Ag	H phase II Ag
2-A	*S. paratyphi* A	1, 2, 12	a	–
4-B	*S. paratyphi* B	1, 4, 5, 12	b	1, 2
7-C1	*S. paratyphi* C	6, 7 (Vi)	c	1, 5
9-D	*S. typhi*	9, 12 (Vi)	d	–

Q.3. ***What is Typhim Vi?***

Ans. (1) It is purified Vi Ag from *S. typhi* Ty 2.

(2) It is given by intramuscular route.

(3) Single dose of 25 µg.

(4) Efficacy 64% to 72%.

(5) Protection starts after 2-3 weeks and lasts for at least 3 years.

Q.4. ***What is Oral Vaccine of Typhoid?***

Ans. Typhoral is an oral vaccine containing stable mutant of *S. typhi* strain — Ty 21a lacking enzyme UDP-galactose 4-epimerase.

(1) It is an enteric-coated capsule that contains viable lyophilised mutant bacilli.

(2) Following ingestion, it initiates infection but

Table 12.4 : Classification of *Shigella*

Group	Species	Number of serotypes	Serotype	Synonymus (Earlier designation)
	Mannitol not fermented			
A	*S. dysenteriae*	12	1	A 1. *S. shiga*
			2	A 2. *S. schmitzi*; Possible some strains of *B. ambiguus* (Andrewes).
			3 to 7 8 to 12	Large-Sachs Group
	Mannitol usually fermented			
B	*S. flexneri*	8	1 to 5	*S. paradysenteriae*
			6	Boyd 88, Newcastle and Manchester biochemical types
			X variant Y variant	Andrewes and Inman (Both have type antigens)
C	*S. boydii*	18	1 to 18	*S. paradysenteriae*
D	*S. sonnei* (Lactose fermented at 3-8 days)	1	1	*Sonnei bacillus*

self-destructs after four or five cell divisions, hence cannot induce illness.

(3) Schedule : 3 doses of one capsule orally to be taken an hour before food with water or milk on days 1, 3, 5.

(4) Protection starts after 2-3 weeks and lasts for 3 years, thereafter booster may be needed.

BACILLARY DYSENTERY

To confirm diagnosis, *Shigella* (Table 12.4 on previous page) must be isolated in pure culture from an adequate sample. Specimens include fresh stool, mucous flakes, and rectal swabs.

A. Microscopical examination of stool

Cover-slip preparation in saline and iodine shows large number of pus cells (neutrophils) with degenerated nuclei, RBC, and macrophages. The presence of protozoa, cysts or helminthic ova is excluded. The normal bacterial flora is considerably diminished. Fluorescent antibody technique is of some help in rapid diagnosis of a case but it is not usually practised.

B. Bacteriological examination

I. Culture

Media : MacConkey's agar, DCA, S-S agar, Selenite-F broth.

A loopful of material is inoculated on selective media like MacConkey's agar or S. S. agar media.

Selenite-F broth (0.4%) is used as enrichment and transport medium which permits rapid growth of enteric pathogens while temporarily (for 9-12 hours) inhibiting the growth of *E. coli*. Organisms from selenite-F broth are subcultured in MacConkey's agar after 24 hours incubation at 37°C.

Colourless colonies appear on MacConkey's agar medium after 12 to 18 hours incubation which are further tested by smear examination, motility preparation and biochemical reactions. Shigellae are gram-negative, non-motile bacilli.

II. Biochemical reactions

Urease, citrate, H_2S and KCN negative; indole and M R positive organism is suggestive of a shigella strain (Fig. 7.34, Table 7.19 on p. 79). *S. sonnei* is a late lactose fermenter.

III. Slide agglutination test

It is done by using polyvalent antisera of three groups (A, B and C) of shigella and antiserum of group D (*S. sonnei*), one by one against the isolate. Monovalent antisera are used for the group for which agglutination has occurred with polyvalent antisera. Then type specific antisera for strains belonging to group A, B or C is used for agglutination test.

Occasionally, agglutination may not occur due to masking of O antigen by K antigen, which can be removed by boiling the bacterial suspension at 100°C for 60 minutes.

IV. Colicin typing

It is done for group D strains.

V. ***Sereny*** test may be done to confirm the invasiveness of the isolated strain of shigella, although, it is seldom practised.

QUESTIONS RELATED TO BACILLARY DYSENTERY

Q.1. ***Which Shigella does produce exotoxin and how the same acts ?***

Ans. (i) It is produced only by *Sh. dysenteriae* type I. (ii) It acts as both enterotoxin and neurotoxin. (iii) Enterotoxin acts on intestinal mucosa causing transudation of fluid in lumen. (iv) Neurotoxin damages endothelial cells of small blood vessels of central nervous system, which result in neurological complications like polyneuritis, coma, meningism. (v) Certain strains of *Sh. dysenteriae* also produce cytotoxin, which acts on Vero cells and is known as Verocytotoxin.

Q.2. ***How to control Shigella infection?***

Ans. Prevention and control of Shigellosis can be achieved by : (a) Improvement of environmental sanitation. (b) Improvement of personal hygiene. (c) Protection of food from flies.

DIARRHOEAL DISEASES

Aetiology of infective diarrhoea :

Bacterial diarrhoea can be divided into two groups, those caused by invasive and those caused by non-invasive microorganisms :

(A) **Non-invasive bacterial pathogens** : Gastroenteritis or food poisoning caused by the undermentioned organisms are **toxin-mediated** *(toxin type)* :

1. *V. cholerae.*
2. Enteropathogenic and enterotoxigenic *Esch. coli* (EPEC, ETEC).
3. Verotoxin-producing *Esch. coli* (VTEC *E. coli* O157 : H7).

4. *Clostridium perfringens* type A.
5. *Staphylococcus aureus* (some strains).
6. *Bacillus cereus.*
7. *Clostridium difficile.*
8. *Shigella dysenteriae* – 1.
9. *Vibrio parahaemolyticus.*

B. **Invasive bacterial pathogens :** These organisms cause gastroenteritis or food poisoning by **invasive mechanism** and not by toxin (*non-toxin* type) :

1. *Salmonella* species.
2. *Campylobacter* species.
3. *Shigella* species.
4. Enteroinvasive *E. coli* (EIEC).
5. Enterohaemorrhagic *E. coli* (EHEC).
6. *Yersinia enterocolitica.*
7. Yersinia *pseudotuberculosis.*

A simplified flow chart is shown in Fig. 12.2 outlining the important steps of examination.

A. Specimens :

1. *Faecal sample* is examined for detection of the offending agent.

2. *Enzyme immunoassay* (EIA) of faecal samples is useful in rapid detection of organisms.

3. Blood cultures are indicated only with constitutional symptoms.

B. Microscopy : Saline and iodine preparations when examined microscopically, causative parasitic agents (*E. histolytica, Giardia lamblia,* and *Cryptosporidium*) can be detected.

C. Culture : Specimen is inoculated in MacConkey's agar (or in TCBS, thiosulphate-citrate-sucrose-bile salt agar in suspected cases of cholera) and incubated at 37°C overnight.

D. Identification : Isolated organism is identified by biochemical and agglutination test.

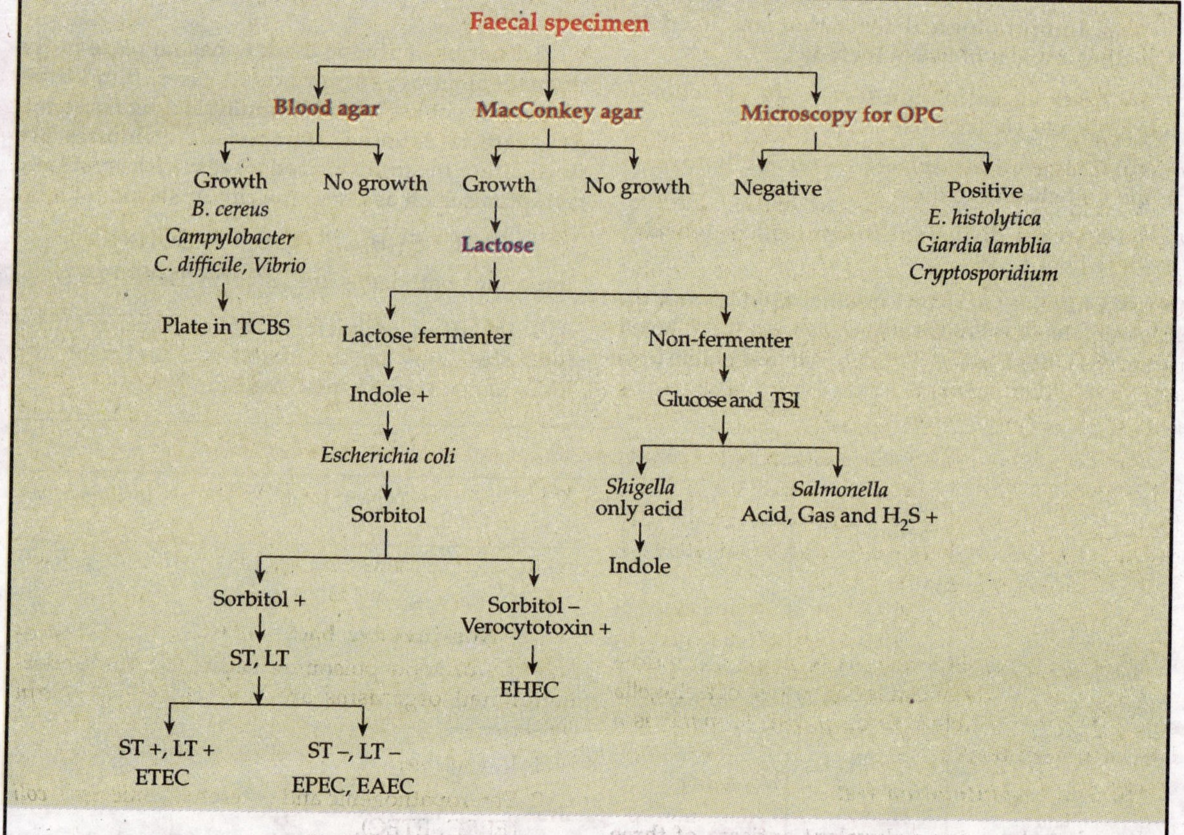

Fig. 12.2 : Steps for identification of enteropathogenic bacteria
OPC = ova, parasite, cyst. TCBS = thiosulphate-citrate-sucrose-bile salt agar

QUESTIONS RELATED TO DIARRHOEAL DISEASES

Q.1. ***Name the transport media for transport of specimens.***

Ans. (i) Stool sample — should be collected in a clean sterile container.

(ii) Rectal swabs — collected if faeces are not readily obtainable.

(iii) Vomit — is less useful.

The specimen should be transported immediately. When more than two hours' delay is expected, the faecal specimen should be collected in suitable transport media such as :

(a) Cary-Blair transport medium.

(b) Stuart's transport medium.

(c) 0.33 M phosphate buffer mixed with equal parts of glycerol (pH 7.0).

Q.2. ***Name the tests employed to detect antigen in diarrhoeal faeces.***

Ans. Immunological tests that are used for detecting antigen in faeces include :

(a) **Latex agglutination test** — for detection of rotavirus and cholera toxin.

(b) **Coagglutination test** — for labile toxin of *E. coli* and cholera toxin.

(c) **Agar gel diffusion (Biken test)** — for labile toxin (LT) of *E. coli.*

(d) **ELISA** — to detect organisms or toxins, e.g. (i) Antigens of rotavirus. (ii) *G. lamblia.* (iii) Cholera toxin (CT). (iv) *E. coli* (LT). (v) *E. coli* heat stable toxin (ST). (vi) Other agents.

(e) **Other tests** : (a) DNA probes. (b) PCR.

Q.3. ***How do you treat diarrhoeal diseases?***

Ans. The following treatment measures are adopted :

1. Major idea in the management of diarrhoea is early replacement of water and electrolytes to prevent or treat dehydration and maintenance of adequate nutrition. Specific treatment is not immediately needed except for protozoal diarrhoea :

- WHO introduced oral rehydration fluid. Revised formula (2004) with reduced osmolarities :

Sodium chloride (NaCl)	...	2.6 g
Potassium chloride (KCl)	...	1.5 g
Tri Sodium citrate, dihydrate	...	2.9 g
Glucose, anhydrous	...	13.5 g
Water	...	1 Lt.

- This fluid compensates electrolyte loss in diarrhoea and helps to control diarrhoea. Intravenous fluids are needed in severe cases of dehydration.

2. Routine antibiotic therapy has no place in the management of uncomplicated cases. Blind drug therapy is not useful due to multiple drug resistance in bacteria causing diarrhoea. Antibiotics are indicated in complicated cases with systemic symptoms such as fever, toxicity or shock.

BACTERIAL FOOD POISONING

Important pathogens are listed in Table 12.5.

1. **Isolation of bacteria** : Faeces, and remnant food stuff may be inoculated in blood agar and Robertson's cooked meat medium (RCM).

Table 12.5 : Bacterial food poisoning : Clinical and epidemiological features

Organism	Incubation period (hrs)	Clinical features	Type of food	Incidence (%)
Infection				
B. cereus	6-12	Watery diarrhoea	Meat, poultry, vegetables	1-2
C. perfringens	9-15	Watery diarrhoea	Meat, poultry	5-15
Salmonella	6-48	Dysentery	Poultry, eggs, meat, vegetables	10-13
Shigella	12-48	Dysentery	Variable	
Intoxication				
B. cereus	1-6	Vomiting	Re-warmed fried rice	1-2
C. botulinum	12-72	Neuromuscular paralysis	Canned food of all types	
S. aureus	2-4	Vomiting, diarrhoea	Meats, custards, salads	15-25
V. parahaemolyticus	10-24	Watery diarrhoea	Shell fish	1-2

2. **Detection of toxin** in specimen of suspected food and in patient's serum may be made by toxin-antitoxin neutralisation in mice.

NON-BACTERIAL INFECTIVE DIARRHOEA

Causative agents are shown in Table 12.6 :

Table 12.6 : Causes of non-bacterial infective diarrhoeal diseases

Causative agent	Usual source	Transmission
Viruses		
Rotavirus, *Astrovirus*, *Calcivirus*, *Adenovirus*	Faeces	Faecal-oral
Protozoa		
Entamoeba histolytica	Faeces	Faecal-oral
Giardia lamblia	Faeces	Faecal-oral
Cryptosporidium	Faeces of domestic animals	Faecal-oral
Balantidium coli	Faeces	Faecal-oral

Specimen : Faeces.

1. **Microscopy** : Saline and iodine preparation of faeces are examined microscopically which will reveal cysts and trophozoites of *E. histolytica*, cysts of *Giardia lamblia* and oocysts of *Cryptosporidium*.

2. **Immunoassays** and gene probes help to detect viruses.

3. **Serological tests** : ELISA of serum is useful.

CHOLERA

Vibrio species associated with human infections are shown in Table 12.7 :

Table 12.7 : Vibrio species associated with human infections (in order of relative frequency)

Clinical disease	Species	Sources of infection
Gastroenteritis	1. *V. cholerae* serotype 01	Water, food
	2. *V. cholerae* non-01 (Non-01 to non-0139)	—do—
	3. *V. parahaemolyticus*	Shell fish, sea water
	4. *V. fluvialis*	Sea food
	5. *V. mimicus*	Water
	6. *V. furnissii*	Unknown
	7. *V. hollisae*	Shell fish
Wound infection	8. *V. alginolyticus*	Sea-water
	9. *V. vulnificus*	Shell fish, Sea-water
	10. *V. damsela*	Sea-water
	11. *V. harveyi* (carchariae)	Sea-water
Sepsis	*V. cholerae* non-01	
	V. vulnificus	
	12. *V. cincinnatiensis*	Unknown
Ear infection	*V. alginolyticus*	
	V. cholerae non-01	
	V. mimicus	
	V. parahaemolyticus	

Table 12.7 contd. next column

Specimens :

1. Watery stool and mucous flakes from stool.

2. Rectal swabs from contact and carriers.

Faecal samples are the best source of culture material.

Transport media : If there are chances of delay, 2–3 gms of faeces are emulsified in 10 to 15 ml V R fluid medium or in bile peptone transport medium or in Cary-Blair medium.

Microscopy

Rapid diagnosis by direct **fluorescent-antibody staining** of smears from liquid stool has been used for identifying *V. cholerae* 01.

Culture

1. Stool sample is directly plated to one or more selective media like BSA, TCBS, or Monsur's GTTA medium.

2. The specimens received on holding transport medium are first inoculated into enrichment media such as alkaline peptone water and incubated for 6-8 hours before plating on a selective medium.

Plating media : Thiosulphate-citrate-bile salt-sucrose agar (TCBS) (Fig. 12.3) and bile salt agar (BSA) are more frequently used plating media. The inoculated plates are generally examined after overnight incubation at 37°C. On TCBS medium, *V. cholerae* strains appear as yellow sucrose fermenting colonies. The colonies are moist, translucent, round, about 1-2 mm in diameter, with a bluish tinge in transmitted light.

Identification

1. Vibrios are oxidase-positive and ferment

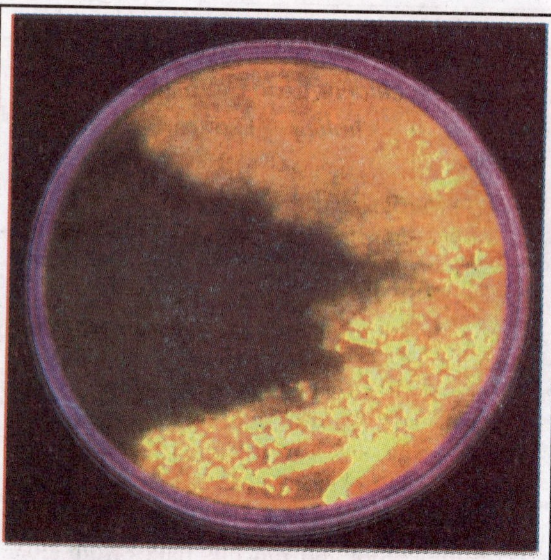

Fig. 12.3 : Colonies of *V. cholerae* on TCBS agar appear yellowish which is virtually diagnostic of *V. cholerae*. Yellowish colour of colonies result from citrate utilisation and production of acid from sucrose.

glucose which distinguish them from the family *Enterobacteriaceae*. Vibrios should be differentiated from other related genera — *Aeromonas* and *Plesiomonas*.

2. Direct detection of *V. cholerae* by FAT or coagglutination test if facilities are existing.

3. Culture and agglutination and biochemical tests.

Biochemical tests

The El tor biotype is usually haemolytic, V.P. positive, haemagglutinate chick red cells and resistant to polymyxin B and group IV cholera phage (Table 12.8) :

Table 12.8 : Distinguishing features of classical and El Tor cholera vibrios

Feature	Classical	El Tor
1. Haemolysis of sheep RBC	–	+*
2. Haemagglutination of chick RBC	–	+
3. V P reaction	Usually weak or –	Usually strongly +*
4. Susceptibility to polymyxin B‡	+	–
5. Sensitivity to phage V (Mukherjee and Basu)	–	+
6. Sensitivity to Mukherjee phage IV	+	–

Table 12.8 contd....

Table 12.8 (continued from previous column)

* Strains isolated after 1961 give variable results
‡ 50 i.u. per disc

Agglutination test

Colonies from selective media are picked up with a straight wire and tested wth *V. cholerae 01* antiserum. If positive, the test is repeated using monospecific *Ogawa* and *Inaba* sera for serotyping. Hikojima strains react equally well with Ogawa and Inaba sera. When the agglutination test becomes negative with one colony, the test is to be repeated with at least 5 colonies as *V. cholerae-01* and non-01 *V. cholerae* may coexist in the same specimen.

When the isolated strain of organisms are not agglutinated by *V. cholerae-01* antiserum, it should be tested with other O antiserum to establish their identity as belonging to one of 02-0139 serogroups.

Any *V. cholerae* or suspected to be *V. cholerae* should be sent to State Reference Laboratory (Cholerae Research Centre, Beliaghata, Kolkata) for confirmation and phage typing.

Serological tests : It is of little use in diagnosis of cholera but of great help in assessing the incidence of endemic foci. O suspension of cholera vibrios are used for agglutination, indirect haemagglutination, vibriocidal tests and antitoxin assay of serum.

Detection of carriers :(i) Repeated stool culture is necessary as the vibrio is excreted intermittently.

(ii) It gives better result if stool is collected after administration of a purgative (magnesium sulphate 15-30 g or mannitol 30 g). Bile may be examined after duodenal intubation.

(iii) Serological test is useful in detecting *chronic carriers*.

QUESTIONS RELATED TO CHOLERA

Q.1. ***What transport media are used in diarrhoea?***

Ans. Transport media include :

(a) **Venkatraman-Ramakrishnan medium (V-R**

medium) — It preserves vibrio for several weeks and prevents over-growth of other organisms.

(b) **Cary-Blair medium**— It is used for *Salmonella, Shigella* and *Vibrio.*

(c) **Autoclaved seawater.**

Q.2. ***Name the enrichment media and their advantages.***

Ans. Enrichment media include :

(a) **Alkaline peptone water** : High pH suppressed growth of commensal bacteria and allows growth of vibrios. Can also be used as a transport medium.

(b) **Taurocholate tellurite peptone water** : Incubation of 6-8 hours in enrichment media is sufficient.

Q.3. ***Name the antigens of V. cholerae.***

Ans. Antigen of *V. cholerae* :

(1) **Somatic O Ag.** On the basis of O Ag, there are 139 serogroups.

(2) **Flagellar H Ag.**

Q.4. ***What is String test?***

Ans. See text.

Q.5. ***How to distinguish biotype of V. cholerae?***

Ans. See text.

URINARY TRACT INFECTIONS

Important causative agents of urinary tract infection are listed in Table 12.9 :

Table 12.9 : Important causative agents of UTI

Organism	Domiciliary	Hospital
1. *Escherichia coli*	80	50
2. *Klebsiella* spp.	8	12-20
3. *Proteus mirabilis* and other *Proteus* spp.	8-13	12-15
4. *Staph. saprophyticus*	0-1	1-2
5. *Staph. epidermidis*	0-1	1-2
6. *Enterococci*	0-1	1-2
7. *Enterobacter* }		
8. *Citrobacter* spp. }	< 1	< 1
9. *Acinetobacter* spp.		
10. *P. aeruginosa*	0-1	8-12
11. *S. aureus*	0	< 1

Laboratory diagnosis

Pretherapy culture of urine is necessary for identification of the organism, antimicrobial susceptibility test and assessment of the results of treatment.

Specimen collection

Specimen of urine should be adequate and free from urethral or genital tract contamination :

1. *Mid-stream clean-catch technique (MSU)* : Before collecting a sample, the urethral meatus and adjoining areas should be cleaned with soap and water and then dried with a sterile sponge. The patient begins to pass urine and then mid-portion of the stream is collected in sterile wide-mouthed container or test tube.

2. *Catheter specimen* (CSU) : In catheterised patients, urine should be collected directly from the catheter and not from the collection bag. The catheter should not be allowed to touch the container.

3. *Urine specimens from infants* : A clean catch specimen after careful cleansing of genitalia is preferred.

Although a catheter specimen of urine yields excellent result, but catheterisation to obtain urine is not justified because of the risk of introducing infection.

Transport

It is important that specimens after collection should reach the laboratory with the minimum of delay, preferably within 2-3 hours after collection or refrigerated at 4°C.

Dip-slide method : Using dip-slide coated on both sides with culture medium and inoculated by dipping into the freshly passed urine and replacing in a sterile container for transport, which can be read several days after delay.

Specimen is collected in two sterile containers : one for culture and other for routine examination including microscopy.

A. Microscopy

Pyuria is associated with most clinical infections but may be absent in symptomless bacteriuria. Pus cells along with RBCs are usually found in urinary deposit in haemorrhagic cystitis. Pyuria without bacteriuria may be an indication of renal tuberculosis.

B. Culture

1. **Media :** (i) Blood agar. (ii) MacConkey's agar.

2. **Semi-quantitative culture :** Most laboratories use a semiquantitative technique of inoculation by *standard calibrated loop. Dip-slide* techniques is useful examining large numbers of urine specimens.

3. **Incubation :** After 18-24 hours incubation of inoculated plate at 37°C, discrete colonies develop, each corresponding to the growth of a single bacterium.

Semiquantitative methods

Calibrated loop method : A loop delivering 0.001 ml. of urine is used to inoculate blood agar. After incubation of the plate for 18 to 24 hours, plates are examined and colonies are counted. The total number of bacteria per ml of urine is thus obtained as follows :

> Total amount of bacteria per ml of urine = No of colonies × 1,000.
>
> This method is more suitable to study large number of urine samples.

Dip slides

Commercially available plastic slides coated with CLED (Cysteine lactose electrolyte deficient) agar on one side and MacConkey's agar on the other side is dipped into the freshly voided urine and replaced in a sterile container and incubated. Viable count is obtained by comparing growth on the media with the manufacturer's chart. Although dip slide technique is relatively expensive, it avoids problem of transporting specimens to laboratory particularly from general practitioner's side, and are useful in screening for significant bacteriuria in busy outpatient department, such as an antenatal clinic.

Interpretation of results

(i) More than 100,000 (10^5) viable bacteria of a single species per ml : *significant growth*, sensitivity test is to be done.

(ii) Between 10,000 to 100,000 bacteria per ml : of *doubtful significance*, further specimens requires to be cultured.

(iii) Less than 10,000 bacteria per ml : no *significant growth*, regarded as contaminants.

4. **Identification of the organisms :** The organisms are identified by biochemical and/or serological tests.

QUESTIONS RELATED TO URINARY TRACT INFECTIONS

Q.1. ***Name the different types of urinary tract infection.***

Ans. (1) **Upper urinary tract infection** : (a) Acute pyelitis — Infection of pelvis of kidney. (b) Acute pyelonephritis — Infection of parenchyma of kidney.

(2) **Lower urinary tract infection**, in which infection is from bladder downwards : (a) Urethritis — Infection of urethra. (b) Cystitis — Infection of urinary bladder. (c) Prostatitis — Infection of prostate.

Q.2. ***How do you interpret colony count?***

Ans. See text.

Q.3. ***What do you mean by significant bacteriuria?***

Ans. See text.

Q.4. ***What is asymptomatic bacteriuria?***

Ans. In asymptomatic infection or overt bacteriuria, there is active disease process in kidney. Hence, if left untreated, it can develop cystitis and might go to renal failure.

Q.5. ***Name the common aetiological agents.***

Ans. See text.

MENINGITIS

Aetiology

Most bacteria causing pyogenic meningitis are encapsulated and possess specific affinity for receptors in the choroid plexus or meninges :

1. **Common pathogens** : More than 80% infections of pyogenic meningitis beyond neonatal period are caused by : (i) *Streptococcus pneumoniae*, (ii) *Neisseria meningitidis*, and (iii) *Haemophilus influenzae*.

2. **Infrequent pathogens** in remaining 20% cases of pyogenic meningitis include : (i) *Listeria monocytogenes*, (ii) Gram-negative enteric rods (e.g. *Klebsiella*), (iii) *Staphylococcus aureus*, (iv) *Streptococcus pyogenes*, (v) *Staphylococcus epidermidis*.

Laboratory diagnosis

Specimen : CSF is obtained by lumbar puncture. The fluid should be examined immediately after collection or placed in the incubator for examination within an hour. The fluid is collected in 3 separate sterile vials — 1 for cell count, 1 for chemical examination, and one for culture.

1. **Microscopy**

Gram film of centrifuged deposit shows plenty of pus cells and few Gram-positive or Gram-negative organisms as the case may be (Table 12.10).

Table 12.10 : Cerebrospinal fluid in meningitis

Features	Normal CSF	Pyogenic meningitis	Tuberculous meningitis (Enterovirus, mumps virus)	Viral meningitis
Pressure	Normal	Highly increased	Moderately increased	Slightly increased
Chemical				
Total protein	30-45 mg%	Highly increased (100-600 mg%)	Slightly increased (80-120 mg%)	Slightly increased (60-80 mg%)
Sugar	40-80 mg%	Diminished (10-20 mg%) or absent	Diminished (30-50 mg%)	Normal
Cell count				
Total cell per cu. mm.	1-3	500-10,000	50-500	4-10
Type of cell	Lymphocytes	Neutrophils-95% Lymphocytes-5%	Lymphocytes 90% Neutrophils 10%	Lymphocytes
Bacteriological (Smear made from centrifuged deposit)				
Gram film	Nil	Gram-negative or positive cocci or bacilli found	–	–
Acid fast film	Nil	Nil	Acid-fast bacilli may found	–

2. **Chemical analysis**

It shows diminished *glucose levels* and increased *protein* (Table 12.10).

3. **Culture**

(i) *CSF* : Centrifuged deposit is inoculated onto blood agar, chocolate agar and cooked meat broth. The plates are incubated up to 24 hours in an atmosphere of 5-10% CO_2.

The isolated organisms are identified by biochemical and/or serological tests.

(ii) *Blood* : Blood culture is particularly useful in meningitis and may be positive in about 50% of cases of meningitis due to *N. meningitidis*, *H. influenzae* and *S. pneumoniae.*

4. **Demonstration of bacterial products**

(i) *Bacterial antigen* can be detected by latex agglutination, counter-current immunoelectrophoresis (CIEP)and ELISA using specific antisera to the common serogroups of *N. meningitidis* serogroup A, serogroup C, *H. influenzae* and *S. pneumoniae.*

(ii) *Bacterial endotoxin* : The limulus lysate test for detection of bacterial endotoxin is both specific and extremely sensitive.

QUESTIONS RELATED TO MENINGITIS

Q.1. *What are the non-bacterial agents that may also cause meningitis?*

Ans. Non-bacterial agents causing meningitis :

(a) **Viral Agents**:

(i) *Enteroviruses* : ECHO viruses, Coxsackie viruses, Polio viruses.

(ii) *Paramyxoviruses* : Mumps virus, Measles virus.

(iii) *Herpes viruses* : Herpes simplex virus, Varicella zoster virus.

(iv) *Adenoviruses.*

(v) *Arboviruses* : *Flavivirus*, e.g. Japanese B encephalitis virus; *Bunyavirus*, e.g. California encephalitis group viruses; *Arenavirus*, e.g. lymphocytic choriomeningitis virus.

(b) ***Fungal Agents***: (i) *Cryptococcus neoformans*, (ii) *Candida albicans*, (iii) *Aspergillus sp.*, (iv) *Mucor sp.*, (v) *Histoplasma capsulatum*, (vi) *Coccidioides immitis*, (vii) *Blastomyces dermatitidis.*

(c) ***Parasitic Agents***: (i) *Entamoeba histolytica* (ii) *Naegleria sp.*, (iii) *Acanthamoeba sp.*, (iv) *Toxoplasma gondii.*

Q.2. ***Name the aetiologic agents of pyogenic meningitis in children.***

Ans. Bacteria causing pyogenic meningitis in children are shown in Table 12.11 :

Table 12.11 : Aetiologic agents of pyogenic meningitis in children of different ages

Neonatal (< 1 month)	Infant & children (1 month – 12 yrs.)	Adolescents (12-18 years)
*Escherichia coli**	*S. pneumoniae*	*S. pneumoniae*
Streptococcus Group B	*N. meningitidis*	*N. meningitidis*
Klebsiella species	*Haemophilus influenzae* type B	
Listeria monocytogenes		
Streptococcus Group D		

* Strains with K1 capsular antigen are most common

Q.3. ***How do you diagnosis neonatal meningitis?***

Ans. In neonatal meningitis, the characteristic features of meningitis are not seen. Features indicative of neonatal meningitis are :

(a) Baby is unwell.

(b) Failure to feed.

(c) Frequent vomiting.

TUBERCULOSIS

Classification

(i) **Strict pathogens**

(a) ***M. tuberculosis complex***

M. tuberculosis — human type

M. bovis — bovine type

M. africanum — human type

M. microti — murine type

(b) ***Lepra bacilli***

M. leprae — causing leprosy in man

M. leprae murium — causing rat leprosy

(c) ***Other animal pathogens***

M. microti — murine type

M. paratuberculosis — Johne's bacillus.

(ii) **Atypical mycobacteria**

Group I — *Photochromogens*

Group II — *Scotochromogens*

Group III — *Non-chromogens*

Group IV — *Rapid growers*

(iii) **Saprophytic mycobacteria (non-pathogenic)**

(a) *M. smegmatis* — Present in smegma, thermophiles (grow at 52°C).

(b) *M. phlei* — Present in grass

(c) *M. stercoris* — Present in dung

(d) *M. thermoresistible.*

M. tuberculosis complex and *M. leprae* are found in diseased tissue of humans and other warm-blooded animals. Most other species (saprophytes and atypical bacilli) are free-living in soil and water.

Laboratory diagnosis

The diagnosis may be strongly suspected clinically when typical cavitary or calcified lesions are detected radiographically, but confirmation requires isolation of bacilli from the lesions. Important diagnostic tests are shown in **Box 12.1** :

Box 12.1 : Laboratory diagnosis of mycobacterial diseases

I. Detection

Microscopy

- Carbol fuchsin acid-fast stain, or Fluorescent auramine rhodamine stain

Direct nucleic acid probes

Culture

- Solid egg-based (LJ) medium, or solid agar-based (Middlebrook) medium
- Broth-based (Middlebrook broth) or Dubos medium.

II. Identification

Morphological properties

Biochemical reaction

Analysis of cell wall lipids

Nucleic acid probes

Nucleic acid sequencing

III. Skin test

Mantoux test

Specimen : Specimen is collected from the suspected site of lesion.

1. Pulmonary tuberculosis : Sputum— early morning respiratory specimens of 3 consecutive days.
2. Meningitis : CSF.
3. Bone and joints : Aspirated fluid.
4. Renal : Three consecutive morning samples of urine.

Microscopy : Finding acid-fast slender red rods in sputum or any other adequate sample identifies *Mycobacterium* as the cause of the disease.

1. *Ziehl-Neelsen staining*—Smears made from the specimen in new glass slides is stained by *Ziehl-Neelsen* method. The acid-fast bacilli appear as pink brightened rods. Care must be taken in urine sample to exclude commensal smegma bacillus which is only acid-fast but not alcohol-fast whereas tubercle bacilli are both acid and alcohol-fast. It has been observed that there should be 10,000 to 20,000 bacilli per ml of sputum for positive microscopic finding.

2. *Fluorescent staining*—Where large number of smears are to be examined, smears stained by *fluorescent stains* such as auramine phenol or auramine rhodamine are examined under ultraviolet light. The bacilli appear as bright rods against dark background.

Approximately 35-50% of all culture-positive specimens have bacilli detected by acid-fast microscopy. Sensitivity of microscopy is high with respiratory specimens, particularly with cavitation.

Concentration of specimens : The bacteria are decontaminated and concentrated in a small volume without inactivation. Such concentrate is mostly used for culture and animal inoculation test and sometime for smear examination. Several methods of concentration of specimen are in use.

1. *Petroff's method*

It is a simple and widely used technique. Sputum mixed with equal volume of 4% sodium hydroxide is incubated at 37°C for about 30 minutes. The mixture is frequently shaken till it gets liquefied and becomes clear. Sodium hydroxide also kills the contaminating bacteria. After centrifugation at 3,000 rpm for 30 minutes, it is neutralised with 8% hydrochloric acid in presence of a drop of phenol red indicator. The deposit is used for smear, culture and animal inoculation.

2. *Homogenisation method*

The specimen is treated with equal volume of dilute acids such as 6% sulphuric acid, 3% hydrochloric acid or 5% oxalic acid, and then clearing the acid by repeated washing with sterile normal saline. The concentration of acid is reduced to half by mixing equal volume of specimen with equal volume of dilute acid.

3. *Trisodium phosphate method*

Composition :

(i) 2.94% Trisodium citrate, $3H_2O$ (0.1M) — 50 ml

(ii) 4% sodium hydroxide (1N) — 50 ml

(iii) N-acetyl-L–cysteine (NALC) — 0.5 gm

At first mix, trisod citrate with sodium hydroxide solution. NALC is added to that solution just before use. NALC is a mucolytic agent. 4-6% sodium hydroxide (toxic agent) may kill or seriously injure mycobacteria. The NaOH concentration becomes 2% after mixing equal parts with the specimen.

Principle :

NALC, a mucolytic agent without antibacterial activity, liquefies mucus by splitting disulphide bonds. The mycobacteria are released when the mucous is liquefied.

Method :

1. Add NALC digestant mixture to equal volume of specimen (e.g. sputum, urine, etc.) in 50 ml plastic centrifuge tubes. Approximately 10-15 ml sample is processed in each tube. The screw cap of the centrifuge tubes are tightened.

2. Homogenise the mixture with a vortex mixture for approximately a slow count of 15, or for a maximum of 30 seconds.

3. Let the tubes stand at room temperature for 15-20 minutes. The specimen should not be exposed to the digestant for more than 20 minutes, because "overtreated" specimens result in fewer positive cultures.

4. After the digestion-decontamination step, add enough phosphate buffer (pH 6.8) (preferred over sterile water) to reach within 1 cm of the top, screw the cap till tightly closed, and invert the tube to mix the solutions and stop the digestion process.

Phosphate buffer acts in the following ways : (a) it makes strong shifts in pH less likely, (b) serves to wash the specimen, (c) to dilute and neutralise toxic substances, (d) to reduce specific gravity of the specimen so that sedimentation of the bacilli during centrifugation is more effective.

5. Centrifuge all tubes at 3,600 × g for 15-20 minutes.

6. Carefully decant the supernatant into a splash-proof can containing a phenolic disinfectant. Carefully wipe the tip of the tube with cotton soaked with 5% phenol.

7. Resuspend the sediment with a Pasteur pipette in 1-2 ml sterile water or phosphate buffer (pH 6.8).

8. Inoculate the culture media (LJ slants and Middlebrook 7H10 or 7H11 agar plates) and prepare smear on clean microscope slides for Ziehl-Neelsen or fluorochrome staining.

Culture

Culture is a more sensitive method for detection of bacilli and, moreover, it is necessary for antimicrobial drug sensitivity testing.

Inoculation

Concentrate of sputum and urine are cultured in two bottles of Löwenstein-Jensen medium. It is ideal to inoculate into one egg-based (e.g. LJ) and one agar-based (e.g. Middlebrook) media. Specimens like CSF and tissue biopsies do not require decontamination before inoculation as they are unlikely to be contaminated. Bone and joint samples are first disrupted in a sterile grinder before inoculation.

Incubaction

The media are incubated at 36°C-37°C in the dark and light up to 12 weeks. Cultures are examined first after 4 days for rapid growing mycobacteria and then weekly till 8 weeks. The tubercle bacilli usually grow in 2 to 8 weeks. Longer incubation is necessary for strains originating from treated patients.

Identification

The colonies of *M. tuberculosis* on LJ medium are dry, rough, creamy or buff-coloured (Fig. 12.6) (Table 12.12). Smears from colonies stained by acid-fast stain show acid-fast bacilli (red bacilli) (Fig. 12.7). Growth from LJ medium is further processed for differentiation of mycobacteria (Fig. 12.4). When an acid-fast bacilli is slow-growing, non-pigmented and niacin positive, it is regarded as *M. tuberculosis*. Differentiation of strains is done by animal inoculation and biochemical tests.

Use of broth culture medium

It generally takes a long time to grow mycobacteria in LJ or Middlebrook agar media (Fig. 12.5), particularly in cases of *M. tuberculosis*, *M. bovis*,

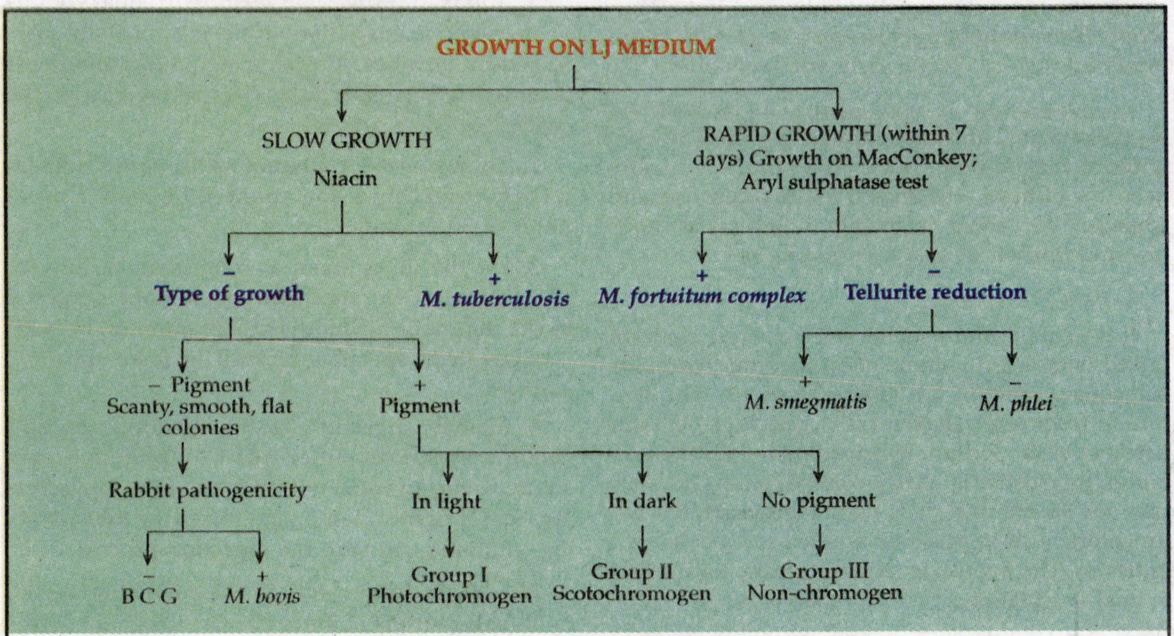

Fig. 12.4. Identification of mycobacteria

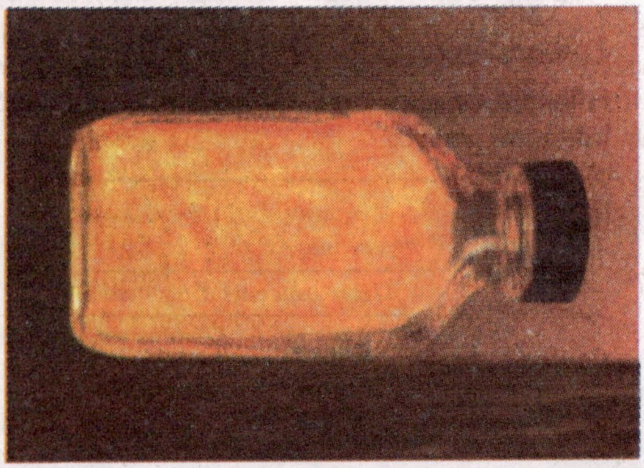

Fig. 12.5. Colonies of *M. tuberculosis* in LJ medium after 22 day's incubation at 35°C. Colonies are rough in consistency and dry; they have more of a yellow colour than the usual buff coloured colonies.

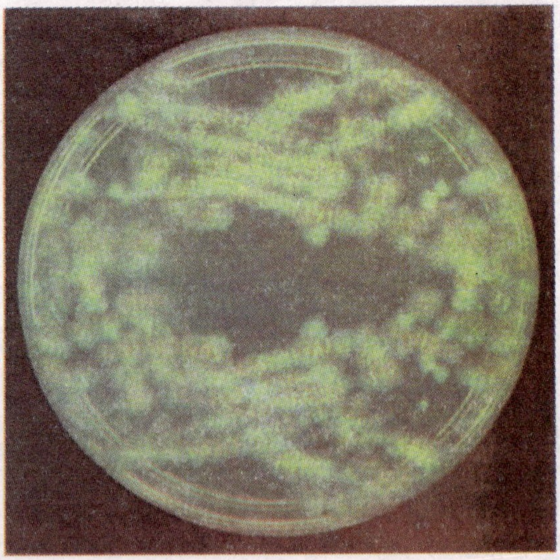

Fig. 12.6. Colonies of *M. tuberculosis* on Middlebrook 7H10 agar after 16 days incubation at 35°C. Colonies are rough and buff coloured.

M. avium-intracellulare and other slow-growing species. However, this time has been shortened through the use of specially formulated broth culture (e.g. BACTEC 12B broth culture) based on radiometric monitoring that support the rapid growth of most of the mycobacteria. Thus, there is a greater rate of recovery of *M. tuberculosis* and other *Mycobacterium* species, and the average time of growth has been decreased from 3 to 4 weeks to 10 to 14 days.

Animal inoculation

Part of the concentrated material (0.5 ml) or the same volume of bacterial suspension from the colonies on culture media is inoculated intramuscularly into the thigh of a tuberculin negative healthy guinea pig

Table 12.12 : Distinguishing points between *M. tuberculosis* and *M. bovis*

Test	*M. tuberculosis*	*M. bovis*
1. Morphology	Slender, long and usually curved	Stout, short and straight
2. Staining	Barred or beaded	Uniform
3. Growth	Eugonic	Dysgonic
4. Action of glycerol in media.	Growth enhanced	Growth inhibited
5. Colony	Dry, rough, raised and wrinkled; consistency tough, tenacious and difficult to emulsify; colour — creamy white or buff-coloured.	Moist smooth and flat; consistency friable; white
6. Biochemical reaction		
(i) Niacin production	+	–
(ii) Nitrate reduction	+	–
(iii) TCH selective action	–	+ (No growth)
7. Animal pathogenicity		
(i) Progressive disease in rabbit	– or mild lesion	+ (Generalised lesion)
(ii) In guinea pig	+ (Progressive and, ultimately, fatal, disease)	+ (Similar action)

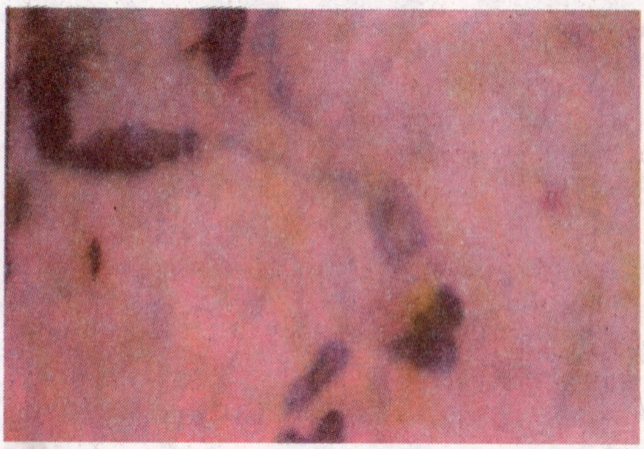

Fig. 12.7. Acid-fast stain of *M. tuberculosis* from colonies in LJ medium. Note relatively thin red acid-fast bacilli.

of 12 weeks old. Inoculation by subcutaneous route is avoided as it causes a local ulcer which may be infectious.

The animal is weighed prior to inoculation and thereafter at weekly intervals. It is tuberculin-tested after 3-4 weeks and autopsied after 6 weeks. The tuberculin-test becomes positive in infected animal and there is progressive loss of weight.

Autopsy shows :

1. *Caseous lesion* at the site of inoculation.
2. Enlarged *caseous inguinal lymph node*. The infection may spread to lumbar, portal mediastinal and cervical lymph nodes depending on the severity of the disease.
3. *Tubercles* may be seen in lungs.
4. *Spleen—enlarged* with irregular necrotic foci.
5. *Peritoneum* may show few tubercles.
6. *Kidneys* unaffected.

Generally, *M. tuberculosis* is highly infectious for guinea pigs and hamsters and virtually non-pathogenic for rabbits, while *M. bovis* is highly pathogenic for both rabbits and guinea pigs. *"Asian type"* of tubercle bacilli and catalase negative and INH-resistant strains of *M. bovis* are less virulent and do not produce progressive disease in guinea pigs.

Sensitivity testing

The isolated tubercle bacilli is tested for drug sensitivity in LJ medium or Middlebrook agar medium after incorporating different concentrations of antitubercular drugs in the media before inoculation (Table 12.13).

More rapid susceptibility testing is achieved by using broth culture medium (BACTEC radiometric system). A *rpo* B gene has been detected in mycobacteria by genetic probe (PCR) in mutation induced rifampicin resistance.

Table 12.13 : Drug concentrations in antimicrobial susceptibility testing for mycobacteria

Drug	Drug concentration (μm/mL)	
	Middlebrook 7H10	Löwenstein-Jensen
Isoniazid	0.2, 1	0.2, 1
Streptomycin	2	4
Rifampin	1	40
Ethambutol	2	2
Ethionamide	5	20
Kanamycin	5	20
Capreomycin	10	20
Cycloserine	20	30
Pyrazinamide	50	–

QUESTIONS RELATED TO TUBERCULOSIS

Q.1. ***How do you report a positive smear with grading?***

Ans. At least 300 oil-immersion fields (OIF) of Z-N stained smears are examined and reported with grading as :

00 AFB in 300 OIF — AFB not seen

1-2 AFB in 300 OIF—doubtful–repeat smear

1-9 AFB in 100 OIF—1+

1-9 AFB in 10 OIF—2+

1-9 AFB in 1 OIF—3+

10 or more AFB in 1 OIF—4+

Q.2. ***How do you identify a positive mycobacterial culture?***

Ans. To identify the mycobacterial isolate, following observations are helpful :

(a) Slow growth at 36°C taking 2-6 weeks.

(b) No pigment production.

(c) No growth on paranitrobenzoic acid (PNB) LJ media.

(d) Niacin—positive.

(e) Weakly catalase—positive.

(f) Nitrate reduction—positive.

(g) Susceptibility to pyrazinamide.

(h) Resistant to TCH.

Q.3. *Name the prophylactic measures available for prevention of tuberculosis.*

Ans. Tuberculosis can be prevented by vaccination; the details of the vaccine administered are : (i) BCG : Bacille Calmette—Guérin. (ii) Type : Live attenuated vaccine.

Q.4. *What is Bactec system?*

Ans. Liquid medium containing drugs are used for antibiotic susceptibility testing (AST) with radiometric growth detection.

LEPROSY

Mycobacterium leprae, the causative agent of leprosy (also called Hansen's disease) was first described by Hansen in 1874 in Norway.

Laboratory diagnosis

Diagnosis of leprosy is based primarily on clinical signs and symptoms.

Specimens : Skin biopsy and scrapings from lesion and nasal mucosa.

Direct evidences

I. Direct slit-skin smear and acid-fast staining : Slit-skin smears made from skin scraping from patches and ear lobes and punctured material from nodules and nasal mucosal scrapings are stained by modified Ziehl-Neelsen method using 4 to 5% sulphuric acid as decolourising agent. Smear shows acid-fast bacilli arranged in parallel bundles within macrophage (*Lepra-cell*). The living bacilli stain uniformly while the dead bacilli look fragmented and irregular or granular in Ziehl-Neelsen stained smear.

Bacteriological index : It is defined as number of viable bacilli in a lesion which is assessed from stained smear by oil-immersion lens (× 100) of microscope.

Calculation of bacterial index : Internationally agreed bacteriological index ranges from 1 to 6+ as shown :

1-10 bacilli in 100 fields = 1+

1-10 bacilli in 10 fields = 2+

1-10 bacilli per field = 3+

10-100 bacilli per field = 4+

100-1,000 bacilli per field = 5+

More than 1,000 bacilli, clumps and groups in every field = 6+.

Morphological index : It is the percentage of uniformly stained bacilli out of the total bacteria present in tissue. It is useful in assessing the prognosis and response to treatment.

II. Skin and nerve biopsy : Skin biopsy is collected from active edge of the patches and nerve biopsy from the thickened nerve for histological confirmation of tuberculoid leprosy when acid-fast bacilli cannot be demonstrated in direct smear.

Microscopically : (a) Tuberculoid leprosy shows infiltration of lymphocytes around the centre of epithelial cells; presence of Langhan's giant cells; few or no acid-fast bacilli. (b) Lepromatous leprosy shows predominantly foamy macrophages (lepra cell) with few lymphocytes and no giant cell.

Indirect evidences

(i) **Lepromin test** : The test is helpful in assessment of prognosis of the disease.

(ii) **Serological test** : Serodiagnosis of leprosy involves detection of antiphenolic glycolipid 1 (anti PGL-1) antibodies. Various serological tests like latex agglutination, *Mycobacterium leprae* Particle Agglutination (MLPA) test (Grade *et. al*, 1993) and ELISA have been described.

QUESTIONS RELATED TO LEPROSY

Q.1. *How do you cultivate M. leprae?*

Ans. (1) Lepra bacilli does not grow in artificial culture media.

(2) Animals are used for isolation and culture.

(3) Generation time is 13-15 days.

(4) Animals used include :

(a) **Mice** — (i) Footpads of mice are used for inoculation. (ii) After intradermal inoculation of specimen granuloma develops at the site of inoculation in 1-6 months.

(b) **Nine-banded armadillo** : (i) Following inoculation of infected material, extensive multiplication of bacilli occurs, hence yield is more than that of human leproma and is sufficient for research purposes. (ii) Lifespan is long (12-15 years), hence it is suitable to study pathogenesis of leprosy.

Q.2. *How M. leprae can survive in environment for long?*

Ans. (1) *M. leprae* can survive in humid climate

for 9-15 days. (ii) They survive exposure to sunlight for 2 hours.

Question 3 and other relevant questions include :

(i) ***What is bacteriological index?***

(ii) ***Name the clinical types of leprosy and difference between tuberculoid and lepromatous leprosy.***

(iii) ***Lepromin test.***

(iv) ***Lepra reaction.***

Ans. See Text book.

BRUCELLOSIS

Classification

A. Major Species :

(1) *B. melitensis* — typically infects goats and sheep, commonly found in Malta and other Mediterranean countries. It is the causative agent on Malta fever.

(2) *B. abortus* — typically infects cattle. It is the most important cause of human brucellosis (undulant fever) in U. K.

(3) *B. suis* — usually infects pigs and is the most important cause of human brucellosis in swine-rearing areas of USA, Latin America and Denmark.

B. Additional species :

(1) *B. canis* — infects dogs in USA and humans are occasionally infected.

(2) *B. ovis* — is responsible for testicular infection of rams in Australia.

(3) *B. neotomae* — infects desert rodents in USA.

Laboratory diagnosis

Specimen : Blood culture in acute stage of the disease is the most definite method of diagnosis. Urine, sputum and breast milk may yield positive culture as the organisms are intermittently excreted in these specimens. Biopsied lymph node or **bone marrow** aspirate culture is done in chronic cases. Serology is useful in diagnosing acute infection. Multiple samples of blood should be collected for culture and serological testing.

Culture and isolation

(1) **Blood cultures** : Because of the systemic nature of infection, blood cultures are first tried.

(2) When the disease has reached an advance stage, **bone marrow aspirate** or **liver biopsy** may be necessary to obtain adequate samples of culture.

Since the organisms may be scanty, at least 10 cc blood (or biopsied material) is cultured in a bottle of liver infusion or glucose serum broth of Trypticase Soy Broth and incubated at 37°C under 5-10% CO_2. *B. abortus*, but not other species, must be incubated under 5-10% CO_2 environment. Sub-cultures are made on liver infusion agar or Trypticase Soy agar every 3-5 days. As growth may often be delayed, culture is retained for six weeks. Brucellae grow faster when the blood culture is transferred to agar medium (e.g. biphasic cultures as in **Castaneda's method**).

(1) **Castaneda's method** of blood culture provides both liquid (liver infusion broth) and solid media (3% nutrient agar slope) in one bottle. Its use reduces chances of contamination and risk of infection to laboratory personnel. Since the bottle contains both liquid and solid media, the broth flows over the surface of agar slant when the bottle is tilted. This results in automatic sub-culture. The bottle is kept in the incubator in upright position. In positive cases, colonies develop on the slant. Blood culture comes positive in 30-50% of cases. *B. melitensis* is more readily cultured than *B. abortus*.

2. **Trypticase Soy broth** : Specimen of blood is inoculated in Trypticase Soy broth and then subcultures on serum dextrose agar every 3-5 days.

3. **BACTEC** is a rapid and automated diagnostic system for culture in which results are obtained in 5-6 days.

Identification

Isolated organism is identified by :

1. requirement of CO_2 for growth.
2. production of urease and H_2S.
3. sensitivity to the dyes basic fuchsin, thionin.
4. agglutination with monospecific sera, and
5. lysis by bacteriophage.

Serology

Because of the difficulty of isolating brucellae, many cases of *Brucella* infection are diagnosed by serological tests which include : the **standard agglutination test** (SAT), and an **ELISA procedure** for detection of Brucella-specific IgM, IgG.

1. ***Standard agglutination test* (SAT)** : Diluted serum of patients is tested by slide or tube method against a brucella suspension. This test usually turns positive 7-10 days after infection. Both IgM and IgG antibodies continue to rise during acute stage of

infection. A presumptive diagnosis can be made when there is a **four-fold** rise in the titre or a single titre greater than or equal to 80. Most patients with active brucellosis show SAT titres of 160 or higher, these titres subsequently fall with adequate therapy. Antigen employed in ST is from *B. abortus*. Antibodies to *B. melitensis* or *B. suis* cross react with *B. abortus* antigen, however, there is no cross-reactivity with *B. canis*. Hence, specific *B. canis* antigen is to be used for diagnosing *B. canis* infections.

Prozone phenomenon (absence of agglutination in low dilution of serum due to high concentration of antibodies) is common and, hence, a serial dilution of serum is to be tested.

(2) ***ELISA and RIA*** : These tests are valuable and very sensitive and can distinguish IgM, IgG and IgA brucella specific antibodies and are helpful to distinguish acute and chronic brucellosis.

Brucellin test (skin test) : It is an intradermal test done by extract of brucella for detection of delayed hypersensitivity. Positive reaction shows an area of erythema and induration of 6 mm diameter within 24 hours.

Detection of animal infection

Milk ring test : It detects brucella agglutinins in the milk of infected dairy cattle and is sufficiently sensitive for testing the bulked milk supply from a herd.

***Technique* (Fig. 12.8)**

1. One ml. column of well-mixed milk is taken in a 3 × 3/8 inch test tube.

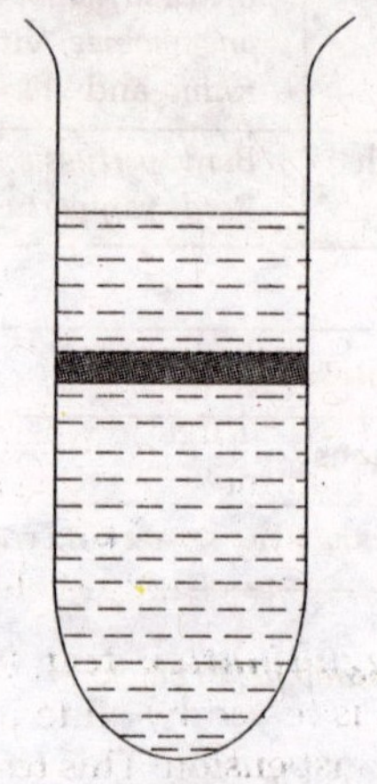

Fig. 12.8 : Milk ring test

2. A drop of concentrated suspension of *B. abortus* or *B. melitensis* stained with haematoxylin is added to the column of milk and mixed thoroughly by shaking.

3. The test-tube with milk and bacterial suspension is incubated in a water-bath at 37°C for 40-50 minutes, i.e. sufficient time for the cream to rise.

Result : In a positive test, the bacteria are agglutinated and rise with the cream to form a blue line above the white skimmed-milk. When brucella agglutinins are absent, the cream line is white and lies above a blue milk column.

QUESTIONS RELATED TO BRUCELLOSIS

Q.1. *Name the results of biochemical tests of Brucella.*

Ans. (1) They utilise carbohydrates oxidatively.

(2) Catalase — Positive.

(3) Urease — Positive.

(4) Oxidase — Positive.

(5) Reduce nitrates.

(6)

Indole	Methyl red	Voges-Proskauer	Citrate
–	–	–	–

(– = negative)

Q.2. *Name the antigen-structure of Brucella.*

Ans. Somatic Ag of Brucella, has 2 antigenic determinants — A and M.

(a) *B. abortus* has 20 times A as M.

(b) *B. melitensis* has 20 times M as A.

(c) *B. suis* shows intermediate pattern.

This feature is important in species identification by agglutination.

Q.3. *What is Brucellin test?*

Ans. (a) It is a skin test in which Ag is injected on the flexor aspect of forearm and observed for reaction after 24 hours. Positive reaction shows raised erythematous plaque 2-6 cm in diameter.

(b) It is used to detect delayed hypersensitivity to *Brucella* antigen.

(c) It is of no use in diagnosis of infection.

(d) It indicates past exposure to *Brucella* infection.

Q.4. *What is milk ring test?*

Ans. See Fig. 12.8 and Chapter 17.

STREPTOCOCCAL SORE THROAT

Streptococcus pyogenes causes streptococcal sore throat. Other organisms causing sore throat are listed in Table 12.14 :

Table 12.14 : Pathogens causing infection of throat and pharynx

Syndrome	Organisms
Sore throat	*Viruses* — more than 2/3rd cases; in remaining 1/3rd of cases. *S. pyogenes, S. aureus, H. influenzae.* Rare pathogens – *Mycoplasma pneumoniae*
Diphtheria	*Corynebacterium diphtheriae*
Candidiasis	*Candida albicans*
Vincent's angina	*Borrelia vincentii* and *Fusobacterium* species
Infectious mononucleosis	*Epstein-Barr virus*

Laboratory diagnosis

Specimen : Throat swab from fauces.

Culture : Blood agar incubated aerobically and anaerobically.

Identification :

(i) Colonies — small, dry, beta-haemolytic.

(ii) Lancefield grouping.

Latent period : 2-3 but up to 6 weeks after throat infection.

Rheumatogenic serotypes : Any serotype, M types 5, 18, 24 more frequently incriminated.

Serology : ASO titre 200 (significant) or more.

RF prone to repeated attacks, hence prophylaxis with penicillin is necessary on a long-term basis and is mandatory to eliminate streptococci.

Laboratory diagnosis of other causes of sore throat — e.g. Diphtheria, Vincent's infections — has been discussed in relevant chapters.

INFECTIONS OF MIDDLE EAR AND SINUSES

Important causative agents of sinusitis and otitis media are listed in Table 12.15.

Laboratory diagnosis

Specimen : Swabs or pus, antral washings (collected carefully for anaerobic culture by disposable sterile syringe, needle of which bent at right angle immediately after collection).

A. *Microscopy* : Gram-stained film is not helpful.

B. *Culture* : Blood agar, nutrient agar, RCM. Incubation – aerobically and anaerobically.

C. *Other tests* : Coagulase test – *S. aureus*, Oxidase test – *Ps. aeruginosa*, urease test – *Proteus* spp. Biochemical tests help to distinguish different species.

INFECTIONS OF THE LUNGS

Causative agents of laryngitis and tracheitis are shown in Table 12.16 :

Table 12.16 : Causative agents of laryngitis and tracheitis

Syndrome	Infective agent
Acute epiglottitis (Acute *laryngotracheobronchitis*, croup)	*H. influenzae*, type b, *Parainfluenza* virus 1, 2, 3
Bronchitis	*H. influenzae, Str. pneumoniae, Br. catarrhalis, Mycoplasma pneumoniae;* viruses – *influenzae, Rhino* and *Adenoviruses*
Whooping cough	*Bord. pertussis, Bord. parapertussis*

Table 12.15 : Bacterial pathogens of sinusitis and otitis media

Syndrome	Pathogens
Acute otitis media and sinusitis	*H. influenzae, S. aureus, S. pyogenes, S. pneumoniae,* Anaerobic cocci, Rhinovirus
Chronic suppurative otitis media and sinusitis	**Aerobes** *S. aureus, P. aeruginosa, Proteus* spp. *(Pr. mirabilis, P. vulgaris)* **Anaerobes** *Bacteroides (B. fragilis, B. melaninogenicus), Fusobacterium,* Anaerobic cocci *(Peptococcus, Peptostreptococcus)*

Laboratory diagnosis

Specimen : **Sputum** : Early morning sample which is most purulent. A properly taken specimen with minimal salivary contamination is to be sent to the laboratory as early as possible. Specimen of blood for culture may be useful in diagnosis of lobar pneumonia.

Microscopy

1. *Gram-film* : Adequate number of pus cells and presence of predominant organisms gives a clue to the probable pathogen.

2. *Ziehl-Neelsen or Auramine film* : Presence of acid and alcohol—fast bacilli offers a presumptive diagnosis of tuberculosis.

3. *Silver methenamine stain* of bronchial lavage and washings for *P. carinii*.

Culture

Purulent portion of sputum is best for culture. If the sputum is too viscid, it may be homogenised by treatment with a liquefying agent that also allows semiquantitative culture :

1. *Blood agar* : It is incubated aerobically at 37°C to look for predominant isolate after assessment of the normal bacterial flora.

2. *Chocolate agar* : It is a selective medium for *H. influenzae*. The inoculated media is incubated at 37°C in air with 5-10% CO_2.

3. *Blood agar* : Inoculated medium is incubated at 37°C anaerobically with 5-10% CO_2.

Culture for mycobacteria : It is done only where indicated. The material is inoculated on egg containing media in screw-capped containers to preserve moisture over the long incubation period of 6-8 weeks. Three samples of sputum to be collected on successive days for culture on Löwenstein-Jensen medium which are then incubated for 6-8 weeks.

Detection of bacterial antigens

A rapid diagnosis of *Pneumocystis carinii* and *Legionella pneumophila* can be made by fluorescent antibody staining of bronchial lavage and respiratory secretions, respectively.

Serological tests

Since the isolation of some causal organisms are difficult to make, all suspected cases should be serologically investigated by demonstration of antibody in the patient's serum (Table 12.17). Most often, such cases are diagnosed by stationary high titres, although demonstration of a four fold rising titre of antibody is better.

Table 12.17 : Results of serological tests in some atypical bacterial pneumoniae

Causative bacteria	Type of antigen-antibody tests	Diagnostic (stationary titre)
Mycoplasma pneumoniae	Complement fixation	256
Coxiella burnetii	Complement fixation	256
Legionella pneumophila	Indirect immuno-fluorescence	256
Chlamydia pneumoniae	Complement fixation and ELISA	256
Chlamydia psittaci	Complement fixation and ELISA	256

KERATITIS

Causes : Mostly herpes virus and foreign body with secondary infection due to bacteria or fungi.

Laboratory diagnosis

1. *Bacterial infections except chlamydiae* : Specimen consists of exudate, collected by a sterile platinum loop directly from the patient's eye.

Diagnosis : Microscopy of Gram-stained smear and culture in blood and chocolate agars are useful to detect the organism.

2. *Chlamydial infections* : Specimen includes scrapings from conjunctiva.

Diagnosis : Microscopy of Giemsa staining or immunofluorescent staining of smear shows cytoplasmic inclusions. Chlamydia grows in tissue culture (McCoy cells).

3. *Mycotic infections* : Specimen consists of scrapings from the base of edge of corneal ulcer.

Microscopy : In 10% KOH mount and methenamine silver or PAS staining, the fungi appear as branched septate hyphae.

Culture : Scraping material is inoculated on Sabouraud dextrose agar.

PYREXIA OF UNKNOWN ORIGIN (PUO)

Causes : Sometimes the cause of a febrile illness (temperature greater than 38°C) remains uncertain in spite of investigations and such a case is known as PUO (pyrexia of unknown origin). In the classic studies of PUO, only patients with persistent fever for 3 weeks or longer were included. According to some, the patient with PUO must have persistent fever for at least one week; usually longer, and often three weeks. The important causes are shown in Table 12.18.

Laboratory diagnosis

(i) **Haematology** : Rarely specific.

(ii) **Biochemistry** : Liver function tests reveal liver damage in relevant cases.

(iii) **Bacteriology** :

(a) *Blood culture* – serial culture should be done.

(b) *Anaerobic culture* of pus.

(c) *Mycobacterial culture.*

(d) *Urine culture.*

(iv) **Serology** : Useful in infectious mononucleosis (Paul-Bunnell test), enteric fever, hepatitis A, B infection, Lyme disease, CMV infections and sometimes in amoebiasis.

(v) **Skin tests** : Mantoux test and tests for histoplasmosis, coccidioidomycosis, sarcoidosis (Kveim-Siltzbach skin test).

(vi) **Other tests** :

(a) *Immunologic tests* such as LE cell phenomenon, antinuclear antibody test in SLE, etc.

(b) *Biopsy* of lymph node or other tissues.

QUESTIONS RELATED TO PYREXIA OF UNKNOWN ORIGIN (PUO)

Q.1. ***Name the serological tests commonly done in PUO.***

Ans. The serological tests which are commonly performed in PUO are :

- Widal test — for enteric fever.
- VDRL test — for syphilis.
- Weil-Felix test — for rickettsial infections.
- *Brucella* agglutination test and complement fixation test (CFT) — for brucellosis.
- Paul-Bunnell test—for infectious mononucleosis.
- ASO test—for streptococci.
- RA test— for rheumatoid arthritis.
- Neutralisation test — for viral infections.
- ELISA and Western-blot test—for AIDS.
- ELISA, RIA, indirect immunofluorescence tests, CFT, etc. — used in various infectious and noninfectious diseases.

Q.2. ***What are the causes of PUO?***

Ans. See text.

Q.3. ***How do you define PUO?***

Ans. See text.

Q.4. ***What is the pathogenesis of PUO?***

Ans. The agents that produce PUO are called pyrogens which are of two types : (i) Exogenous pyrogens, and (ii) Endogenous pyrogens.

Exogenous pyrogens are the products that are released from microorganisms, which interact with host cell and release endogenous pyrogens that stimulate the thermoregulatory centre in the hypothalamus — resulting in fever.

Endogenous pyrogens are products released from monocytes, macrophages, neutrophils, eosinophils, certain tumour cells, etc. which induce fever. They

Table 12.18 : Causes of PUO

Cause		Percentage
Infections	Bacterial, viral fungal and parasitic diseases	35
Neoplasms	Especially lymphoma (both Hodgkin's and non-Hodgkin's lymphoma), leukaemia and also other forms of cancer, e.g. hypernephroma, hepatoma, disseminated malignancy	20
Connective tissue diseases	Systemic lupus erythematosus, polyarteritis nodosa, temporal arteritis.	20
Granulomatous diseases	Sarcoidosis, Crohn's disease, granulomatous hepatitis.	15
Miscellaneous	Drug-induced fevers, cryptic haematomas, psychogenic fever (fictitious fever).	10

were initially called by different names, but recently the name Interleukin I is proposed for these molecules.

Principle of action :

Exogenous pyrogen
↓
Endogenous pyrogen
↓
Prostaglandin in hypothalamus
↓
Depression of pyrogen-sensitive neurons
↓
Hyperthermia

SEPTICAEMIA

Causative organisms

Septicaemia as complications of more localised lesions is much more common than the generalised infections.

Organisms most commonly isolated from cases of septicaemia include :

1. ***Gram-negative bacilli (60-70% cases)***
   - (i) *Salmonella* : (a) *S. typhi.* (b) *S. paratyphi A.* (c) *S. paratyphi B.* (d) *S. paratyphi C.*
   - (ii) *Brucella* spp.
   - (iii) *Haemophilus influenzae.*
   - (iv) *Escherichia coli.*
   - (v) *Klebsiella pneumoniae.*
   - (vi) *Proteus mirabilis* and *P. vulgaris.*
   - (vii) *Enterobacter* spp.
   - (viii) *Bacteroides* spp.
2. ***Gram-positive cocci (20-40% cases)***
   - (i) *Staphylococcus aureus.*
   - (ii) *Streptococcus pneumoniae.*
   - (iii) *Streptococcus pyogenes.*
   - (iv) *Streptococcus faecalis.*
3. ***Gram-positive bacilli***

Laboratory diagnosis

Blood culture is the main diagnostic procedure. Sample should be collected before initiating antimicrobial therapy.

1. **Specimen** : Three to six samples of blood, 10 ml each to be collected from antecubital vein over 24 hours. Sample of blood should be directly inoculated into a large volume (50-100 ml) of medium (glucose broth). One culture should be obtained from each vein puncture, using anaerobic as well as aerobic techniques. Addition of pyridoxal hydrochloride improves the chances of isolating nutritionally deficient variant streptococci.

Utility of larger volume of blood and media : Following are the advantages :

(i) Number of organisms in the blood may be very few, even as few as one/ml.

(ii) Dilution of bactericidal substances present in blood.

2. **Culture** :

Processing of culture : (a) After collection of blood in blood culture bottles these are incubated aerobically and blind subcultures are made after 24 hours, 48 hours, 72 hours, on 6th day and 10th day.

(b) Subcultures are made on :

(1) Blood agar.

(2) MacConkey's agar.

(3) Chocolate agar.

(4) Anaerobic supplemented blood agar for anaerobes.

(5) Sabouraud's dextrose agar for fungi.

(6) Other selective media as indicated.

One blood agar is to be incubated anaerobically, chocolate agar under 5-10% CO_2 and other media under ordinary laboratory conditions. Colonies obtained on solid media after incubation are studied further for identification by the help of biochemical reactions and antibiotic susceptibility by Kirby-Bauer's disc diffusion method.

Cultures should be incubated at 37°C and to be observed daily for early signs of growth making periodic (daily or on alternate days) blind Gram-stains and subcultures. Cultures should not be discarded as negative for at least 3 weeks. Subculture is made on blood agar aerobically and anaerobically.

Castaneda's method of culture of blood is likely to yield better result.

Identification

The isolated organism is identified by biochemical and agglutination tests.

3. **Antibiotic sensitivity test**

Laboratory monitoring of therapy is necessary for which the minimum inhibitory concentration (MIC) and minimum bactericidal concentration (MBC) of the antimicrobial agent for the isolated organism must be determined. The routine disc diffusion technique with a fixed concentration of drug is not adequate for guiding treatment of infective endocarditis. The measurement of MIC and MBC of antibiotic helps to determine adequate dose of the antibiotic to be used for ensuring the serum levels that can penetrate the valves and kill the organisms.

Culture negative endocarditis : In about 10-20% cases, blood culture yields persistently negative result, several reasons are suggested for the same :

(i) Recent antibiotic therapy.

(ii) Infection by fastidious or slow-growing organisms, e.g. *Haemophilus* spp., *Bacteroides*, *Actinobacillus* spp. or nutritionally–variant streptococci will not grow on standard medium.

(iii) Bacteraemia is intermittent.

(iv) Infection with *Coxiella burnetii* or *Chlamydia psittaci* : Blood cultures may be negative but the diagnosis is established by serological tests (CFT) for both Phase I and Phase II antigens. Titres are usually above 250 and even greater.

4. Other tests

(i) *Echocardiograms* demonstrate the vegetations and valve changes in 75-80% cases of native valve endocarditis.

(ii) *Leucocytosis* and elevated ESR are common but not invariable. Measurement of *C-reactive protein* in blood is sometimes more reliable than ESR in making assessment of progress.

QUESTIONS RELATED TO SEPTICAEMIA

Q.1. *Name the causative agents of septicaemia.*

Ans. See text.

Q.2. *What is bacteraemia?*

Ans. *Bacteraemia* may be defined as a condition of simple presence of bacteria in blood without any multiplication which is often silent and transient.

Q.3. *What is septicaemia?*

Ans. *Septicaemia (sepsis)* is a condition in which bacteria circulate and either continuously poured in the blood stream from a focus in the body or may actively multiply in the blood.

Q.4. *What is Pyaemia?*

Ans. *Pyaemia* is essentially septicaemia with metastatic infection. When bacterial endotoxin circulates in the blood, the condition is called *endotoxaemia.*

Q.5. *What is toxaemia?*

Ans. Toxaemia refers to formation of toxic products in blood. When bacterial endotoxins circulate in the blood, the condition is called endotoxaemia. Endotoxaemia can occur in absence of bacteria in the blood stream, e.g. from Gram-negative bacteria present in the gut, endotoxin passes across the gut wall.

Q.6. *Name the predisposing factors of septicaemia.*

Ans. Predisposing factors of septicaemia

Impaired Host Defenses :

(a) Deficiency of cell-mediated immunity.

(b) Deficiency of humoral immunity.

(c) Decreased complement level.

(d) Diminished phagocytic activity.

(e) Poor natural killer cell activity.

(f) Diminished inflammatory response.

(g) Malignancy. (h) Diabetes mellitus.

(i) Congenital inflammatory response.

(j) Severe neutropenia

(k) Intravenous drug abuse.

(l) Prematurity and low birth weight.

(m) Old age. (n) Splenectomised patients.

(o) Immunosuppressive therapy.

(p) Uraemia. (q) Aplastic anaemia.

(r) Hepatic failure.

(s) Nephrotic syndrome. (t) Myeloma.

Pre-existing infections :

(a) Abdominal sepsis—peritonitis, liver abscess.

(b) Pneumonia due to Gram-negative bacteria.

(c) Gram-negative infections of burns, wounds, abscesses, etc.

(d) Meningitis.

(e) Gynaecological sepsis—puerperal sepsis, pelvic abscesses, salpingitis.

(f) Food poisoning.

(g) Osteomyelitis, septic arthritis, etc.

(h) Urinary tract infections.

Instrumentation and surgery examples : After surgery on urinary tract, gastrointestinal tract, etc. radiological invasive techniques—catheterisation, cystoscopy, prosthetic devices, endotracheal tubes, etc.

Other factors : Like difficult delivery, exposure to infected incubators, exposure to infected ventilators, etc.

Laboratory Diagnosis of Viral Diseases

13

INTRODUCTION

The choice of materials and methods for laboratory confirmation of viral infection depends on the stage of illness (Table 13.1).

The following methods are commonly employed :

(a) *Microscopy* : Cytopathic effect, inclusion bodies.

(b) *Culture and isolation* : Laboratory animals, chick embryo, tissue culture, cell culture.

(c) *Serology* : HI, CFT, EIA, Western blot test.

(d) *Detection of viral proteins and genetic material* : DNA probes, PCR.

Table 13.1
Preferable materials and methods in different stages of viral infection

Stage of illness	Detection of Virus/antigens	Detection of* Specific antibody
Incubation	Rarely	No
Prodrome	Occasionally	No
Onset	Frequently	Occasionally
Acute phase	Frequently	Frequently
Recovery	Rarely	Usually
Convalescence	Very rarely	Usually

* In vaccinated individuals, antibody may be detected in the very early stage.

Specimens

Specimens to be collected early in the acute phase of the disease before the virus ceases to shed (Table 13.2).

Collection and transport of specimens

Ideally all specimens for detection of virus should be processed by the laboratory immediately because many viruses are labile and the samples are also susceptible to bacterial and fungal overgrowth. Specimen should be placed in ice and transported in special media (***Stuart's viral transport media***) containing proteins.

Blood for serological test is transported to laboratory in sterile test tube. Serum is separated as soon as possible. Blood for viral culture is to be transported in a sterile vial containing anticoagulant. Blood should be refrigerated at 4°C until processing, and can be stored for months at –20°C or below. Virus specific IgM should be tested before freezing since IgM may form insoluble aggregates upon thawing.

A. Microscopy (cytology)

Viruses produce cytopathic effect (CPE) which include : change in cell morphology, cell lysis, vacuolation, syncytia formation and inclusion bodies (Table 13.3).

1. Cytopathic effect (CPE): Viruses cause cell degeneration or cell death which can be seen by microscopical examination of cultures. Each infectious virus particle gives rise to a localised focus of infected cells (a focus of cytopathology) that can be seen with the naked eye (Fig. 13.5). Such foci are called plaques and each plaque represents an infectious virus. Cell degeneration is manifested by certain changes.

(a) ***Syncytium formation (Fig. 13.1)***: Syncytium or multinucleated giant cells result from fusion of contiguous cells in the monolayer as seen in measles virus.

(b) ***Cell necrosis and lysis***: Infected cells become pyknotic and granular, e.g. enteroviruses.

(c) ***Cellular clumping***: The cells do not fuse but produce large clumps resembling clusters of grapes, e.g. adenovirus.

Table 13.2
Recommended specimens for viral culture/diagnosis

Common pathogenic viruses	Specimens for culture	Comments
Respiratory tract		
Adenovirus, influenza virus, enterovirus (picornavirus), rhinovirus, paramyxovirus, rubella virus, HSV	Nasal washing, throat swab, nasal swab, sputum	Enterovirus is also shed in faeces
Gastrointestinal tract		
Reovirus, rotavirus, adenovirus, Norwalk virus, calcivirus	Stool, rectal swab	Samples are investigated by electron microscopy and antigen detection (ELISA); viruses are not cultivated
Maculopapular rash		
Adenovirus, enterovirus (picornavirus)	Throat swab, rectal swab	—
Rubella virus, measles virus	—	Rubella and measles virus may be detected in urine
Vesicular rash		
Coxsackie virus, echovirus, HSV, VZV	Vesicle fluid, scraping or swab, enterovirus in faeces	Initial diagnosis of HSV andVZV can be made from vesicle scraping (Tzanck smear)
Central nervous system		
(Aseptic meningitis/encephalitis)		
Enterovirus (picornavirus)	Stool	—
Arboviruses (e.g. togaviruses, bunyavirus)	Rarely cultured	Diagnosis by serological tests
Rabies virus	Tissue, saliva, brain biopsy	Diagnosed by immunofluorescent study for antigen.
HSV, CMV, mumps virus, measles virus	CSF, brain	Virus isolation and antigens are analysed by immunofluorescence
Urinary tract		
Adenovirus, CMV	Urine	CMV may be shed without apparent disease
Blood		
HIV; human T cell leukaemia virus; hepatitis B, C and D viruses	Blood	Serological test : Antigen or antibody detection (ELISA), PCR and reverse transcriptase PCR

Table 13.3 : Viral cytopathic effect (CPE)

CPE	Features
Change in cell morphology	Cell rounding Degeneration Aggregation Loss of attachment of substrate
Histologic changes	Inclusion bodies in the nucleus or cytoplasm. Migration of chromatin
Syncytia formation	Multinucleated giant cells caused by virus-induced cell—cell-fusion
Changes in cell surface	Viral antigen expression Haemadsorption (haemagglutinin expression)

(d) ***Inclusion bodies*** : Inclusion bodies are virus-specific intracellular globular masses produced during replication of virus in host cells and visible under the light microscope. They are far larger than a single mature virus particle (elementary body), size ranges from 20-25 μm and can be seen by light microscope. Inclusion bodies formed by different viruses show distinct shape, size, location and staining properties and their presence in an infected cell is a presumptive histological evidence of viral infection. These are generally **acidophilic** (eosinophilic) structures, appear pink when stained by Giemsa's or eosin-methylene blue stain and examined under light microscope. Some viruses produce **basophilic** inclusions (adenovirus). They may appear round, globular, oval or irregular.

Site of occurrence : Inclusion bodies may be formed in the nucleus, cytoplasm or both (Figs. 13.2 & 13.3) :

(i) *Intracytoplasmic bodies* : Small pox (*Guarnieri bodies*), rabies (*Negri bodies*), yellow fever (*Councilman bodies*). Inclusion bodies produced in fowl-pox virus infections are called Bollinger bodies which are larger than that formed in vaccinia virus infections. Intracytoplasmic *molluscum bodies* (20-30 µm) are large.

(ii) *Intranuclear bodies* : These were classified by Cowdry (1934) into two types : *Cowdry A* includes inclusion bodies of variable size and of granular appearance (herpes virus, yellow fever virus) and *type B* of more circumscribed inclusion (adenovirus, poliovirus). Large intranuclear inclusion is also seen in CMV infection of cell.

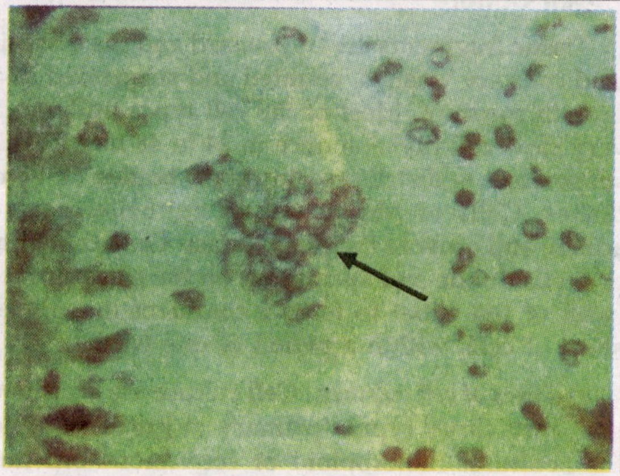

Fig. 13.1 : Syncytium (multinucleated giant cell) formation caused by measles virus (lung biopsy tissue of a case of viral-induced giant cell pneumonia).

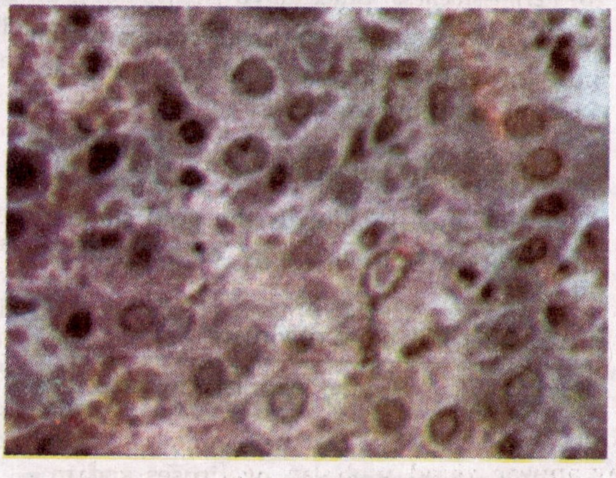

Fig. 13.2 : CPE produced by HSV (Liver biopsy tissue) showing an eosinophilic Cowdry type A intranuclear inclusion body.

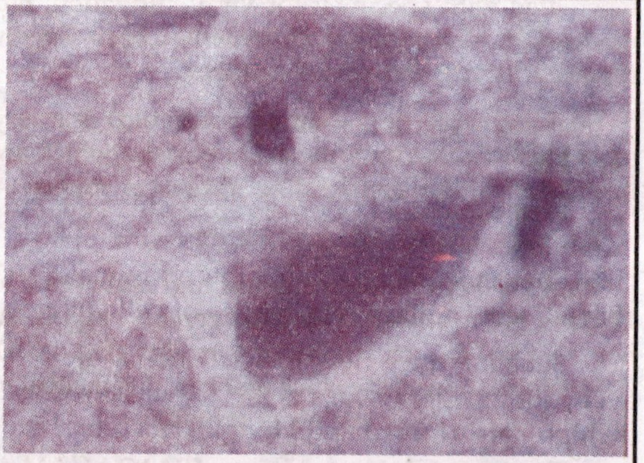

Fig. 13.3 : Negri bodies in rabies (brain tissue)

(iii) *Inclusions formed in both nucleus and cytoplasm* : Measles virus infection.

(e) ***Discrete focal degeneration*** : It is found in herpes virus infections.

(f) ***Transformation*** : Oncogenic virus transforms cells and causes loss of contact inhibition and the cell growth appears in a piled-up fashion producing "microtumours" (Fig. 13.1).

2. **Immunoelectron microscopy** : When virus-specific antibody is added to a sample, the virus particles clump and thereby facilitate the detection and simultaneous identification of virus. This technique is useful in diagnosis of enteric and rota viruses which are found in abundance and have a characteristic morphology.

B. Culture and isolation

Culture and isolation is the gold standard for proving a viral aetiology of a syndrome (Table 13.4) :

Table 13.4 : Cultivation of viruses

Animals	Suckling mice, rats, monkeys, chimpanzees
Embryonated eggs	Chorioallantoic membranes, allantoic cavity, amniotic sac and yolk sac
Tissue culture	Organ culture Explant culture Cell culture [primary cell culture, diploid cell culture, continuous or immortalised (tumour) cell line]

1. **Laboratory animals** :

In the past, white mice and chimpanzees were

inoculated with specimen for viral cultivation, but inoculation of laboratory animals has been largely replaced by the use of cell cultures.

Suckling mice (less than 48 hours old) are very susceptible to toga and coxsackie viruses, which are inoculated by intracerebral or intranasal routes.

2. **Chick embryo (embryonated egg) :**

Eggs are kept in the incubator and embryos 7 to 12 days old are used. The embryonated egg is inoculated by one of the several routes (Fig. 13.4). After inoculation of the chick embryo, it is incubated and examined daily for virus growth :

(a) ***Chorioallantoic membrane (CAM)*** : CAM is inoculated mainly for growing poxvirus. Viral replication produces visible lesions (pocks), gray-white area in the transparent CAM. Each pock is derived from a single virion. Pocks produced by different viruses have different morphology.

(b) ***Allantoic cavity*** : Allantoic inoculation is done mainly for production of vaccine of influenza virus. Other allantoic vaccines include yellow fever (17D strain) and rabies (flury strain) vaccines. Duck's egg, being larger, provide better yield of rabies virus than hen's egg.

(c) ***Amniotic sac*** : It is mainly inoculated for primary isolation of influenza virus.

(iv) ***Yolk sac inoculation*** : It is inoculated for cultivation of some viruses as well for some bacteria (chlamydiae and rickettsiae).

3. **Tissue culture :**

There are three types of *tissue culture* — *organ culture, explant culture* and *cell culture*. Small bits of organs (*organ culture*) from man and animal are maintained in tissue culture growth medium. Organ cultures are done mainly for highly specialised parasites of certain organ, e.g. tracheal ring culture for isolation of corona virus. Explant culture is rarely done nowadays.

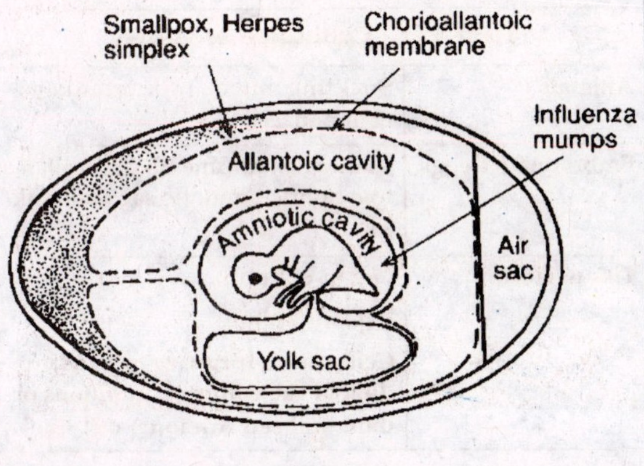

Fig. 13.4 : Embryonated egg of 10 days old showing different routes of inoculation

The *cell culture* method is routinely employed nowadays for identification and cultivation of viruses. The growth medium for tissue culture is basically a balanced salt solution and contains 13 essential amino acids, glucose, salts, buffering system, protein supplement (lactalbumin hydrolysate), calf serum (5%), antibiotics (penicillin, streptomycin) and phenol red (indicator).

Cell Culture

Tissue fragments are trypsinised and the dissociated cells are washed, counted and suspended in a growth medium. Most of the cell types undergo a very slow cell division once in 24 to 48 hours. Cell suspension is distributed in tubes, bottles or Petri dishes. Cells of fibroblastic or epithelial nature adhere and grow in the glass surface. On incubation, the cells divide and spread out on the glass surface (wall of test tube) to form a confluent monolayer sheet of cells within a period of one week :

(a) *Types of cell cultures* : Cell culture are classified into three types (primary cultures, diploid cultures, heteroploid or continuous cell line cultures) on the basis of their origin, chromosomal characters and the number of generations through which they can be maintained (Table 13.5).

(b) *Permissiveness* : Since all viruses do not grow in all cell lines, as a virus does not grow in a cell unless it carries receptor for the virus. Hence, specimen is to be inoculated in 3 to 4 cell lines with the hope that at least one of them will be permissive for the unknown virus.

(i) ***Primary cell culture*** : These are normal cells obtained from fresh organs of animal or human being and cultured. Once the cells get attached to the vessel surface, they undergo mitosis until a confluent monolayer of cells covers the surface. These cells are capable of only limited growth in culture and cannot be maintained in serial culture. They are commonly employed for ***primary isolation*** of viruses and in ***preparation of vaccine***. The examples of primary culture include monkey kidney cell (Fig. 13.5), and human amnion cell culture.

Table 13.5 : Cell cultures commonly used

Type	Cell derived from
Primary cell culture	Rhesus monkey kidney cell culture, Human amnion cell culture, Chick embryo fibroblast cell culture
Semicontinuous cell lines (diploid cell culture)	Human embryonic lung strain, Rhesus embryo cell strain
Continuous cell lines	HeLa (Human carcinoma of cervix cell line); HE_{P-2} (Human epithelioma of larynx cell line), KB (Human carcinoma of nasopharynx cell line), Vero (Vervet monkey kidney cell line), BHK-21 (Baby Hamster kidney cell line)

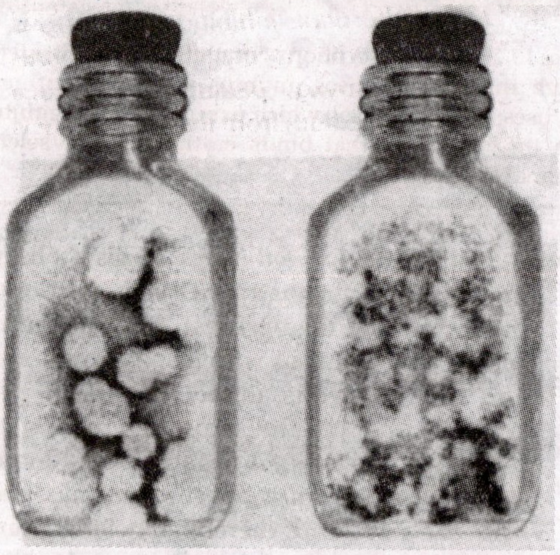

Fig. 13.5 : Monkey kidney cell cultures; left plaques produced by poliovirus, right plaques produced by echovirus. Progeny of a single viral particle are located in each clear area.

(ii) ***Diploid cell cultures*** (Semicontinuous cell lines) : These cells of a single type, usually *fibroblasts*, contain the same number of chromosomes as the parent cells and are *diploid*. The diploid cell strains can be subcultured for limited number of times. There is a rapid growth rate and after about 50 serial subcultures they undergo "*senescence*" and the cell strain is lost. The diploid cell strains are susceptible to a wide range of human viruses. They are also used for isolation of some fastidious viruses and production of viral vaccines. The fibroblasts are usually derived from *embryo* tissues (*human embryo lung strains*).

(iii) ***Heteroploid cultures*** (Continuous tumour cell lines) (Fig. 13.6) : These are cells of a single type capable of infinite growth *in vitro*. They are derived from immortalised cell lines (cancer cells), often of epithelial origin. These cells grow faster and their chromosomes are *haploid*.

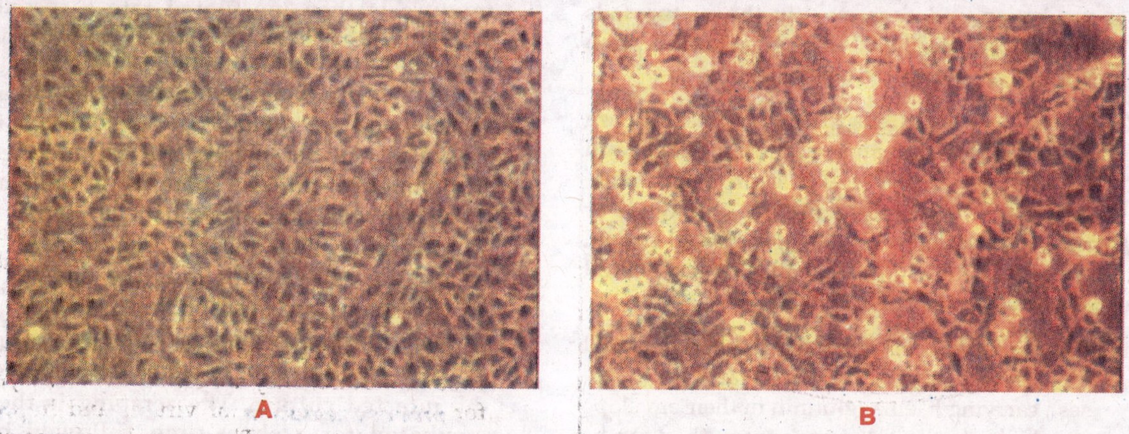

Fig. 13.6 : CPE of HSV infection : (A) Uninfected vero cell (*continuous cell lines*); (B) HSV-infected vero cells showing rounded cells, multinucleated cells, and loss of the monolayer.

They are termed *continuous cell lines* as they can be serially cultivated indefinitely. The standard continuous cell lines have been derived from human cancers, such as HeLa (derived from cervical cancer of a lady, Hela by name), HEp2 and KB cells. Continuous cell lines are maintained either by serial subculture or by storing in deep freeze at –70°C so that these can be used when necessary. These are not used for preparation of viral vaccines, as vaccines prepared in cancer cells is considered unsafe for human use.

Primary cell cultures are generally best for virus isolation and rhesus monkey kidney cell cultures are widely used, which are sensitive to a wide range of viruses.

Identification : For precise identification of a virus grown in cell cultures, several additional tests have to be performed :

1. **Morphologic examination** : Morphological study of a virus can only be made by electron microscopy which is technically difficult and expensive. Moreover, this may not lead to successful identification of the virus.

2. **Serological test** : Serologic tests help in most cases for precise identification of the virus :

(i) *Neutralisation* : It can be performed with any virus producing CPE. Standard known antiviral serum is mixed with the unknown virus recovered from the cell culture medium. After incubating the antibody-virus mixture, it is inoculated into a fresh cell line. Specific antiserum neutralises virus activity during incubation, and, consequently, the mixture fails to produce specific CPE. The haemadsorption viruses are typed by neutralisation test.

(ii) *Haemadsorption* : Cells infected with influenza virus, parainfluenza virus, mumps virus, and toga virus express a viral glycoprotein (haemagglutinin) in the cell membrane that binds or adsorbs red blood cells of defined animal species to the infected cell surface (called haemadsorption) (Fig. 13.7).

(iii) *Haemagglutination* : When the above-mentioned viruses-orthomyxo, paramyxo and togaviruses), carrying haemagglutinin in their envelope are shed into the culture medium, they can be detected by the agglutination of erythrocytes, a process called haemagglutination.

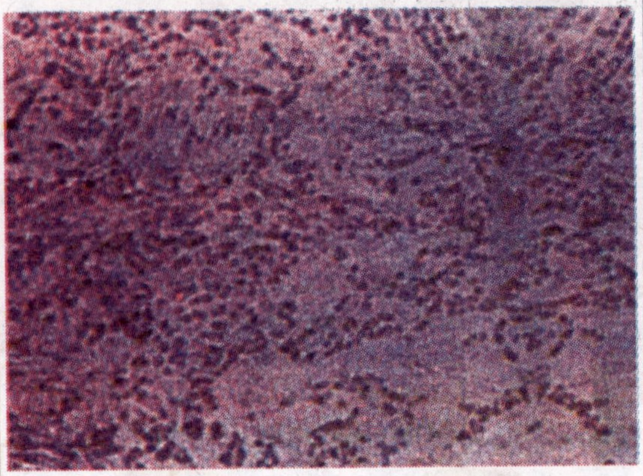

Fig. 13.7 : Haemadsorption of erythrocytes to cell infected with influenza viruses, mumps virus, parainfluenza viruses, or togaviruses which express a haemagglutinin on their surfaces that binds erythrocytes of selected animal species

(iv) *Haemadsorption inhibition test* : This is observed with haemagglutinating viruses (orthomyxo; paramyxo and togaviruses). Medium from the cell culture is mixed with a specific antiserum, and the mixture is added to a fresh culture. After incubation, the second culture is tested for haemadsorption. A negative result indicates that the antiserum is specific and has reacted with the virus and, thereby, blocking haemadsorption.

(v) *Cytopathogenic effects interference inhibition test* : Specific antibody to the unknown interfering virus (e.g. rubella virus, when it is the suspected identity of the unknown virus) is added to medium obtained from the cell culture. The mixture is then inoculated into a second culture. After incubation for 2–3 days, the cytopathic virus (e.g. echovirus) is added to the second cell culture and incubated for 1–2 days. If cytopathogenic effects have occurred, it is concluded that the first culture was infected with the interfering virus against which the antiserum was employed.

(vi) *Direct immunofluorescence* : A cell culture is inoculated with a specimen and incubated. After 24–48 hours the virus can be identified by adding a fluorescent monoclonal antibody to the suspected virus to a scraping obtained from the infected culture. The scraping is then incubated for a short time, followed by washing to eliminate unreacted antiserum, the scraping is examined — under the fluorescent microscope. When the cells fluoresce, the virus in question is responsible for the infection of the monolayer.

(vii) *Immunoelectron microscopy (IEM)* : Although a virus can be visualised by electron microscope, but precise identification of a virus (e.g. herpes simplex, VZ, CMV and Epstein—Barr) is not possible on a mere morphological basis. IEM uses a specific antibody labelled with electron-dense tag to specifically identify the virus. The technique is very expensive and not useful for routine purpose.

C. Serology

Serology is useful and simpler in diagnosis in many cases. The course of the infection (acute or chronic) can also be determined by serology.

1. General considerations :

Total antibody assays are done, usually to observe a significant rise of specific antibodies to a suspected virus on two paired samples, first when the patient is ill and second during convalescence (2 to 3 weeks later). There is usually a four-fold rise in antibody titre. The diagnosis is usually retrospective and mainly useful in epidemiological study.

2. Techniques :

(a) ***Haemagglutination inhibition*** (HI) is used for the measurement of antibodies directed against haemagglutinating viruses, e.g. influenza viruses. Antibodies to the viral haemagglutinins in serum prevents a standardised amount of virus binding to and agglutinating erythrocytes.

(b) ***Complement fixation test*** (CFT) is the mainstay for some viral diseases. However, it can only detect CF-antibodies (i.e. IgG and IgM) and cannot differentiate between the two.

(c) ***Direct immunofluorescence test*** : A fluorescein —Conjugated antiserum of the suspected virus is mixed with the infected tissue sample and examined under a fluorescent microscope for pale green fluorescent areas on the slide.

(d) ***Enzyme immunoassay (EIA)***

(i) *Measurement of antibody by EIA* : A known antigen is adsorbed to a solid phase-like test tube, microtitre plate well to which proper dilution of patient's serum is added and then incubated. If there is antibody in patient's serum, it will attach to the antigen. The solid phase is washed off the unreacted immunoglobulins. After washing enzyme-labelled anti-human immunoglobulin (AHIG) is added to the solid phase. The solid phase is again washed off to remove unreacted antibody (AHIG). Then a substrate is added to the solid phase. The enzyme-labelled antibody (AHIG) binds to the patient's antibody that has reacted with the immobilised antigen.

The enzyme splits the substrate to a colour compound. The intensity of the colour is proportional to the quantity of antibody present in the patient's serum. The colour is measured by ELISA reader. These tests are rapid (takes 10–15 minutes) and easy.

(ii) *Measurement of antigen* : A known specific antibody is adsorbed to the solid phase (e.g. well in microlitre plate). Patient's serum is added, and if viral particles or viral antigens are present in the circulation, they will be bound by the immobilised antibody. The solid phase is washed. Then enzyme-labelled antibody (e.g. AHG) of the same specificity to the solid phase is added. After incubating and washing off unbound reactants, a chromogenic substrate is added. A positive reaction is indicated by the development of colour.

(e) ***Western blot (immunoblot) test*** : It is a most widely used confirmatory test for detection of positive HIV antibody immunoassay. The test is done as follows :

(i) HIV antigens are separated by electrophoresis on polyacrylamide gel which is blotted onto nitrocellulose paper strips.

(ii) The strip is incubated with patient's antibody.

(iii) After washing to remove the unbound antibody, an enzyme labelled anti-human globulin (AHG) antiserum is placed on the strip. The labelled antibody binds to any antibody captured by the viral antigens. When a chromogenic substrate is added subsequently, the antigen-antibody complexes are revealed as stained bands which represent the major antigenic proteins of HIV.

D. Detection of viral genetic material

(1) **Nucleic acid probes** : Nucleic acid probes are short segments of DNA complementary to specific regions of a viral genome. DNA probe analysis is especially useful to detect slowly replicating or non-productive viruses, e.g. CMV, human papilloma viruses and HIV (during window period).

(2) **Polymerase chain reaction (PCR) and reverse transcriptase PCR** : PCR is a method that duplicates short DNA segments thousand to a million fold. When the viruses are present in low concentrations, they can be duplicated (amplified) using PCR.

Viral Assays

1. Total particle count

Total count of viruses irrespective of whether they are viable or nonviable is estimated by electron microscopy and haemagglutination :

(a) *Electron microscopy* : The virus particles in a negatively stained suspension can be counted directly. The commonest method is to mix virus suspension with known concentration of latex particles and studied under the electron microscope. The number of virus particles in the suspension are calculated from the ratio of latex spheres to virus particles.

(b) *Haemagglutination* (HA) : Although it is not a very sensitive method, yet HA titre gives an approximate count. About 107 influenza viruses are necessary to bind erythrocytes (0.5 ml of 0.5% suspension) into a lattice-like aggregates of macroscopic size.

2. Infectious virions assay (assay of infectivity)

Quantitative infectivity assay

The quantitative infectivity assay measures the number of viable infectious particles in a suspension. This can be measured by two methods :

(i) *Plaque assay* : Serial dilutions of a virus suspension are inoculated into confluent monolayers of culture cells in a Petri dish or bottle. After allowing time for adsorption (1 to 4 hours), the monolayer is covered with agar gel which prevents diffuse spread of the viruses readily through the fluid medium. Moreover, the agar gel layer restricts spread of the released progeny particles in such a way that only neighbouring cells are infected. Each infectious particle gives rise to a localised focus of infected cells, called a plaque, which can be seen with the naked eye (Fig. 13.5). The titre of viruses is expressed in plaque forming units (PFU) per volume. Since each plaque represents an infectious virus, the plaque titre is the infectivity titre.

(ii) *Pock assays* : Since each pock in CAM arises from infection by a single virus particle, the number of pocks formed corresponds with the number of viruses present in the inoculum.

Antiviral Susceptibility Testing (AST)

It is done for defining mechanisms of antiviral resistance and to assess the frequency with which drug-resistant viral mutants emerge in clinical practice. There are two types of AST :

(i) *Phenotypic assays* : These are *in vitro* susceptibility tests. Cell culture is incubated with several dilutions of the drug to which a constant amount of virus has been added. The test measures the reduction in the number of plaques, inhibition of viral DNA synthesis, and reduction in the yield of viral structural proteins (e.g. gp 24 of HIV).

(ii) *Genotypic assays* : These analyse viral nucleic acids to detect specific mutations responsible for drug resistance. CMV shows UL 97 (phosphotransferase) and UL 54 (polymerase) mutants with ganciclovir resistance. These are detected by PCR amplification and sequencing of entire UL 54 gene and fragment of UL 97 gene.

QUESTIONS RELATED TO LABORATORY DIAGNOSIS OF VIRAL DISEASE

Q.1. *How are viruses cultivated?*

Ans. Viruses are obligate intracellular parasites, hence they can be grown in living cells only.

Three types of methods have been developed for their cultivation :

(a) Animal inoculation.

(b) Embryonated eggs.

(c) Tissue culture.

Q.2. *What are the tissue cultures (cell lines)?*

Ans. Three types of tissue cultures are available :

(a) Organ culture — whole organ.

(b) Explant culture.

(c) Cell culture — most commonly used.

Q.3. *How to prepare monolayers?*

Ans. (1) Desired tissue is cut into small pieces.

(2) Tissue is dissociated into the component cells by treating with a proteolytic enzyme (e.g. trypsin) and by mechanical shaking.

(3) Dissociated cells are washed, counted and suspended in a suitable growth medium containing all essential nutrients (amino acids, vitamins, salts, glucose, etc.) and supplemented with up to 5% of calf or fetal calf serum.

(4) Cell suspension is distributed in a glass or a plastic container.

(5) The cells adhere to glass or plastic surface on incubation and divide to form a confluent monolayer sheet of cells within a week.

SPACE FOR NOTES

Laboratory Diagnosis of Fungal Infections

14

CLASSIFICATION OF FUNGAL INFECTIONS

A. Superficial mycoses

Dermatophytosis caused by : *Trichophyton, Epidermophyton* and *Microsporum species.*

Pityriasis versicolor : *Malassezia furfur.*

White piedra : *Trichosporon beigelii.*

Black piedra : *Piedraia hortaie.*

Tinea nigra : *Exophiala werneckii.*

Candidiasis : *Candida albicans* and other species of *Candida.*

The **specimens** from this group include — skin, hair and nails.

B. Subcutaneous mycoses

Eumycetoma caused by : *Madurella mycetomatis, Madurella grisea.*

Black or dark grains : *Leptosphaeria senegalensis, Exophiala jeanselmei, Pseudallescheria boydii.*

White or yellow grains : *Acremonium species.*

Eumycetomas require to be differentiated from actinomycotic mycetomas.

- Chromoblastomycosis : *Fonsecaea pedrosoi* (Pigmented fungi).
- Sporotrichosis : *Sporothrix schenckii.*
- Rhinosporidiosis : *Rhinosporidium seeberi.*

Specimens from this group include pus from abscesses, exudate from lesions, aspirated fluid from sinus tracts and tissue from biopsy.

C. Systemic mycoses caused by 'Pathogenic fungi'

- Histoplasmosis : *Histoplasma capsulatum.*
- Blastomycosis : *Blastomyces dermatitidis.*
- Paracoccidioidomycosis : *Paracoccidioides brasiliensis.*
- Coccidioidomycosis : *Coccidioides immitis.*

D. Systemic Mycoses caused by 'Opportunistic fungi'

- Cryptococcosis : *Cryptococcus neoformans.*
- Aspergillosis : *Aspergillus fumigatus* and other aspergillus species.
- Zygomycosis : *Mucor, Rhizopus* and *Basidiobolus* species.
- Systemic candidiasis : *Candida albicans.*

Specimen from this group include pus or exudate, cerebrospinal fluid, respiratory secretions, bone marrow, blood, urine and tissue from biopsy or autopsy.

LABORATORY DIAGNOSIS

I. Specimens

1. Skin scrapings, nail clippings and hairs can be transported in an envelope, Petri dish, or other convenient conveyance.

2. Specimens from mucous membrane may be directly inoculated in culture medium or smeared on clean slide by swab or culture loop.

3. Scrapings, crusts, aspirated pus and tissue biopsies are to be collected aseptically from subcutaneous infections.

4. In suspected systemic infections, specimens are to be collected from as many sites as possible, such as blood and CSF.

Specimen processing : The specimen is divided into two parts, one for microscopy and other for culture. Yeasts are handled in the same way as bacteria. Moulds, however, require some special procedures.

II. Examination

Microscopy

1. **Potassium hydroxide (KOH) mount** : KOH dissolves keratin and cellular material but does not affect fungi. Specimens are placed on a slide to which a drop of 10-20% potassium hydroxide is added and then covered by a cover slip and left for 20 minutes in incubator at 37°C to digest keratin. Microscopical examination shows fungal structure.

2. **Staining technique** : Gram stain, Papanicolaou (usually performed in cytopathology laboratory), Periodic acid-Schiff (PAS) staining and methenamine silver staining stain most fungi well.

Giemsa staining is useful for yeasts and cells of *Histoplasma capsulatum* because of their small size. All fungi are gram-positive though of little value.

3. **Direct immunofluorescence** : DFAT is useful to identify fungi in tissues and smears.

4. **Histology** : Examination of biopsy specimens of tissue provide firm evidence of invasive disease. Tissue sections prepared from paraffin block are stained by Gomori methenamine silver and periodic acid-Schiff stain. Such staining indicates only the presence of fungi in tissues and not the species.

Antigen detection

Detection of cryptococcal polysaccharide antigen in CSF and serum by latex agglutination test is routinely done. The test is sensitive, specific and simple to perform. Methods for detection of Candida and Histoplasma antigens have also been described.

Culture and isolation

1. **Culture media** : Pathogenic fungi grow on **Sabouraud** dextrose agar (pH 5.6, slight acidic pH which does not allow bacterial growth) contains 4% dextrose, 1% peptone, and 2% agar. Chloramphenicol (50 mg/L), cycloheximide (500 mg/L), or other antibiotic is often added to the medium to further prevent bacterial or saprophytic fungal contamination.

2. **Technique** : Two cultures with the specimens are done and incubated at room temperature (25°C) and at body temperature (37°C) to reveal dimorphism. Tube, Petri dish and slide are used for culture. Slide culture is useful for studying morphology of fungus.

Cultures are incubated for at least 2 to 3 weeks and in some cases up to 6 weeks.

3. **Identification** : Culture provides an unequivocal evidence of fungal infection.

(a) **Macroscopic appearance** (colony character) (Fig. 14.1) : (i) Dimorphic fungi produce colonies of 1-2 mm diam, delicate hyphae which give the mould form of the colonies a cobweb or hair-like appear-

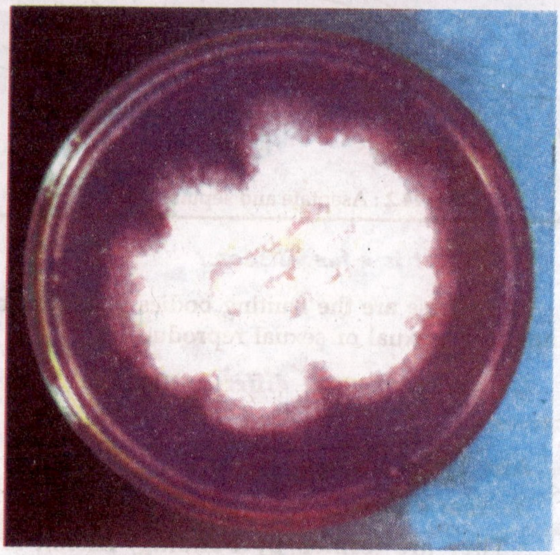

A

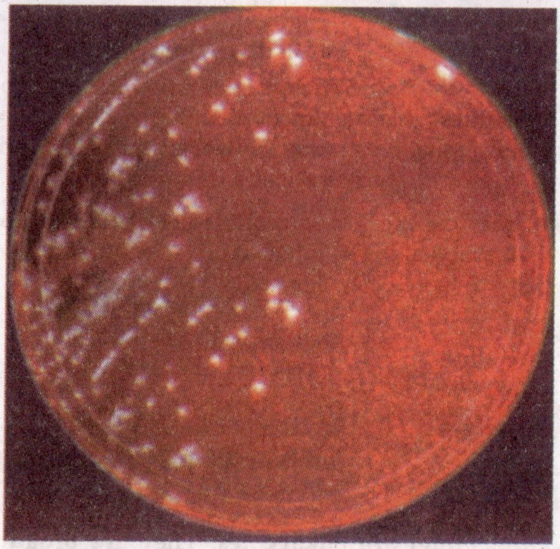

B

Fig. 14.1 : A. Dimorphic fungus, colonies in Sabouraud dextrose chloramphenicol agar (incubated at 37°C for 145 days) showing yeast form centrally and mould form peripherally. B. *Candida albicans* in 5% sheep blood agar.

ance (Fig. 14.1A). (ii) Trichophyton rubrum produces wine-red diffusible pigment.

(b) **Microscopic morphology** (Tease mount) : A small portion of the colony including some of the surface agar is dug out with a pair of dissecting needles or pointed applicator sticks. The colony fragment is placed on a microscope slide in a drop of lactophenol aniline blue. The colony is teased apart using dissecting needles, and then a cover slip is positioned over the drop and gently pressed on the surface with the eraser end of a pencil to facilitate microscopic examination.

Findings : Yeasts are unicellular. On the other hand, moulds are filamentous (hyphae), produce specialised conidia, and grow slowly.

The following fungal structures may be seen :

(i) Mycelium : Presence of septate or aseptate hyphae (Fig. 14.2), or pseudohyphae.

(ii) Mycelium may be vegetative (portion extending into culture medium) or aerial (portion above the medium/substrate).

(iii) Presence of specialised structures, e.g. chlamydospores, or yeasts, etc. may be present.

(c) **Nucleic acid probes** : Genetic probes are available for detection of *Blastomyces dermatitidis*, *Coccidioides immitis*, *Cryptococcus neoformans*, and *Histoplasma capsulatum*.

Indirect methods based on host immune response

(a) **Skin testing** : Skin test once a popular diagnostic test is now almost abandoned because of false-positive results. However, those tests are useful to study patient's immune status.

(b) **Serologic tests** : Serologic tests like ELISA for histoplasmosis, latex agglutination test and CFT have been devised.

QUESTIONS RELATED TO LABORATORY DIAGNOSIS OF FUNGAL INFECTIONS

Q.1. What are fungi? How are they broadly divided?

Ans. Fungi are eukaryotes. They are broadly divided into following two groups :

(i) **Yeast** : These are ovoid or ellipsoidal cells and they reproduce by sexual process known as budding. Budding is an asexual method of reproduction of yeast. Daughter bud arises from parent bud, enlarges and separates from parent cell.

(ii) **Mould** : These are filamentous fungi. They reproduce sexually and/or asexually by forming spores.

Q.2. How do you define hypha and pseudohypha? How to differentiate the two?

Ans. Hypha : It is an elongated tubular, thread-like branching filament of even width.

Pseudohypha : A chain of elongated cells is known as pseudohypha.

Differences between Hypha and Pseudohypha

Hypha	Pseudohypha
It is formed by apical elongation	It is formed by budding
Cell walls are parallel to each other	Cell walls are constricted at septa
Septa are straight and perpendicular	Septa are curved
Septum and constriction is absent at origin of branches	Septum and constriction is present at origin of branches

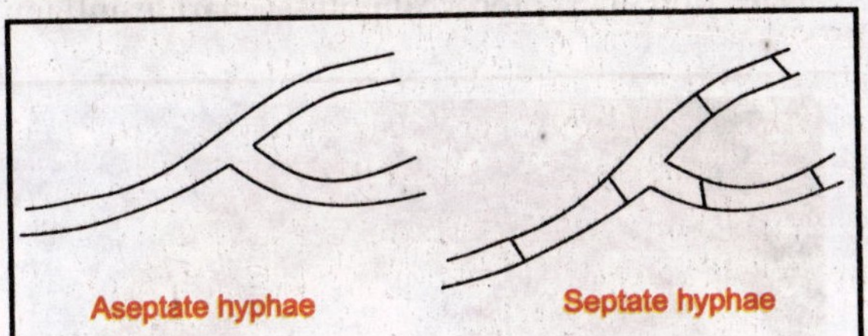

Fig. 14.2 : Aseptate and septate hyphae

Q.3. What is a fungal spore?

Ans. These are the fruiting bodies produced by fungi for asexual or sexual reproduction.

Q.4. What are the different types of fungal spores?

Ans. Types of fungal spores :

Asexual spores

- They are formed by budding, fission and mitosis (Fig. 14.3).
- Asexual spores are of following types :

1. **Chlamydospores** — These are asexual spores

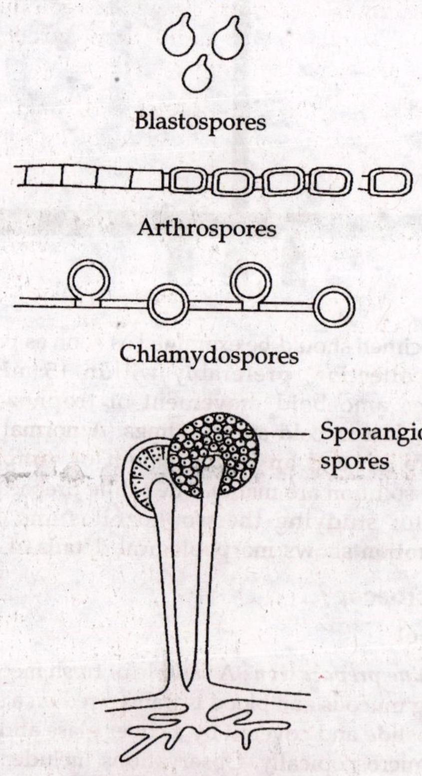

Fig. 14.3 : Asexual spores

which are large with thick double refractile wall produced from hyphal cell. They are resistant and store nutrients and function as spores. Spores may be formed in groups or occur singly and may be terminal or intercalary.

2. **Arthrospores** — These are asexual spores produced as a result of fragmentation of hyphae. They are cuboidal, rectangular spores formed in chains, with a slightly thick wall and are released at maturity.

3. **Blastospores** — These are asexual spores produced as a result of budding.

4. **Sporangiospores** — These are asexual spores present inside the sporangium.

Conidia :

- These are asexual reproductive structures borne exogenously on specialised hyphae called conidiophores.
- Two types of conidia exist — macroconidia and microconidia.

Sexual spores :

- They are produced as a result of meiosis.
- Following types of sexual spores are seen :

(1) **Ascospores** are sexual spores inside a sac-like structure called ascus.
Example : Ascomycetes.

(2) **Zygospores** are sexual spores formed by sexual conjugation of two fungi.
Example : Zygomycetes.

(3) **Basidiospores** are sexual spores formed on basidium. *Example* : Basidiomycetes.

Q.5. *What are the surface infections or superficial mycoses?*

Ans. Surface infections : Infections of outermost epithelial tissue producing cosmetic effects only. These fungi do not elicit allergic response because they are not in contact with living tissue.

- Tinea versicolor. • Tinea nigra. • Piedra.

Cutaneous infections : Infections of cornified layer of the skin and its appendages.

- Dermatophytoses.

Q.6. *What is the current systemic classification of fungi?*

Ans. Method of sexual reproduction forms the basis for the systemic classification. Thus there are four groups of fungi which include :

- *Zygomycetes* — sexual fusion forms zygospores.
- *Ascomycetes* — sexual fusion forms ascus and ascospores.
- *Basidiomycetes* — sexual fusion forms basidium and basidiospores.
- *Fungi imperfectii* — these are fungi in which sexual process is not observed.

Q.7. *What are the common antifungal agents?*

Ans. Common antifungal agents are :

- *Antifungal antibiotics* :
  – Amphotericin B – Nystatin – Griseofulvin
- *Synthetic antifungal agents* :
  – Tolnaftate.
  – Imidazoles such as clotrimazole, ketoconazole
  – Triazoles such as fluconazole, itraconazole.
- Miscellaneous antifungal agents :
  – Flucytosine – Potassium iodide
  – Selenium sulphide – Gentian violet.

Laboratory Diagnosis of Parasitic Diseases

15

AMOEBIC INFECTIONS

Definitive diagnosis of amoebiasis is made by detection of *E. histolytica* in tissues or discharge from the lesions. Cultures are not employed for diagnosis of intestinal amoebiasis and serological tests are sometimes useful in extra-intestinal amoebiasis.

ACUTE AMOEBIC DYSENTERY

Laboratory diagnosis

Specimen : Stool, blood-stained mucous, colonic scrapings from edge of ulcerated areas.

Macroscopically the stool is blood and mucous mixed, copious, dark red and smells offensive, acidic and does not adhere to the container.

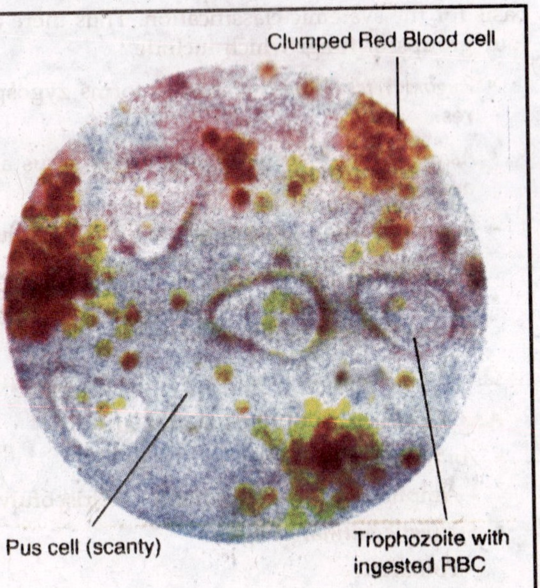

Fig. 15.1 : Unstained wet preparation (saline) of stool showing trophozoites with pseudopodia and ingested RBC. There is also a leucocyte and epithelial cell.

Specimen should be examined as soon as possible after collection, preferably within 15 minutes, because amoeboid movement of trophozoite is rapidly lost in cold surroundings. A normal saline preparation and an iodine mount of sample (2% iodine solution are made). The saline preparation is used for studying the trophozoites and iodine preparation shows morphological details of cysts.

Microscopy

Stool

Saline preparation : A sample of fresh faeces containing mucous and blood is transferred on a slightly warm slide and covered by a cover glass and examined microscopically. Observations include :

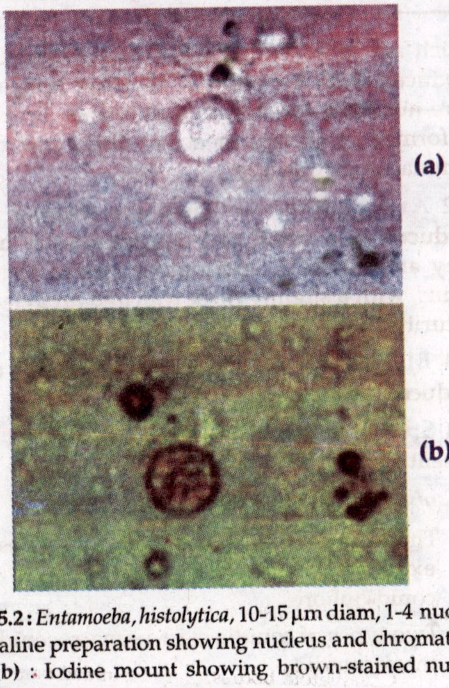

Fig. 15.2 : *Entamoeba, histolytica*, 10-15 µm diam, 1-4 nuclei. **(a)** : Saline preparation showing nucleus and chromatoid bar. **(b)** : Iodine mount showing brown-stained nuclei (× 400).

(a) Motile trophozoites throwing pseudopodia and containing red blood cells found in large number. Endoplasm is bluish or ground glass appearance and nucleus is not visible but a faint outline may be detected (Fig. 15.1).

(b) Cyst has a smooth and thin cell wall and contains round, refractile chromatoid bars. Glycogen mass is not visible (Fig. 15.2a).

(c) Red blood cells and pus cells are found in fair number.

(d) Charcot-Leyden crystals, diamond-shaped, clear and refractile structures and often present in faeces.

Iodine preparation : It is rarely necessary for diagnosis :

(a) Trophozoite stains yellow to light brown. Nucleus is clearly visible with a central karyosome.

(b) Cyst : Cytoplasm shows a smooth and hyaline appearance. Nucleus is clearly seen and no more than 4 nuclei are present (Fig.15.2). Glycogen mass stains brown while chromatoid bars are not stained.

The morphological differences of *Entamoeba histolytica* and *Entamoeba coli* are shown in Table 15.1, Figure 15.3 and that between *E. histolytica* and other intestinal amoebae are shown in Table 15.2 and Figure 15.3.

Microscopical differentiation of *E. histolytica* from the non-pathogenic *E. dispar* is difficult as they are morphologically indistinguishable. The exceptions are absence of ingested RBCs in their cytoplasm. Zymodeme analysis requires culture and difficult. Antigen detection kits are now commercially available to distinguish the two strains.

Mucosal scrapings : Mucosal scrapings obtained by sigmoidoscopy serve as an useful adjunct to conventional stool examination for ova and cyst (O and C) in cases of suspected amoebiasis.

(i) At least six samples of mucosa are to be sampled for accurate results.

(ii) Examination methods include a direct wet mount, a permanently stained smear and immunostained smears (employing either immunofluorescent or immunoenzymatic staining).

Table 15.1 : Morphological differences of *E. histolytica* and *E. coli*

Stages	***Entamoeba histolytica***	***Entamoeba coli***
Trophozoite form		
Fresh preparation		
Size	15-30 mm	20-40 µm
Motility	Very active	Sluggish
Cytoplasm	Clearly defined into ectoplasm and endoplasm	Not defined, ectoplasm scarcely seen
Cytoplasmic inclusions	Red cells, leucocytes and tissue debris but no bacteria	Bacteria and other materials, but never RBC
Nucleus	Not visible in unstained preparation	Visible in unstained preparation
Stained with iodine		
Nuclear character	Central karyosome; fine chromatin granules line the delicate nuclear membrane	Eccentric karyosome; coarse chromatin granules line the thick nuclear membrane
Cyst form		
Stained with iodine		
Size	10-15 µm	15-20 µm
Nucleus	1-4, central karyosome	1-8, eccentric karyosome
Glycogen mass	Visible in uninucleate stage	Large and visible in the binucleate stage
Fresh preparation		
Chromatoid bodies	Rounded bars	Filamentous, thread-like with square or pointed ends

Table 15.2 : Differential features of cysts of intestinal amoebae

Species	Size (μm)	Nuclei	Chromatoid body	Glycogen inclusion
Entamoeba histolytica	10-15	1-4	+ Blunt immature cyst	Diffuse
Entamoeba hartmanni	7-9	1-4	+ Blunt immature cyst	Diffuse
Entamoeba coli	15-30	1-8	Rare needle-like	Diffuse
Iodamoeba butschlii	9-15	1	Karyosome surrounded by refractile globes	Compact mass
Endolimax nana	7-9	4	Large mass of karyosome at periphery connected with a small mass	—

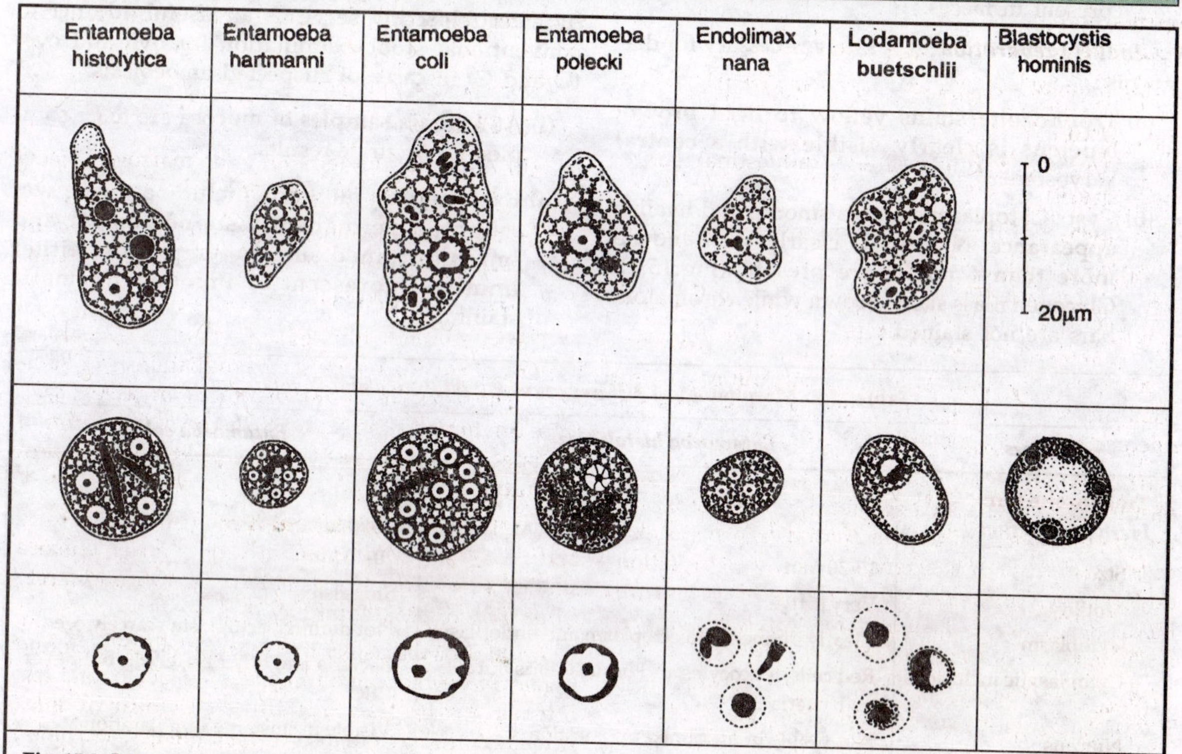

Fig. 15.3 : Intestinal amoebae of humans. As amoeboid form of *B. hominis* is rarely seen and difficult to see, hence not shown here. Top row : Trophozoites; Middle row : Cysts; Bottom row : Trophozoite nuclei in relative proportion (schematic).

CHRONIC AMOEBIASIS AND CARRIERS

Emphasis is made on detection of cyst of *E. histolytica* in faeces for establishment of diagnosis.

Identification of cyst-passers is necessary to diagnose chronic amoebiasis, detect carriers and in epidemiological survey.

EXTRAINTESTINAL AMOEBIASIS

Liver, lung or brain biopsy samples are subjected to routine histology (H and E section) and Giemsa-stained touch preparation which will reveal trophozoites of *E. histolytica* in extraintestinal lesions. Trophozoites can be detected in the scraping material from the wall of amoebic abscess, and rarely from aspirated anchovy sauce like pus or expectorated sputum.

AMOEBIC LIVER ABSCESS

The pus of amoebic liver abscess is distinctive red brown "anchovy-sauce"-like appearance. Since the amoebae actively multiply in the walls of abscesses, the last material aspirated is likely to contain trophozoites and may be detected by direct microscopic examination or in HE or PAS stained smears.

Serological test

Serological tests become positive only in invasive amoebiasis. Tests for antibodies of *E. histolytica* in blood assist in diagnosis of extraintestinal infections. Serological tests include Indirect haemagglutination assay (IHA), Enzyme-linked immunosorbent assay (ELISA), Latex agglutination (LA) test, Gel diffusion precipitation (GDP), and Counter—current immunoelectrophoresis (CIE), etc. While LA and ELISA are highly sensitive, but they often give false-positive results. Serological tests remain positive for several years even after successful treatment.

(a) *Indirect haemagglutination assay (IHA)*

Titre :

1 : 256 to 512 – Possible extraintestinal amoebiasis.

1 : 1,024 or over – Extraintestinal amoebiasis.

(b) *ELISA* : Results comparable to IHA.

(c) *Cellulose acetate precipitin (CEP) test* : It has got high specificity in extra-intestinal amoebiasis.

Culture : Cultures are not done routinely, but sometimes proved positive in cases negative by microscopy. The following media are in use :

(i) *Boeck and Drbohlav's media* of Lock's-egg-serum medium or Lock's-egg-albumin medium. This media has been modified by Laidlaw replacing glucose with starch. It is extensively used for isolation and maintenance of *E. histolytica*. Other culture media of this type include *Cleverland* and *Sander's medium, Nelson's medium*, etc.

(ii) *Monoxenic medium* : It is obtained by growing *E. histolytica* with *Trypanosoma cruzi*.

(iii) *Diamond's axenic medium* is useful in the studies on pathogenicity, antigenic characterisation and drug sensitivity. It does not require presence of other microorganisms.

Growth is obtained in all these media by inoculation with a small amount of stool following incubation. Supernatant fluid is examined microscopically for presence of trophozoites of *E. histolytica*.

NOTE :

Immunity : Infection with invasive strains of *E. histolytica* induce both humoral and cellular response. The immune response is greater in persons having extraintestinal amoebiasis. Infection offers some degree of protection as evident by very low frequency of recurrency and recurrence of invasive colitis and liver abscess in endemic areas.

KALA-AZAR
(Old World Visceral Leishmaniasis)

Visceral leishmaniasis (VL) is caused by *L.d. donovani* and *L.d. infantum* in Old World. VL caused by *L. donovani* was first characterised in India where it is also known as Kala-azar (meaning black sickness), Dum Dum fever or tropical splenomegaly. The two main species tend to cause similar disease, although *L. infantum* infects mainly young children, and has a greater tendency to cause lymph node enlargement.

Specimen :

(i) Peripheral blood.

(ii) Aspirated material of bone marrow, spleen or enlarged lymph node.

The various laboratory procedures adopted in diagnosis of kala-azar are summarised in Fig. 15.4.

A. Direct evidence

The demonstration of Leishmania is a most important conclusive evidence of diagnosis of kala-azar. The parasite is demonstrated in **amastigote** form on microscopic examination on stained film of the specimen from patient and **promastigote** form on culture.

1. **Microscopy of stained film** : Amastigote form of *L. donovani* is detected in Leishman or Giemsa stained smears of **bone marrow or spleen** and rarely from that of peripheral blood.

(a) **Blood** : Occasionally amastigotes can be found in peripheral blood mononuclear leucocytes and less often in neutrophils in buffy coat smear or thick smear stained by Giemsa or Leishman stain. Blood collected in an anticoagulant (EDTA) is centrifuged in an Wintrobe tube. The uppermost layer of white cells (buffy coat) is carefully withdrawn by a Pasteur pipette and smear made. A thick film prepared by a large drop of blood may show amastigotes in monocytes.

(b) **Bone marrow aspiration biopsy** : It is the **most common** and **useful** technique for direct demonstration of the parasite in kala-azar, particularly in the early cases where spleen is not sufficient enlarged to be punctured.

(c) **Splenic puncture** is one of the most valuable methods for confirming the diagnosis of kala-azar.

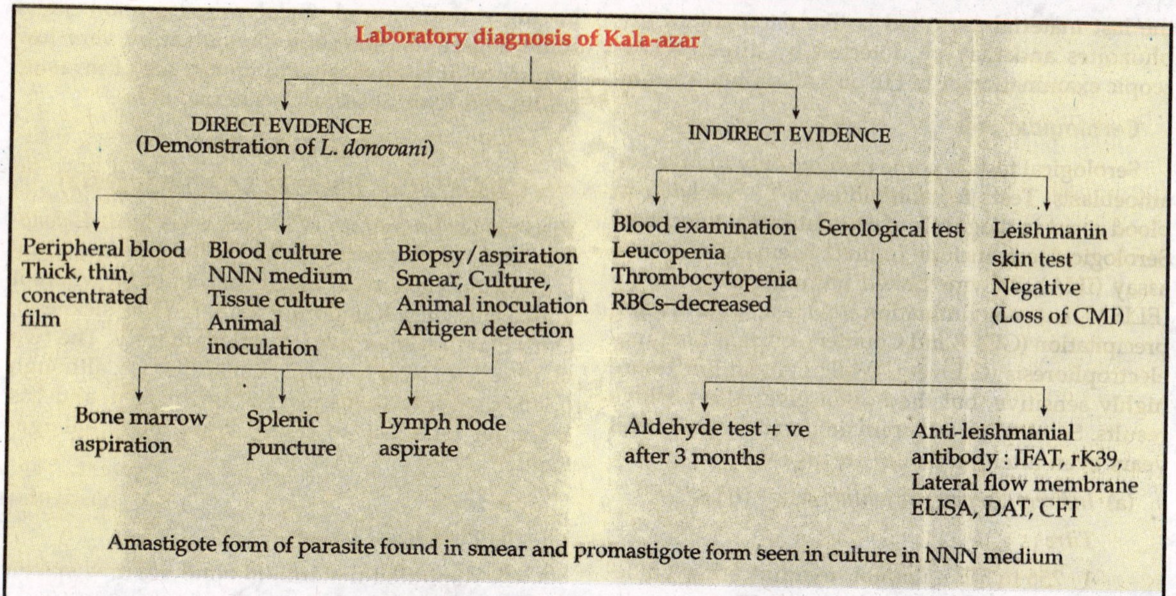

Fig. 15.4 : Laboratory diagnosis of kala-azar

Bone marrow puncture is a safer procedure compared to spleen puncture as there is risk of haemorrhage in splenic puncture. However, other workers consider the procedure of spleen puncture to be safe when performed by an expert and the patient's platelet count is not less than 40,000/cumm and prothrombin time is normal. Amastigote forms of parasite are found in stained films.

Result of aspiration biopsy : The positive result of examination of aspirates by stained smear and culture for amastigotes is :

Spleen	–	98%
Bone-marrow (sternum or iliac crest)	–	50-85%
Enlarged lymph node	–	65%

Examination of aspirated material : The aspirated material is examined as :

(i) Smear preparation : At least 2 thinly-spread smears are prepared on clean slides immediately after aspiration. Only a small quantity of aspirate is necessary. Dilution of material with blood is to be avoided.

The remaining aspirate is utilised for culture or placed into a tube containing EDTA anticoagulant and mixed. When the aspirate is diluted with blood, centrifuge the EDTA sample and examine the deposit as for peripheral smear.

(ii) The smears are rapidly air-dried and fixed in a few drops of absolute methanol.

(iii) Fixed smears are stained by Giemsa or Leishman stain.

(iv) When dry, add a drop of oil on smear and examine the smear microscopically under a 100 × oil-immersion objective to identify the amastigote.

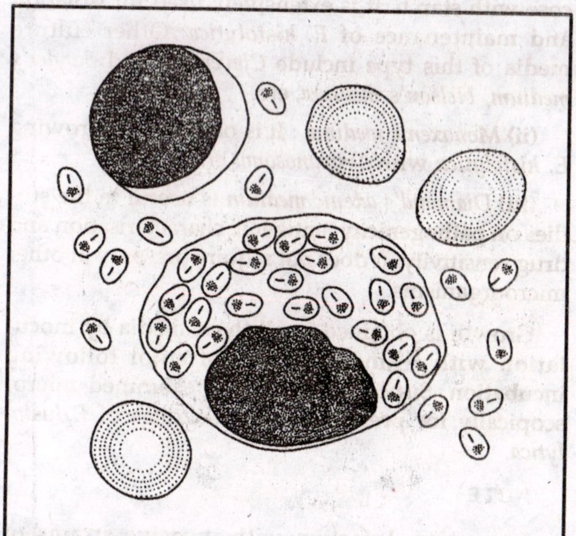

Fig. 15.5 : Schematic representation : *L. donovani* amastigotes in mononuclear (macrophage) cells

Amastigote of Leishmania species (Fig. 15.5 to 15.7)

(i) Small round to oval bodies, 2-4 μm in diameter, depending on species.

(ii) Usually found in groups inside mononuclear phagocytic cells or lying free between cells.

(iii) Nucleus and rod-shaped kinetoplast in each amastigote stain dark reddish-mauve. Both structures must be observed.

(iv) Cytoplasm of the amastigote takes pale staining and is often difficult to see especially when the parasites are present in groups.

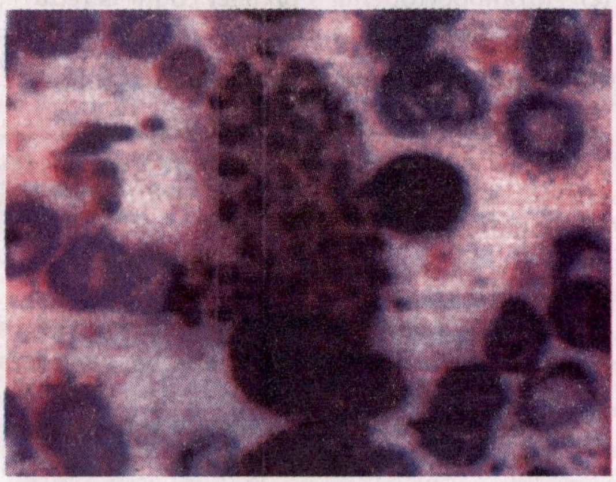

Fig. 15.6 : *Leishmania donovani* : Amastigotes *L. donovani* in macrophage cells in smear made from bone marrow aspirate (Giemsa skin)

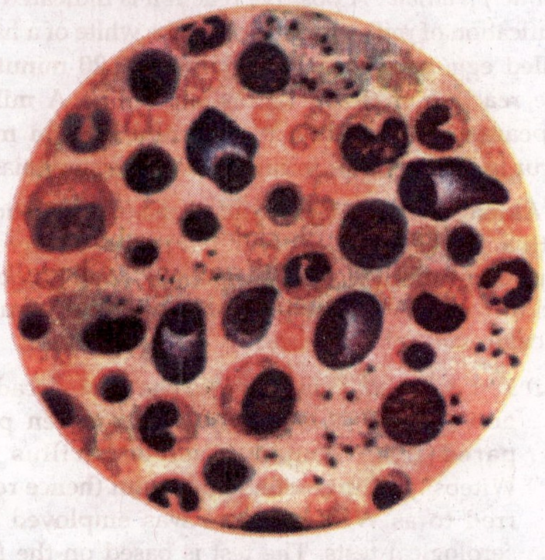

Fig. 15.7 : Smear of bone marrow fluid obtained by sternal puncture (Leishman staining) — Free and phagocytosed *L. donovani*

The amastigotes of different species of *Leishmania* are structurally similar. There are, however, variations in size between species.

LD bodies should be distinguished from *Toxoplasma gondii* and *Histoplasma capsulatum*, both of which are also intracellular organisms of monocyte-macrophage lineage of cells. The most distinguishing structure is kinetoplast of LD body which is lacking in *T. gondii* and *H. capsulatum*.

Isolation (culture): Culturing of aspirates in visceral leishmaniasis is useful in detecting light infections. In Indian kala-azar, blood culture may establish a diagnosis without the need of spleen aspiration. Moreover, culture is also useful in checking for infection during and after treatment. The form of parasite found in culture is promastigote (Fig. 15.8).

Choice of culture medium : Both Novy-Nicolle-McNeal (NNN) medium and Schneider's enriched insect tissue culture medium are recommended for the *in vitro* culture of *Leishmania*. Tissue culture medium is more sensitive than NNN medium.

1. NNN medium

Preparation of medium

Difco blood agar base	–	8 gm
Glass distilled water	–	200 ml
Defibrinated rabbit blood (10%)	–	20 ml

Add the agar base in water, dissolve in a water bath and then sterilise in autoclave at 121°C for 15

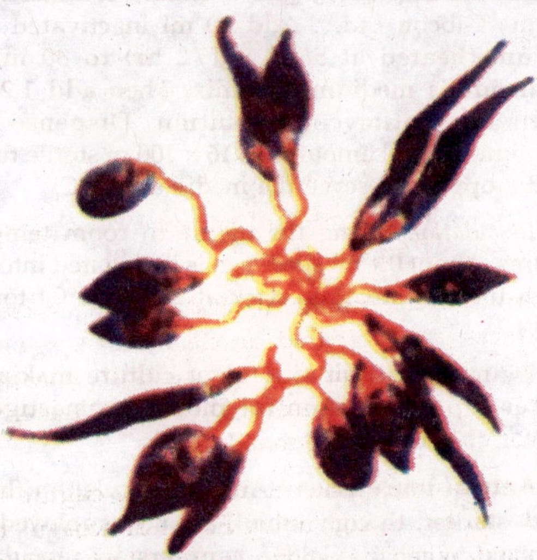

Fig. 15.8 : *Leishmania donovani* : Promastigote forms from culture (Giemsa stain × 100)

minutes. Allow the agar to cool to 45°-50°C. Add aseptically 20 ml defibrinated rabbit blood. Mix gently and dispense the medium in 5 ml amounts into 20 ml sterile screw-capped bottles (MCcartney type are preferable). Allow the medium to solidify with the bottles in a sloped position.

Inoculation : Specimen must be collected aseptically as bacterial contamination kills Leishmanial parasites :

(a) Two bottles of culture are aseptically inoculated with 0.1 ml of specimen in each.

(b) Incubate at 24°C (±2°C) for 4 weeks.

(c) Using a sterile wire loop transfer a drop of the culture to a slide every 4 days and examine after placing a cover glass by 40 × objective. Look for motile flagellated promastigotes of leishmania (Fig. 15.8).

(d) Subcultures are made from negative cultures after 8 days into fresh medium. The primary culture is examined every 4 days for promastigotes for a further period of 3 weeks.

2. Schneider's insect tissue culture medium

Preparation of medium

Schneider's Drosophila tissue culture medium	80 ml
Foetal calf serum	20 ml
Antibiotic-antimycotic soln.	1.2 ml

All the ingredients are available commercially from "Gibcon Ltd.". Add 20 ml inactivated calf serum (heated at 56°C × 1/2 hr) to 80 ml of Schneider's medium and mix. Then add 1.2 ml antibiotic-antimycotic solution. Dispense the medium in 3 ml amounts in 16 × 100 m sterile tubes and stopper. Preserve the media at –20°C.

Inoculation : Bring the media to room temperatures. About 0.1 ml specimen is inoculated into the each tube. Incubate in dark at 24°C (±2°C) for 14 days.

Examine daily a loopful of culture making a cover-slip preparation for motile promastigotes under 40 × objective.

Animal inoculation : Animal inoculation (hamster) studies, though useful, are not employed for routine diagnosis. Golden hamsters are inoculated intranasally for cutaneous and mucocutaneous leishmaniasis and peritoneally for visceral leishmaniasis with specimen, and killed after 2 to 3 months. Parasite can be seen in smears taken from the organs (liver and spleen).

Demonstration of antigen : Immunoblotting (Western blot test) PCR have been developed for detection of leishmanial antigens.

B. Indirect evidence

1. **Blood examination** : The blood picture in an established case of kala-azar include :

(a) Leucopenia with neutropenia, average leucocyte count – 3,000/cumm.

(b) Erythrocyte count is also decreased.

(c) Thrombocytopenia – platelet count is reduced to about 100,000/cumm.

(d) Serum globulin level is increased.

2. **Serological test** : Important serological tests comprise of a non-specific aldehyde test, specific test for detection of antileishmanial antibodies and leishmanial skin test.

(a) Non-specific tests

(i) *Napier's aldehyde test* (Formal-gel test) : The test depends on increase of non-specific polyclonal serum globulin in the patient's serum. The aldehyde test becomes positive only when the disease is more than 3 months' duration.

Test : Take 1-2 ml of serum in a test tube, add 2 drops of concentrated formalin (40% v/v) and mix well. Allow to stand up to 20 minutes.

Interpretation : A positive reaction is indicated by jellification of milk-white opacity like white of a hard boiled egg, usually in the course of 2-20 minutes. The reaction is called strongly positive. A milky appearance of serum without solidification may occur in 5-20 minutes in early visceral leishmaniasis.

Aldehyde test is also found positive in infections with *S. japonicum* and *T. brucei*. It is also positive in other hypergammaglobulinaemia *Multiple myeloma* and *Cirrhosis liver*. Aldehyde test is negative in cases of cutaneous leishmaniasis.

(ii) *Test with WKK antigen* : In the past decades, non-specific (non-leishmanial) antigen prepared from human tubercle bacillus by Witebsky, Klingenstein and Kuhn (hence referred to as WKK antigen) was employed for serological tests. The test is based on the fact that all mammal leishmaniae share some antigens between themselves as well as with some mycobacteria.

Complement fixation test with WKK antigen becomes positive early in disease. However, the test also becomes positive in some other conditions, e.g. tuberculosis, leprosy and tropical eosinophilia. The test is only of historic interest and is no more in use.

(b) Specific tests

Serological test for anti-leishmanial antibodies : In active visceral leishmaniasis, there is production of specific as well as non-specific polyclonal IgG and IgM antibodies.

Specific antileishmanial antibodies can be detected in patient's serum by indirect immunofluorescence test (IFAT), counter immunoelectrophoresis (CIE) and enzyme-linked immunosorbent assay (ELISA).

3. **Leishmanin skin (Montenegro) test**: Intradermal injection of 0.1 ml of killed promastigote suspension on the dorsoventral aspect of the fore arm shows negative result after 48-72 hrs in active visceral leishmaniasis and in diffuse cutaneous leishmaniasis (DCL). Positive result is indicated by an induration of 5 mm or more.

Leishmanin test is a delayed hypersensitivity reaction, useful for epidemiological surveys of a population to find out groups at risk for infection.

A combination of tissue smears (bone marrow, aspiration from spleen or lymph node), culture and animal inoculation may be required to optimise the laboratory diagnosis of leishmaniasis.

MALARIA

Causative agents of malaria

1. *Plasmodium vivax*, cause benign tertian malaria.

2. *Plasmodium falciparum*, causes malignant tertian malaria.

3. *Plasmodium malariae*, cause benign quartan malaria.

4. *Plasmodium ovale*, cause benign tertian malaria.

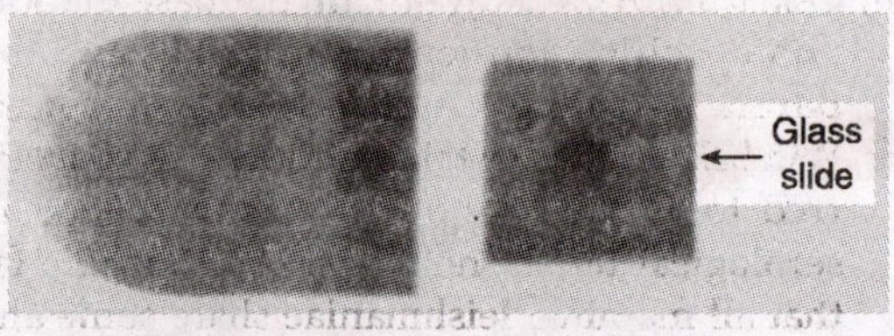

Fig. 15.9 : Preparation of thin and thick blood smear

Malarial parasites of animals

Several species of *Plasmodium* cause natural infection in animals and birds. Parasites other than those of primates cannot infect man and that too occurs rarely :

1. Monkey malarial parasites include *P. cynomolgi, P. inui, P. knowlesi, P. shortti, P. brasilianum.*

2. Malarial parasites of birds are *P. gallinaceum* (fowl), *P. relictum* (passerine birds).

Laboratory diagnosis

I. Demonstration of parasite

A. Examination of thin and thick blood film

Microscopic demonstration of parasites in the blood smears is the definitive method of diagnosis of malaria. Examination of both thin and thick smears or films of blood is recommended (Fig. 15.10). Thin film is useful for identifying the specific species and thick film is a concentration method in more volume of blood to detect the presence of organisms.

Specimen: Blood films should preferably be prepared directly from capillary blood. In case of EDTA anticoagulated blood, smears are to be made within an hour of collection of blood. Although blood films can be taken at any time over the course of infection before starting treatment, but the best time is the midway between paroxysm of chills and fever (a few hours after the peak of the fever), when the greatest number of intracellular organisms are present. It may be necessary to take repeated films at intervals of 5 to 6 hours.

(a) *Thin smear* : Wipe off the first drop of blood. The next drop of blood is touched with a clear dry glass slide, near one end. The blood is spread evenly and thinly with the edge of a spreader slide. The film should stop before it reaches the edge of the slide. The thin, feathered end should be at least 2 cm long, and the film should occupy the central area of the slide. Thin smears are one blood cell in thickness. The film is dried in air (Fig. 15.9).

(b) *Thick smear* : Usually 2 to 3 drops of capillary blood are directly placed from the finger prick to other end of the same slide as for thin smear or onto another slide. With the corner of another slide produce a square or circular patch of about 10 mm diameter. Continue stirring for 30 sec to prevent the formation of fibrin strands that may obscure the plasmodia after staining (Fig. 15.9). The optimum thickness of thick film is that which will just allow printed letters to be read through it.

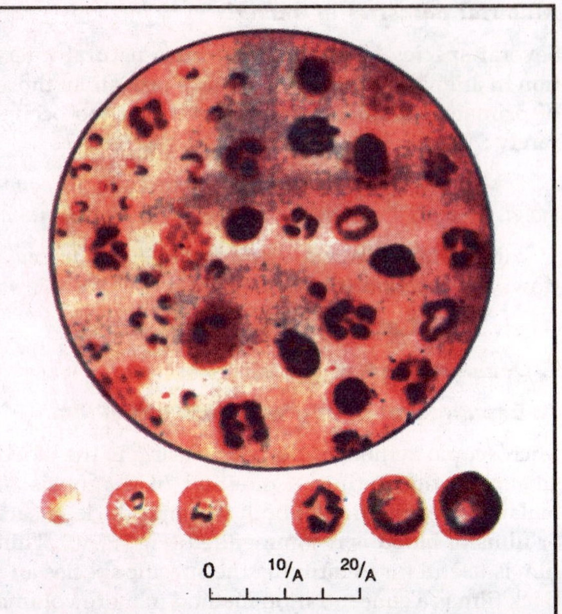

Fig. 15.10: *P. vivax* in thick blood film (Leishman stained). Blood smear shows trophozoite stage and gametocytes

Staining : Both films are air dried. The thick film is dehaemoglobinised by placing the film in distilled water in a vertical position in a glass cylinder for 5 to 10 minutes and then dried in air in upright position.

Both the films are now stained with Leishman's or Giemsa's stain. Other stains like Wright's or Field's stain or JSB (Jaswant Singh and Bhattacharji) stain may also be used.

Examination : All asexual erythrocytic stages, as well as gametocytes can be seen in the peripheral blood in *P. vivax* (Fig. 15.10), *P. ovale* and *P. malariae* infections, but in *P. falciparum* infection, only ring form and gametocytes can be seen (Fig. 15.11).

The typical text book presentation of the blood smears may not be always seen. A thin film is examined first and if parasites are found, there is no need to examine the thick film. If parasites are found in thick film, the thin film is reexamined thoroughly to determine the species :

1. **Ring form** (young trophozoites) of all species appear as streaks of blue cytoplasm with detached nuclear dots but species cannot be differentiated from their appearance.

2. Thick and thin blood films should be examined carefully for presence of characteristic rings of *P. falciparum* (Fig. 15.11), which frequently occur in multiples within a cell, as well as in the accole position. The presence of distinctive crescentic gametocytes in RBC is diagnostic of *P. falciparum*.

3. **Schizonts** and **gametocytes** more or less retain their normal appearances although, they appear smaller and less regular in outline. Presence of Schuffner's dots is also useful identifying point.

(a) Banana-shaped intraerythrocytic gametocytes (crescents) identify *P. falciparum* infection.

(b) Enlarged RBC with intracellular, coarse, brick-red stippling (Schuffner's dots) are characteristic of *P. vivax* infection.

(c) Schuffner's dots in oval-shaped RBCs are characteristic of *P. ovale* infection.

4. **Mixed infection** : Careful search in blood films should be made for mixed infections. Although, mixed infections can occur with any combination of the four species, most frequently the combination is *P. falciparum* and *P. vivax*.

Approximate quantitation of parasites : When parasites (trophozoites, schizonts and gametocytes) are found, an approximate number of parasites per thick film field (100 × objective) is :

+ = 1-10 parasites per 100 thick film fields.
++ = 11-100 parasites per 100 thick film fields.
+++ = 1-10 parasites per thick film field.
++++ = More than 10 parasites per thick film field.

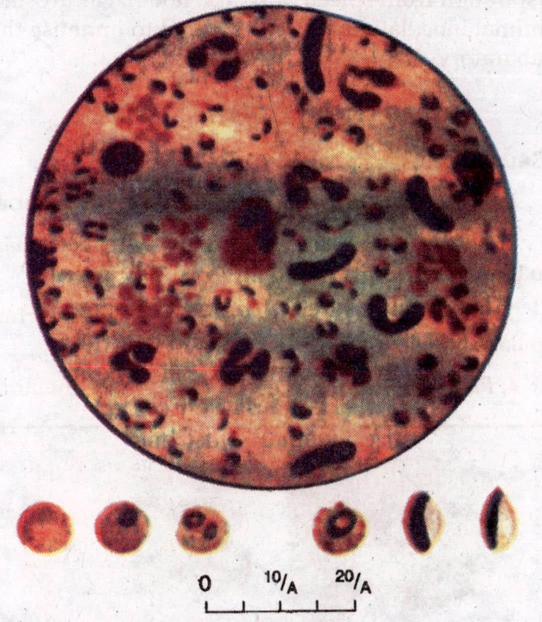

Fig. 15.11 : *P. falciparum* in thick blood film (Leishman-stained)

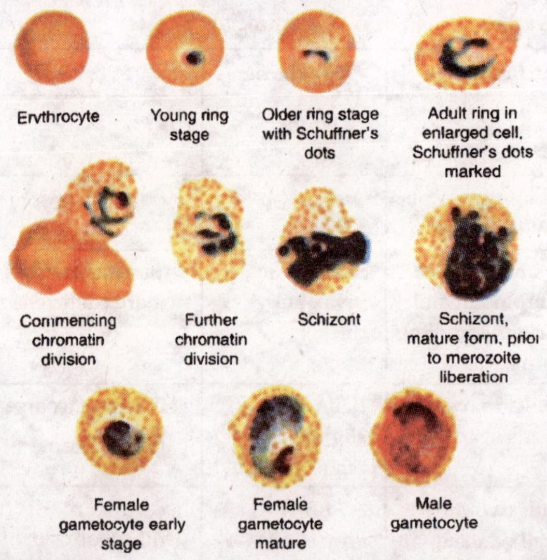

Fig. 15.12 : *Plasmodium vivax* : Erythrocytes stages. 1. Normal red cell; 2. Ring form (early trophozoite); 3. Older ring form, red cell contains Schuffner's dots; 4. Amoeboid trophozoite; 5, 6, 7. Early schizont; 8. Mature schizont; 9. Female gametocyte (early); 10. Female gametocyte (mature); 11. Male gametocyte.

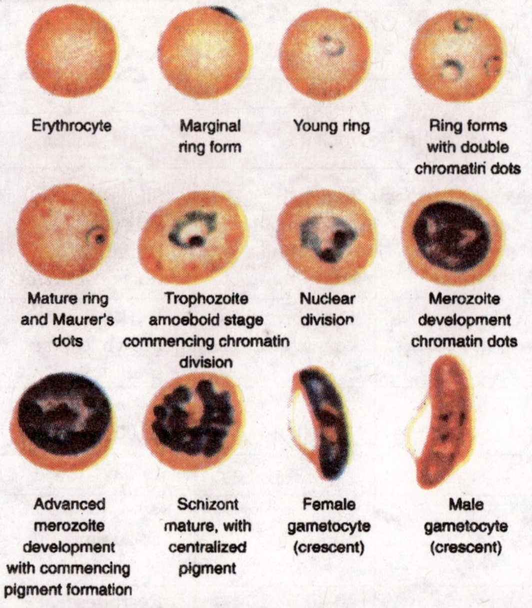

Fig. 15.13 : *Plasmodium falciparum* : Erythrocyte stage

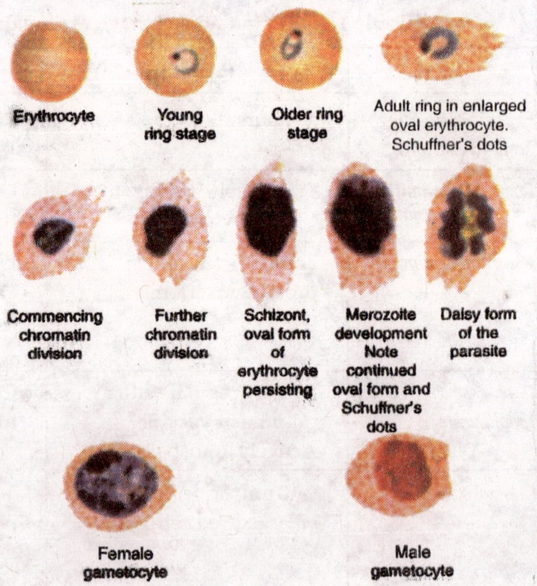

Fig. 15.14 : *Plasmodium malariae* : Erythrocyte stage × 2,000

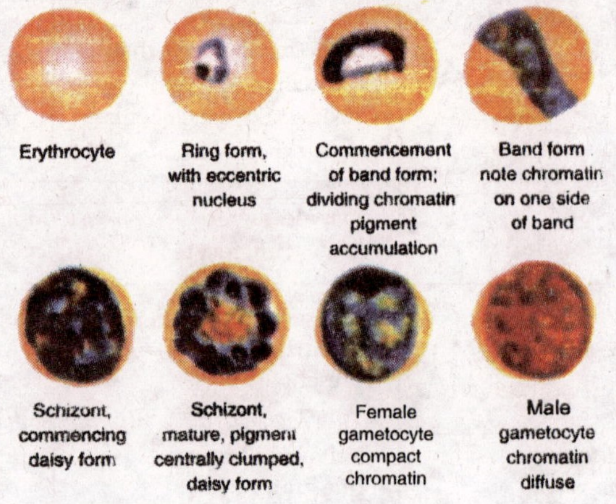

Fig. 15.15 : *Plasmodium ovale* : Erythrocyte stage × 2,000

The morphology of the four species of *Plasmodium* that infect humans in thin films are demonstrated in Figures 15.12 to 15.15 and summarised in Table 15.3. Identification is not difficult when abundant organisms are found.

B. Quantitative buffy coat smear

Parasites may be concentrated by microhaematocrit centrifugation using glass capillary tube and closely fitting plastic insert (QBC malaria blood tubes, Becton Dickinson, Sparks, Md, USA). The QBC (quantitative buffy coat) tube is a specially prepared glass haematocrit tube, precoated internally with acridine orange stain and potassium oxalate.

Table 15.3 : Differential characters of malarial parasites of man during erythrocytic phases

	P. vivax	*P. falciparum*	*P. malariae*	*P. ovale*
Erythrocytic schizogony (duration)	48 hours	48 hours	72 hours	48 hours
Forms of parasite in peripheral blood	Trophozoites, schizonts, Gametocytes	Only ring and crescents (gametocytes)	As in vivax	As in vivax
Ring form in a RBC	Large 2.5 μm, single prominent chromatin	Delicate, small, 1.5 μm, Double chromatin and multiple rings common. Accole forms found	Same as in vivax but thicker	Same as in vivax, more compact.
Late trophozoite	Large, irregular with a prominent vacuole. Actively amoeboid	Compact, seldom seen in blood smear	Band-like slightly amoeboid	Compact, coarse pigment.
Schizont	9-10 μm, large, fills an enlarged red cell	4-5 μm, fills two-thirds of a red cell which is not enlarged. Usually not seen in blood smear	6-7 μm, almost fills a normal-sized red cell	6.2 μm, fills three quarters.
Number of merozoites	12-24, arranged in irregular grape-like cluster	18-24, arranged in grape-like cluster	6-12, daisy-head, or rosette pattern	6-12 irregularly arranged
Gametocytes	Spherical or globular. Size – much larger than a red cell, male 9 μm, female 10-11 μm. Host cell enlarged with Schuffner's dots	Crescentic. Larger than a red cell, male 9-11 μm, female 12-14 μm. Host cell hardly recognisable	As in vivax. (7 μm)	As in vivax. (9 μm)
	Female gametocyte : Blue cytoplasm; small and compact nucleus Male gametocyte : Pale blue cytoplasm; large and diffuse nucleus			
Infected erythrocyte	Enlarged, pale, Schuffner's dots present	Normal size, Maurer's dots (large red spots) sometimes basophilic stippling	Normal, occasionally Ziemann's stippling	Slightly enlarged, Schuffner's dots prominent
Malarial pigment	Yellowish brown, fine granules	Dark brown or blackish, one or two solid blocks	Dark brown, coarse granules	Dark yellowish brown, coarse granules
Maximal parasitaemia	25,000/μl	1,00,000/μl	10,000/μl	25,000/μl
Incubation period	14 days	12 days	30 days	14 days
Duration of first attack, (untreated)	18-20 days	10-20 days	6 months	18-20 days
Relapse period	2-5 years	Recrudescence	10-40 years Recrudescence	Recrudescence, rare
Duration of sporogony in mosquito at 25°C	9-10 days	10-12 days	25-28 days	14-16 days
Drug resistance	No	Yes	No	No

A volume of 56-65 microlitres of blood collected from finger, ear or heel puncture and centrifuged at 12,000 rpm for 5 minutes. RBCs containing malarial parasites are less dense than normal red cells and concentrate just below the leucocytes at the top of the erythrocytic column.

The parasite contains DNA but the mature RBCs do not contain DNA and RNA. Parasitic DNA is detected by acridine orange stain and appear as bright specks of light among the non-fluorescing erythrocytes. When the QBC malaria blood tubes are rotated under a special type of lens (paralens), almost all the plasmodia in the blood sample can be visualised.

C. Microconcentration technique

Blood is collected in microhaematocrit tube and centrifuged at high speed. The sediment is mixed with normal serum and smear prepared. Although, the positivity rate is increased by this technique, but there is change in morphology of the parasite.

II. Immunodiagnosis

Serology cannot match the sensitivity of microscopic detection of malarial parasite, but may assist diagnosis of light infection. It has got limited value in clinical diagnosis because they will not differentiate between an active and a past infection. These antibody test including indirect fluorescent antibody (IFA) test and indirect haemagglutination assay (IHA), ELISA and RIA are useful for epidemiological purposes.

III. Newer approaches to diagnosis

A. Rapid and simple stick test (ParaSight F test, Becton Dickinson, Europe).

This test is based on detection of a monoclonal antibody against *P. falciparum* histidine rich protein 2 antigen. This test is based on antigen capture approach and has been incorporated in a **dipstick** format. Antibodies specific for *P. falciparum* HRP 2 are immobilised in the dipstick (test strip) when dipped in blood. A solid pink line indicates positive test. This test is very useful in treatment and diagnosis of drug-resistant *P. falciparum*.

B. Use of fluorescent dye : Benzothiocarboxypurine (fluorescent dye) intensely stains nucleic acid of malarial parasites after penetrating RBCs. The dye does not stain nuclei of WBCs. This is useful in field laboratory for mass screening because of rapid staining and evaluation but it requires a fluorescent microscope.

C. Detection of parasitic antigen : Detection of malarial antigens by RIA, DNA probes and PCR are under evaluation.

ASCARIASIS

A. Direct evidences

1. **Demonstration of adult worm** : This is sometimes possible in the following situations :

(a) When adult worm is spontaneously passed in stool or vomitus.

(b) Administration of anthelminthics may result in expulsion of worm and its detection.

2. **Detection of egg** : *Ascaris* egg can be detected in stool by direct wet mount and also by concentration method.

(a) *Direct wet mount* : Diagnosis is usually made microscopically by finding of eggs in a direct saline preparation of faeces. Since many eggs are produced, concentration techniques are rarely required. A single female *A. lumbricoides* may account for 3 eggs per mg of faeces. Usually both fertilised and unfertilised eggs are found (Table 15.4). Fertilised eggs may sometimes appear decorticated. Rarely semidecorticated unfertilised egg is encountered (Table 15.4). When a patient harbours only male parasite(s), eggs are not found in the stool.

(b) *Concentration technique* : Occasionally, when the worm infestation is light, concentration technique may be necessary. Unfertilised eggs are not detectable by salt floatation. Sedimentation technique is more sensitive than floatation method.

(c) Duodenal aspirate of an infected patient collected by duodenal intubation also shows eggs.

3. **Demonstration of larva in sputum** : *Ascaris* larvae may be detected in sputum in Loeffler's syndrome along with eosinophils and Charcot-Leyden crystals.

B. Indirect evidences

1. **Blood examination** : Eosinophil count may be increased at the early stage of infection.

2. **Skin test** : Skin test with *A. lumbricoides* antigen gives a positive result, but is unreliable and not used for diagnosis.

3. **Serological test** : Serological tests are of particular use in *Ascaris pneumonitis*. The available tests include ELISA, IHA and microprecipitation on larvae. Although these tests are useful in serosurvey, but is not useful in routine diagnosis.

Table 15.4 : Features of eggs of *A. lumbricoides*

Types of egg	*Main features*	*Diagrams*
Fertilised egg	1. *Shape* : Round or oval in shape 2. *Size* : 60-75 µm × 40-50 µm 3. *Colour* : Bile stained (yellow-brown) 4. *Egg shell* : Surrounded by thick smooth translucent shell consisting of three layers – outer coarsely mammaliated albuminous coat, a thick transparent middle layer, and the inner lipoidal vitelline membrane. 5. *Content* : A large unsegmented ovum of granular mass with a clear space at each pole. 6. *Concentration* : Floats in saturated solution of common salt.	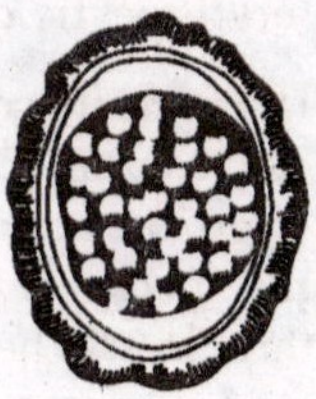
Unfertilised egg	1. *Shape* : Elliptical 2. *Size* : 80 µm × 55 µm 3. *Colour* : Bile stained 4. *Egg shell* : Thinner, with the outer mammillary albumin coat scanty and irregular. 5. *Content* : Contains a small atrophied ovum with a mass of disorganised, highly refractile granules of various sizes. 6. *Concentration* : Does not float in saturated salt solution.	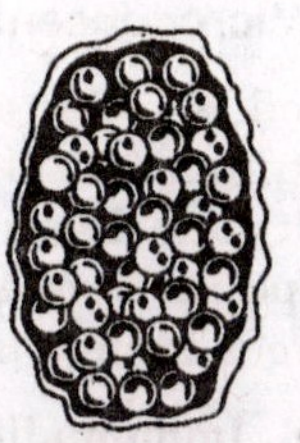
Semidecorticated egg	1. Features are similar as for fertilised egg except that shell is single, smooth, thick and colourless or very pale yellow. 2. *Content* : A round, colourless granular central mass. 3. *Concentration* : Floats in saturated salt solution.	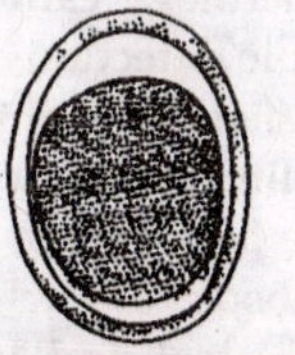
Semi-decorticated unfertilised egg	1. *Shell* : A single thin smooth colourless shell. 2. *Content* : Large roundish refractile granules. 3. *Concentration* : Does not float in saturated salt solution.	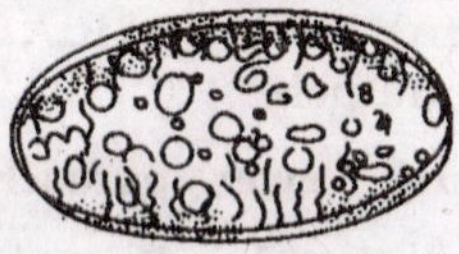

ENTEROBIUS VERMICULARIS

1. **Cellophane tape test** : Diagnosis is made by finding *E. vermicularis* eggs in morning samples collected from perianal skin by applying the adhesive surface of cellophane tape or by NIH (devised by National Institute of Health, USA) swabs (Fig. 15.16). The tape is mounted in water or 0.1 M sodium hydroxide on a slide with the adhesive side down, covered with a cover slip and examined under a microscope. Other methods (e.g. the use of anal swabs) have also been used effectively to demonstrate enterobius infections. The ova (about 55 × 25 µm in size) are oval, flattened on one side and usually contain a larva.

(a) Specimens are to be collected prior to bathing or going to toilet.

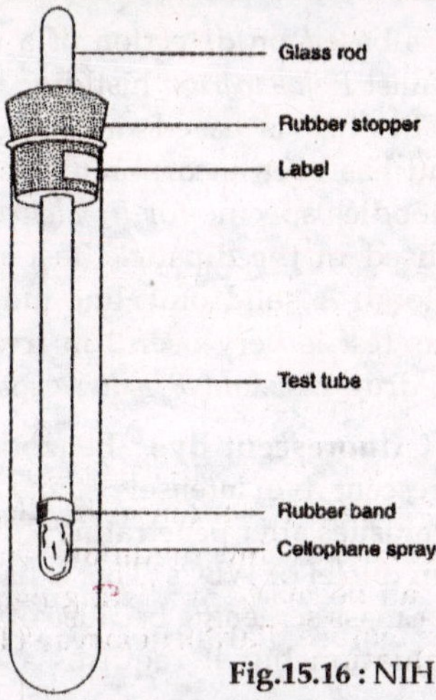

Fig.15.16 : NIH swab

(b) Four to six consecutive negative finding of tape preparations are required to rule out pinworm infection.

2. **Stool samples** :

(a) Eggs may also be found in faeces in patients with heavy worm burdens.

(b) Adult female worms may be found in faeces.

HOOKWORMS

Species

Group I : True human parasites (Anthrophilic)

1. *Ancylostoma duodenale*
2. *Necator americanus*

} Cause ancylostomiasis in man

Group II : True human parasites (Anthrophilic)

1. *Ancylostoma braziliense* found in dogs and cats in Brazil.

2. *A. caninum* — found in dogs and cats in most tropical areas.

3. *A. ceylanicum* (According to some it is nothing but *A. braziliense*) found in civet cat in Sri Lanka.

4. *Uncinaria stenocephala* found in dogs, cats and foxes in Europe and North America.

Ancylostomiasis, caused by these two principal human hookworms, is one of the main causes of anaemia in tropics. Other species of the genus *Ancylostoma* also may produce human infections in various parts of the world. *Necator americanus* is found in USA as well as other parts of the world, but *A. duodenale* does not occur in the USA, although its geographical distribution elsewhere in tropical and subtropical Asia overlaps that of *Necator*. All hookworms have common morphologic characteristics with some minor difference. Infection with *N. americanus* is more common throughout India, South-East Asia, Africa and S. America. *A. duodenale* is found in Middle-East, Mediterranean and in Punjab and UP in India.

The zoophilic (animal) parasites rarely or never mature in man and cause *creeping eruption* or *cutaneous larva migrans*.

Laboratory diagnosis

The diagnosis of hookworm infection is made by demonstration of eggs in the faeces by direct microscopy or by concentration methods. The species identification can be made by distinguishing adult worms and the mature filariform larvae (Table 15.5, Fig. 15.17).

Table 15.5
Differential characteristics of filariform larvae (3rd stage larvae) of *A. duodenale* and *N. americanus*

	A. duodenale	*N. americanus*
Size	720 μm	660 μm
Head	Blunt	Pointed
Sheath	Faint cuticular striations	Prominent striations, especially at posterior end
Intestine	No apparent gap between intestine and oesophagus	Apparent gap between intestine and oesophagus
Oesophageal smears	Not prominent	Prominent
Tail	Long and blunt	Short and pointed

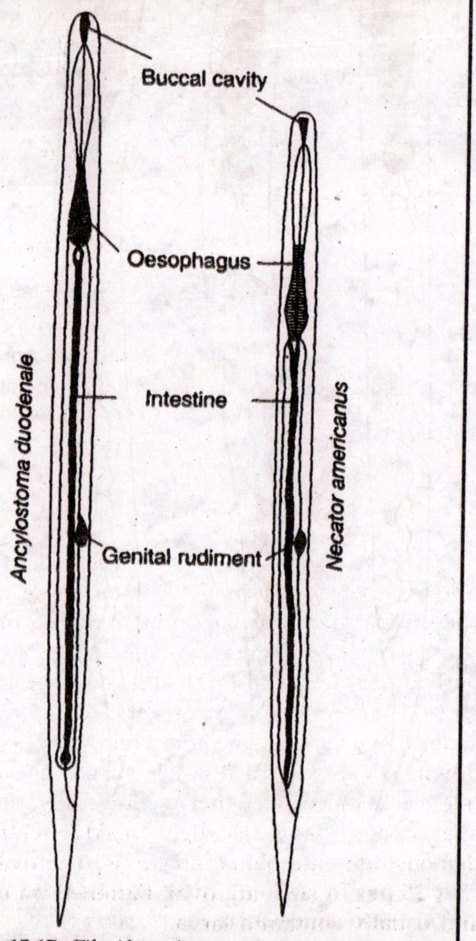

Fig.15.17 : Filariform larvae of *A. duodenale* and *N. americanus*

I. Direct evidence

1. **Examination of stool** : Demonstration of characteristic eggs in direct wet mount of faeces establishes diagnosis. Eggs of *Ancylostoma* and *Necator* are morphologically indistinguishable. However, if direct smear is negative, a concentration smear should be made.

Routine examination : (i) Microscopic examination of a direct faecal smear (saline mount) is made. With counts of fewer than 5 eggs per cover slip preparation indicate light infections unlikely to produce anaemia. Counts above 25 eggs per coverslip indicate heavy infection.

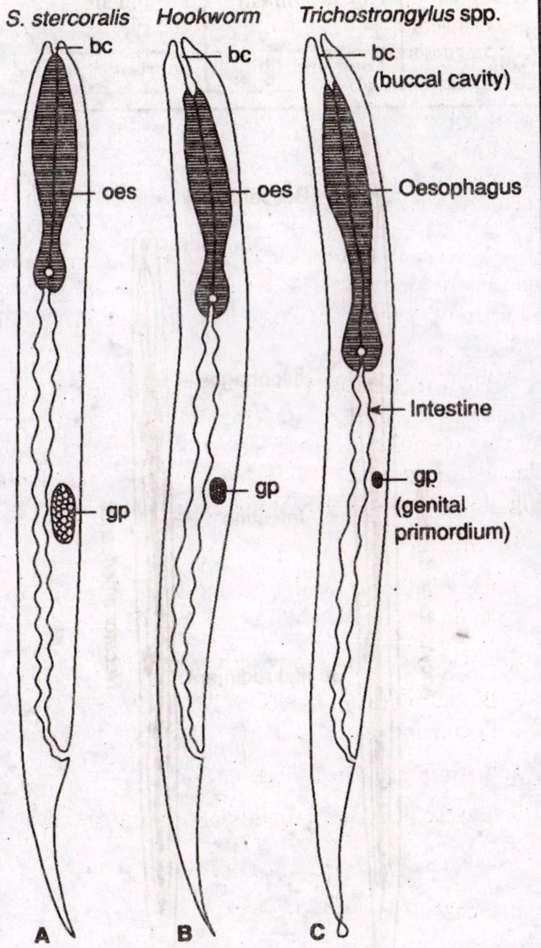

Fig.15.18 : Rhabditiform larvae of (A) *S. stercoralis*; (B) Hookworm; (C) *Trichostrongylus* spp. (Note : Larva of *S. stercoralis* has short buccal cavity, while that of hookworm larva is long).

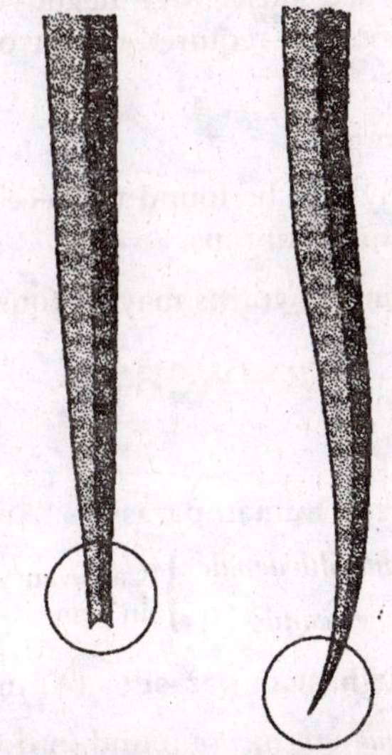

15.19 : Tail of filariform larva : *S. stercoralis* (presence of slit) and hookworm (pointed tail)

(ii) When there has been a prolonged delay in examination of the stool samples (usually more than a day), larvae may develop and hatch. The first-stage rhabditiform larvae) of hookworm has to be differentiated from those of *Strongyloides stercoralis*, the stage typically passed in stool of human strongyloidiasis. The rhabditiform larva of hookworm has a long, narrow buccal chamber and an inconspicuous genital operculum (Fig. 15.18).

(iii) The species differentiation of hookworm can be made by studying adult worms or culturing larval stages to the infective filariform stage with subsequent differentiation of larval forms (Figs. 15.17 and 15.19).

Concentration method

Concentration methods are useful in detection of light infection and to assess the worm load. The following techniques are usually followed.

A. **Formal ether sedimentation technique** : About a gram of faeces is emulsified in 7-10% formol saline (fixative) and left for 10 minutes. It is then strained by an wire gauge (40 meshes to an inch) in a centrifuge tube. Add 3 ml ether to the filtrate and shake vigorously for one minute and then centrifuge at 2,000 rpm for 2 minutes. Allow to settle. Supernatant fluid with debris is decanted leaving 1-2 drops. Cover-slip preparation from the deposit is examined for ova and cyst. In this technique cysts, eggs and larvae are fixed and sedimented. Count the number of eggs which give the approximate number of ova per gram of faeces.

B. Salt floatation technique : Common salt or zinc sulphate are used for concentration of ova, cysts and larvae.

(a) *Saturated sodium chloride technique* : The faecal sample is dissolved in a solution of higher density so that eggs float on surface. Eggs float after 20-30 minutes and begins to sink after 60 minutes :

(i) One quarter of a 20-25 ml test tube is filled with saturated solution of sodium chloride.

(ii) About one gram of faeces is emulsified in the solution using a glass rod or stick and then 12-15 ml salt solution is added.

(iii) The tube is kept in a completely vertical position on a rack. Any coarse matter may be removed.

(iv) Using a Pasteur pipette, further solution is added to ensure that the tube is filled to the brim.

(v) A cover glass is carefully laid on the top of the tube, so that the cover slip is in contact with the fluid.

(vi) The preparation is allowed to stand for 30-35 minutes undisturbed for the cysts and eggs to float.

(vii) The cover glass is lifted carefully from the tube by a straight pull upwards and placed on slide with face downwards.

(viii) Examine under low power (10 × objective) and count the number of ova which gives an approximate idea of the number of ova per gram of faeces.

Application : Common salt floatation method is useful for concentrating *Ascaris* eggs or hookworm eggs in field surveys.

(b) *Zinc sulphate floatation method* : This technique is similar to that of salt floatation method except that 33% zinc sulphate solution is used in place of saturated sodium chloride. Slide is prepared in the same way.

During microscopy, the unstained preparation is first examined, and then a drop of iodine is placed under the cover glass and viewed under high power (40 ×). Cysts of *Giardia lamblia* and *E. histolytica* and some other ova float in the method. The cysts appear distinct in iodine preparation.

Table 15.6 shows the comparative result of the three concentration tests.

Table 15.6 : Comparative analysis of different faecal concentration techniques

Parasite	Formal ether	Sat. NaCl	Zinc sulphate
Cysts			
Giardia lamblia	+	–	+
E. histolytica	+	–	+
Eggs			
Ascaris lumbricoides (fertilised)	+	+	–
Hookworm	+	+	–
Trichuris trichiura	+	–	+
Taenia species	+	–	–
Schistosoma species	+	–	–
Fasciola species	+	–	–
Opisthorcis species	+	–	+
Larvae			
Strongyloides stercoralis	+	–	–

2. **Study of duodenal contents** : Aspirate obtained from duodenum by duodenal intubation (Ryle's tube) may sometimes contain eggs or adult hookworms.

3. **Culture** : Stool culture may be done using Harada-Mori filter paper strip technique or charcoal culture method. It is necessary to distinguish the filariform larvae of *A. duodenale* and *N. americanus* (Fig. 15.17) on epidemiological ground.

II. Indirect evidences

1. Occult blood (benzidine) test of stool is positive.
2. Anaemia — microcytic hypochromic.
3. Blood picture — Hb, PCV, MCV, MCHC all decreased.
4. Eosinophilia in blood.
5. Charcot-Leyden crystals are found in stool.

FILARIAL WORMS

Filarioidea (Filarial worms)

Based on normal habitats of adult worms, filarial infections can be divided into four groups which include :

A. **Lymphatic filariasis**

Wuchereria bancrofti, Brugia malayi, Brugia timori.

B. Subcutaneous filariasis

+ *Loa loa*

Onchocerca volvulus

Mansonella streptocerca

C. Serous cavity filariasis

Mansonella ozzardi (mesentery)

Mansonella perstans

D. Animal tissue nematodes

Dirofilaria

Dirofilaria immitis (dog heartworm)

Dirofilaria tenuis (raccoon parasite)

Dirofilaria repens (dog parasite)

+ *Loa loa* and some animal filaria (e.g. *Dirofilaria conjunctivae)* also infect conjunctivae.

These animal parasites sometimes infect man and cause pulmonary dirofilariasis and erythematous subcutaneous nodules.

Eight species of filarial worms infect humans that cause filariasis, but traditionally the term filariasis refers to lymphatic filariasis attributable to *W. bancrofti, Brugia malayi* and *Brugia timori*. They can be differentiated on the basis of their location in the body and characteristics of microfilaria (Fig. 15.21).

Laboratory diagnosis

Specimens :

(i) Microfilaria begins to appear in **blood** a year or more after an infection. Diagnosis is established by detection of microfilaria of *W. bancrofti* in blood.

(ii) Occasionally, microfilaria can be found in chylous **urine** or hydrocele fluid.

(iii) Sections of adult worms are sometimes detected in **biopsied lymph node.**

The procedures adopted for laboratory diagnosis are shown in Fig. 15.20.

A. Direct evidences

Microscopy : Definitive diagnosis is made by detection of microfilariae in a thick blood smear and chylous fluid.

Examination of blood : It should be remembered that most microfilariae of *W. bancrofti* and *B. malayi* typically exhibit nocturnal periodicity.

Collection time :

(a) For periodic *W. bancrofti* – 22.00-04.00 hrs.

(b) Subperiodic (nocturnal) *W. bancrofti* – 20.00-22.00 hrs.

(c) Subperiodic (diurnal) *W. bancrofti* – 14.00-18.00 hrs.

1. **Blood** : About 5-6 ml venous blood collected in an anticoagulant (Pot. oxalate or Sodium citrate) is centrifuged and the deposit is examined by :

(a) *Thick smear technique* : Smear made from two drops of deposit is stained by Leishman/Giemsa stain and examined microscopically.

(b) *Wet-slide preparation* : Two drops of deposit is mixed with equal volume of water (to lyse the red cells) on a slide. The preparation is covered with a cover slip and examined microscopically using low power (10 × objective).

Larger volumes of blood increase the diagnostic sensitivity. Membrane filtration of microfilariae from 10 ml oxalated or citrated blood is better than the concentrated sediment prepared by centrifugation.

W. bancrofti, B. malayi and *Loa loa* demonstrate a sheath on their microfilaria (Fig. 15.21) and is the first step in the identification of specific types of filariasis. Further differentiation is based on the study of the head and tail structure of microfilariae (Fig. 15.22). *W. bancrofti* does not have nuclei in the tip of the tail, while *B. malayi* has two prominent

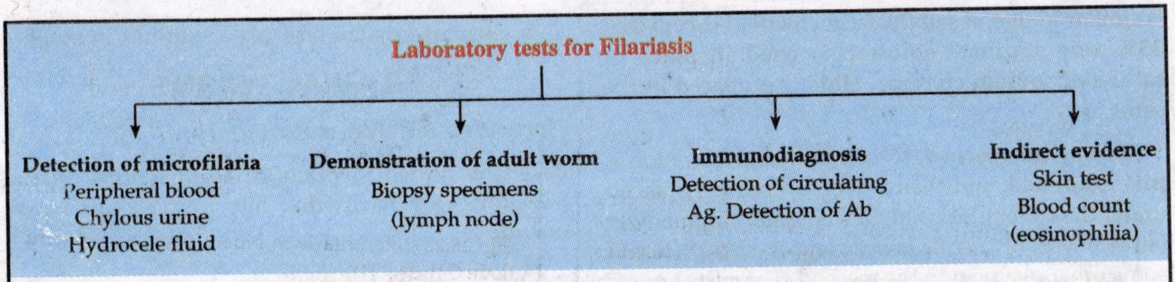

Fig. 15.20 : Schematic presentation of diagnostic tests of lymphatic filariasis

nuclei at the tip of the tail. An exact species identification is not critical from treatment point of view because treatment of all the filarial infections, except *Onchocerca volvulus*, is identical.

DEC provocation test: A small single dose of diethyl carbamazine (2 mg/kg BW) makes microfilaria to appear in peripheral blood even during day time. After 30-50 min of administration of a 100 mg DEC tablet in an adult, blood sample is collected for detection of microfilaria. This is useful in mass screening.

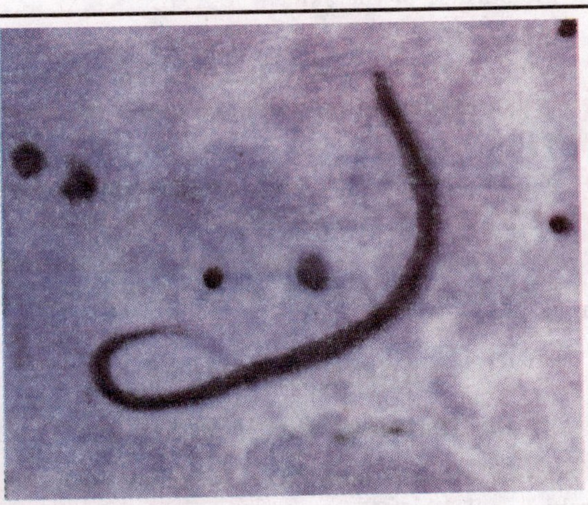

Fig. 15.21. Microfilaria *(W. bancrofti)* in peripheral blood

2. **Examination of chylous fluid**: Chylous fluid is creamy white and opalescent. **Chyle** consists of lymph and particles of digested fat (ether soluble). When blood is also present, the specimen appears pinkish-white. About 10-20 ml of first urine passed by the patient in the morning is collected.

Procedure : Urine is centrifuged at 2,000 rpm for 10-15 minutes. The supernatant is thrown out and the deposit is mixed with equal volume of water and centrifuged again. The supernatant is discarded and wet preparation from deposit is placed on slide, covered by cover slip, examined for the presence of microfilariae. The deposit may be smeared on slide and stained by Leishman or Giemsa stain.

3. **Examination of biopsy specimens**: Adult filarial worms can sometimes be found in sections of biopsied lymph nodes (Fig. 15.23) as incidental finding but this is not done for routine diagnosis.

4. **Detection of circulating antigen**: With the development of monoclonal antibodies, detection of circulating filarial antigen has been done in reference laboratory. The result is promising but the test is not widely available as a diagnostic test.

B. Indirect evidences

1. **Immunological tests**: Specific antibodies against filarial antigen can be detected by serological tests. A hypersensitivity reaction to filarial antigen is often observed.

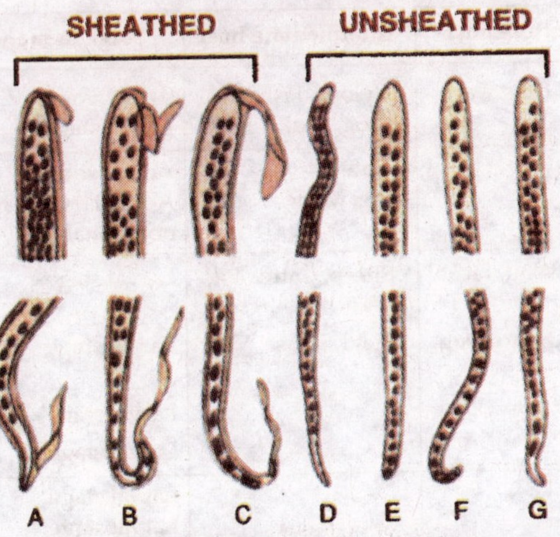

Fig. 15.22. Differential characteristics of human microfilariae: Sheathed microfilariae: *A-W. bancrofti; B-B. malayi; C–Loa loa.* Unsheathed microfilariae : *D-O. volvulus; E-M. perstans; F-M. streptocerca; G-M. ozzardi*

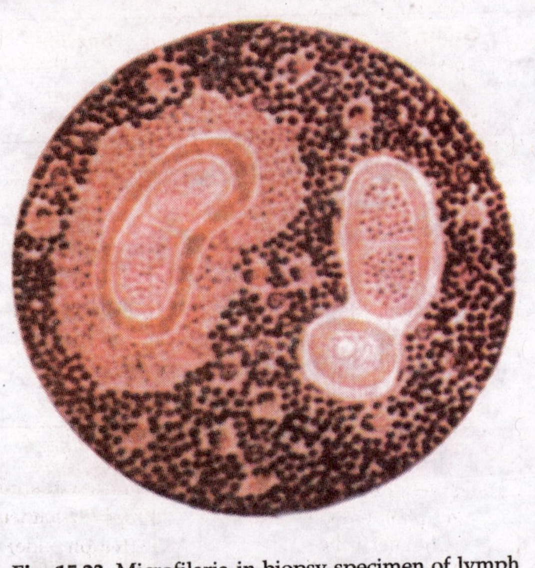

Fig. 15.23. Microfilaria in biopsy specimen of lymph node (HE section)

(a) *Detection of serum antibody* : Using *Brugia pahangi* antigen, fluorescent antibody tests (FAT) and ELISA can detect over 95% of active cases and 70% of established elephantiasis. Cross-reactions are observed in 15% cases of strongyloides and 5% of other intestinal nematodes.

Since microfilaria are often difficult to find in blood in bancroftian filariasis, the antibody detection tests are giving promising results. The test becomes negative 1-2 years after cure.

(b) *IgG subclasses antibodies against B malayi* : There is significantly higher level of filarial IgG4 antibodies in blood of microfilaraemic carriers, acute cases and in occult filariasis suggesting presence of active filarial infection in these patients (Bhunia et al, 2003). Filarial antigen detection shows significantly high level of antigen in this group.

(c) *Skin test* : Intradermal skin tests using filarial antigen (extracts of microfilariae, adult worms and third stage larvae of *B. malayi* or of the dog filaria *Dirofilaria immitis*), show immediate type hypersensitivity which persists for life. The diagnostic value of the test is limited due to high false-positivity.

2. **Blood count** : Eosinophilia (5-15%) is a common finding.

GUINEA WORM

Causative agent

The adult female of *Dracunculus medinensis* (also called guinea worm) resides in the subcutaneous tissue, especially of legs, arms and back. At the site of localisation, the worm sets up an inflammatory reaction producing a papule and then blister.

Laboratory diagnosis

1. **Detection of adult worm** : Diagnosis is made by observing the typical ulcer and the female worm at the surface of the skin.

2. **Detection of embryos** : The affected (ulcer) is flooded with water that induces the release of embryos which can be examined under the microscope.

3. **Intradermal test** with dracunculus antigen leads to a wheal type reaction after 24 hours.

4. **X-ray examination** may show coiled structure or linear density (up to 25 cm) or calcified worm in deeper tissues.

TAENIA SAGINATA

Systemic classification of cestodes

Systemic classification of cestodes has been described in Table 15.7.

Table 15.7 : Systemic classification of cestodes

Group	Genus	Species	Definitive host	Intermediate host	Stage in man
1. Pseudophyllidea	*Diphyllobothrium*	*D. latum* *D. mansoni*	Man, Dog, Cat Dog, Cat	Cylops, Fish Frog, Snake, Man	Adult worm Larval stage
2. Cyclophyllidea	*Taenia*	*T. saginata* *T. solium*	Man Man	Cow Pig, Man	Adult worm Adult, larval stage occasionally
	Echinococcus	*E. granulosus*	Dog, Wolf, Jackal	Sheep, Cattle, Pig, Man	Larval stage
		E. multilocularis	Fox, Dingo, Dog, Wolf	Field mouse, Vole	Larval stage
		E. oligarthus *E. vogeli*	....	....	Larval stage Larval stage
	Multiceps	*M. multiceps* *M. serialis*	....	....	Larval stage Larval stage
	Hymenolepis	*H. nana* *H. diminuta*	Man, Rat Rat (Man)	Not required Rat flea	Adult and larval stages in intestine Adult worm
	Dipylidium	*D. caninum*	Dog, Cat (Man)	Dog flea	Adult worm

Table 15.8 : Distinguishing features of adult worms of *T. saginata* and *T. solium*

Features	*T. saginata*	*T. solium*
Length	5-10 metres	2-3 metres
Scolex	Large, quadrate, four suckers, no rostellum and no hooklets, measures 1-2 mm	Small, globular, four suckers, with rostellum and hooks, measures 1 mm
Neck	Fairly long and narrow (0.5 mm wide). It is quite fragile	Neck is short, about 5-10 mm in length
Proglottids	1,000–2,000 Segments expelled singly and may force anal sphincter	Below 1,000 Segments expelled passively in chains of 5-6
Uterus	Lateral branches 15-30 on each side, thin and dichotomous	Lateral branches 5-10 on each side, thick and dendritic
Vagina	Vaginal sphincter present	Vaginal sphincter absent
Ovaries	2 in number, no accessory lobe	2 in number with an accessory lobe
Testes	300-400 follicles	150-200 follicles
Life span (Adult)	10 years or more	Upto 25 years

Laboratory diagnosis

A. Direct evidences

Laboratory confirmation of diagnosis of *T. saginata* infection is made by demonstration of gravid segments and eggs passed in faeces.

Microscopic examination of stool :

Eggs with characteristic thin shell and six hooked oncosphere, are diagnostic. Since eggs of *T. saginata* and *T. solium* are indistinguishable, the species diagnosis is to be made by examining the gravid segment (Table 15.8). Moreover, eggs are not frequently found in faeces because of absence of uterine openings.

T. saginata segment shows :

(a) 15-30 lateral branches of uterus.

(b) No accessory lobe in the ovary.

(c) Presence of vaginal sphincter muscle.

(d) Typical isoenzyme patterns.

Microscopic examination of segment

Species identification is made by examining gravid segment. The gravid segment pressed between two slides and is examined by a hand lens that will show 15-20 lateral branches of uterus in each segment.

B. Serology

Serodiagnosis by IHA, ELISA and IFA have been used for detection of *T. saginata* and *T. solium* coproantigens which appear to be very promising.

Diagnosis in animals

ELISA and CIEP using oncosphere as antigen have been used with some success. In slaughtered cattle, cysticercus bovis can be seen by naked eye.

TAENIA SOLIUM

MORPHOLOGY

Adult worm

Adult worm lives in the small intestine (upper jejunum) of man and it is 2-3 metres in length and life span upto 25 yrs. Commonly a single worm is present, but several worms up to 25 or more may sometimes be found in a patient.

Scolex (head) : Head measures 1 mm in diameter (pin-head size) and globular, possesses a rostellum armed with double rows of hooklets and 4 circular suckers (Figs. 15.24 and 15.25).

Neck : Short, 5-10 mm long.

Proglottids : Number 800-900, gravid segment measures 12 mm × 6 mm, being twice as long as wide. The proglottids of *T. solium* resemble those of *T. saginata* in general. Gravid uterus consists of a median longitudinal stem with 5-10 compound lateral branches on each side (Figs. 15.26 and 15.27).

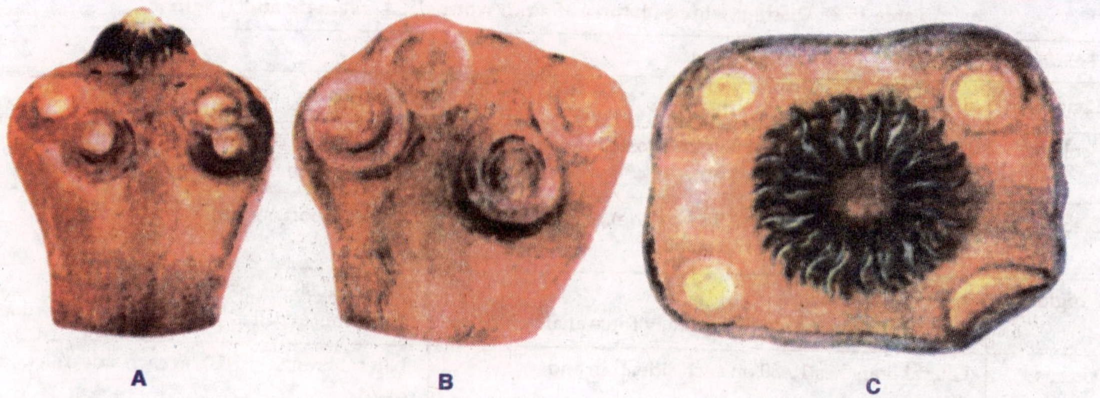

Fig. 15.24. Scolex of *T. solium* and *T. saginata*. A : Armed scolex of *T. solium* with four circular suckers and rostellum with hooklets. B : Unarmed scolex of *T. saginata* with four circular suckers and without a rostellum and hooklets. C : Scolex of *T. solium* when viewed from above.

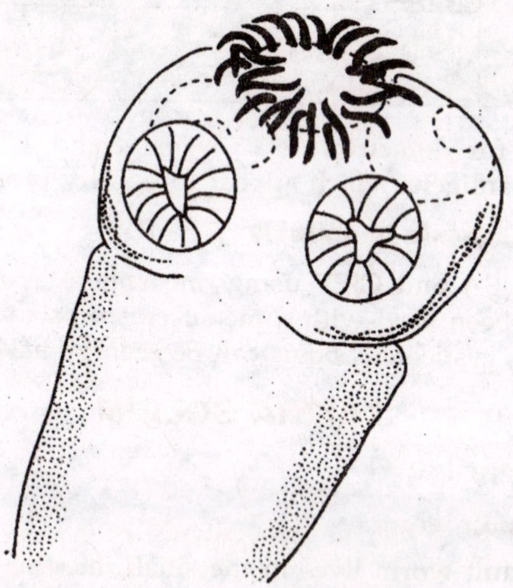

Fig. 15.25 : Scolex of *T. solium*

In mature proglottids, the ovary has 2 lobes and an accessory lobe (in *T. saginata*, accessory lobe lacking), and a vaginal sphincter muscle is lacking (present in *T. saginata*).

Proglottids are not very active. The gravid segments are not passed singly, but pass out passively as short chains.

The differential characteristics of gravid adult *T. solium* and *T. saginata* are shown in Table 15.6.

Laboratory diagnosis

1. Intestinal taeniasis :

Laboratory confirmation of diagnosis is made by

(a) Identifying gravid segments passed in faeces.
(b) Detection of eggs in faeces.

2. Human cysticercosis

(a) Calcified cyst in muscles can be recognised *radiologically* and by *biopsy*.

(b) **CT scans** or **MRI** techniques may reveal the presence of cysticerci in the brain.

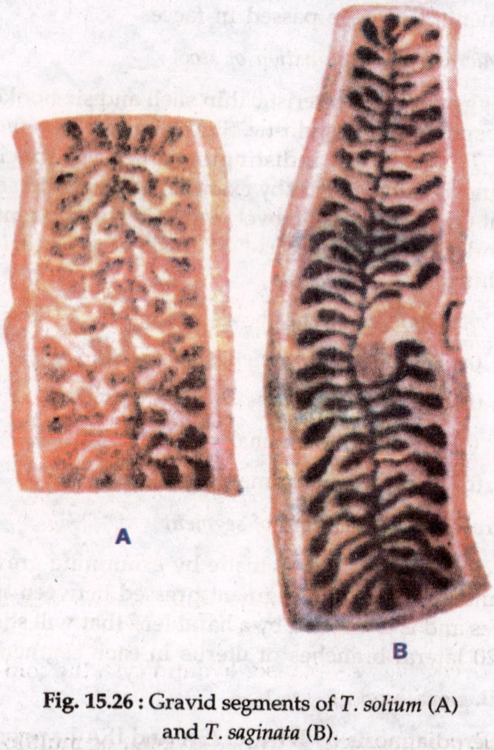

Fig. 15.26 : Gravid segments of *T. solium* (A) and *T. saginata* (B).

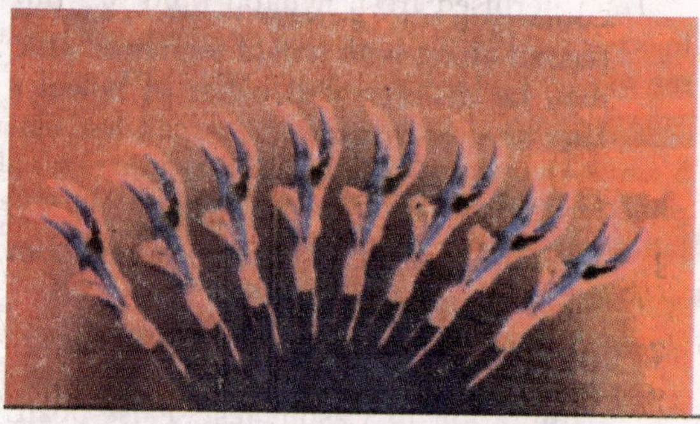

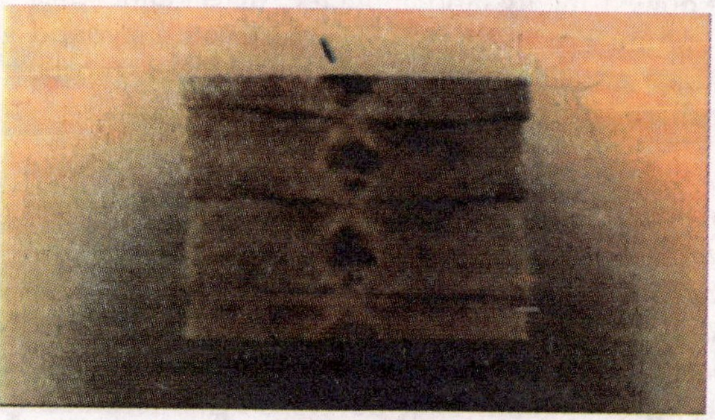

Fig. 15.27 : A. Hooks of *T. solium*. B. Segments of *D. latum*

(c) Fine needle aspiration (FNA) cytology is useful and cost-effective since it eliminates the biopsy.

(d) Serologic tests is helpful in some patients but cross-reactivity is observed between cysticercosis and hydatid infection.

(e) Immunoblot and immunoelectrotransfer blot (EITB) using blood in antibody detection in neurocysticercosis are useful tests.

Eosinophilia usually occurs in the early stage of cysticercosis. An indirect *haemagglutination* test using antigen from cysticercus of pig has been reported to give positive result.

HYDATID CYSTS

Species

A number of cestodes (tapeworms) live as adults in the small intestine of man and animal and larval stages of some of them often occur in human tissues, e.g. **cysticercosis** caused by *T. solium* and *T. saginata;* **sparganosis** caused sometimes by *D. latum.*

In addition to intestinal cestodes, a number of tissue cestodes occur in larval stages in human tissue. The most significant diseases produced by larval stages of tissue cestodes include several forms of **hydatid disease** (*Echinococcus* species), **coenurosis** (*Multiceps* species) and **sparganosis** (*Spirometra* species).

The genus *Echinococcus* has four species which include :

(1) *E. granulosus* — causes hydatid cyst, the commonest echinococcal infection.

(2) *E. multilocularis* — causes alveolar or multilocular disease.

3. *E. oligarthus* — causes polycystic hydatid disease.

4. *E. vogeli* — causes polycystic disease.

There is clear evidence of strain variation in *E. granulosus,* but for other species, clear-cut evidence of strain variation does not exist.

Diagnosis

Diagnosis of hydatid cyst is difficult and depends on clinical, radiographic, aspiration and serological findings.

1. **Radiographic findings**: Radiologic examination (plain X-rays permit the detection of cyst only), ultrasound, CT scan and angiography may provide the first evidence of a cyst's presence.

2. **Exploratory cyst puncture**: Aspiration of cyst contents may reveal the presence of protoscolices (hydatid sand); however, it is contraindicated because of accidental spilling of the contents may cause anaphylaxis and secondary spread of hydatid infection.

Hydatid sand is not always present. Moreover, daughter cysts and/or scolices may disintegrate in old cyst. So only the hooklets are left. This may cause diagnostic problem.

3. **Serologic tests**: Antigen : Specific antigens (8-and 16-kDa antigens) are present in the hydatid fluid. Antibodies to the antigen appear in blood after infection. The source of antigen include sterile hydatid fluid obtained from sheep or man, cyst wall or protoscolices.

Tests:

(a) **Antibody detection**: ELISA, indirect immunofluorescence test (IFT), latex agglutination (LA) test, and indirect haemagglutination assays (IHA) are done using hydatid antigen to detect antibodies in serum. Precipitin and CFT tests with hydatid antigen are also found to be positive. Diagnostic sensitivity varies from 60-90%.

Hydatid antigen dot immunoassay: It is a newer method of diagnosis of hydatid cyst in which serum sample is incubated with a textile colloidal dye and a nitrocellulose stick to which the hydatid antigen has been bound. The presence of *E. granulosus* specific antibodies leads to dying of stick reactive area, and a colour spot develops. This technique shows good correlation with other available methods.

(b) **Antigen detection** : Specific antigen in sera and in CSF (in cerebral hydatid cyst) can be screened by double diffusion and counter immunoelectrophoresis technique.

4. **Casoni test** : Until recently, the Casoni test was the only means of diagnosis of hydatid disease and almost abandoned now. This is an immediate hypersensitivity (Type I) skin test introduced by Casoni in 1911.

Antigen : Hydatid fluid collected from animal or human cysts and is sterilised by Seitz or membrane filtration.

Test : Sterilised fresh hydatid fluid (0.2 ml) is injected intradermally on one arm and equal volume of saline as control on the other arm.

Result : In a positive reaction, a large wheal (about 5 cm in diameter) with multiple pseudopodia-like projections appears within half an hour. The wheal fades away in an hour.

Remarks :

(i) False-positive and false-negative cases may occur. Non-specificity has been the major limitation of Casoni test. False-positive reactions have been observed with other parasitic and nonparasitic diseases.

(ii) Diagnostic sensitivity is limited in patients having intact or hyaline cysts.

(iii) The antigen may sensitise the patient leading to antibody production and anaphylactic reaction. The test is, therefore, rarely used for diagnostic purpose.

PARAGONIMIASIS

Causative agents

Paragonimiasis is a chronic lung infection of lungs of men and carnivores. Important species are shown in Table 15.9. *P. westermani*, commonly known as

Table 15.9 : Paragonimus species infecting man

Species	Distribution	Disease (mode of transmission)	Egg characteristics (size, μm)
P. westermani	Asia	Pulmonary (crabs, cray fish, fresh water shrimp)	85 × 47; abopercular thickening
P. mexicanus (*P. peruvianus*, *P. equadoriensis*)	Central and South America America	Pulmonary (crabs)	79 × 48; undulated shell
P. africanus	Cameroon, Guinea, Liberia, Nigeria, The Gambia	Pulmonary (crabs)	90 × 50; tends to be more narrow, abopercular thickening
P. uterobilateralis	Cameroon, Guinea, Liberia, Nigeria, The Gambia	Pulmonary (crabs)	65 × 40; abopercular thickening
P. heterotremus (*P. tuanshanensis*)	China, Laos, Thailand	Pulmonary (crabs); (raw shrimp salad in Thailand)	86 × 48; uniform thickness
P. kellicotti	North America	Pulmonary (crabs, cray fish)	
P. miyazakii	Japan	Pleural effusion (crabs, raw juice of crabs; cray fish)	75 × 43, uniform thickness, eggs not normally seen
P. philippinensis	Philippines	Pulmonary (crabs)	79 × 50; abopercular thickening
P. skrjabini (*P. szechuanensis*)	China	Pleural, subcutaneous nodules	80 × 48; uniform thickness
P. hueitungensis	China	Pulmonary (crabs)	65 × 40; abopercular thickening

"lung fluke" mostly found in human infection causing an important disease.

Diagnosis : Clinical diagnosis of paragonimiasis is suspected in an individual with chronic cough, vague chest pain and haemoptysis who have resided in an endemic area and is in the habit of eating raw or undercooked crab or cray fish. Chest X-ray films often show infiltrates, nodular cysts and pleural effusion. Since the symptoms closely simulate those of pulmonary tuberculosis, diagnosis should be established by detection of eggs and antibodies.

Specimens: Paragonimus eggs can be detected in sputum and faeces and concomitant examinations of both should be done. In many cases, eggs are intermittently passed in sputum and faeces. Eggs are occasionally found in aspirated pleural fluid.

A. Demonstration of eggs in sputum

Sputum often contains blood, mucus and rusty brown particles in which eggs can be seen.

(a) *Physical examination* : Watery, mucoid or mucopurulent; or red or jelly-like due to haemorrhage.

(b) *Microscopy* :

(i) *Direct microscopy* : Carefully examine any blood tinged flecks for eggs; the egg clusters have been described as looking like iron-filings. Repeated sputum examination, at least for seven consecutive days should be examined. A saline wet mount is preferred. When eggs cannot be found in direct examination, sample should be concentrated.

The eggs possess prominent opercula, the shell is distinctly thickened at abopercular end of the shell, and they are unembryonated when passed in faeces.

(ii) *Concentration method* : Mix equal volumes of sputum and 3 to 4% sodium hydroxide in a centrifuge tube, leave for 10-15 minutes (to dissolve the mucus) and then centrifuge at 2,000 rpm for 5 minutes. Examine the sediment microscopically.

B. Detection of eggs in faeces

(a) Routine microscopy is often negative in mild infection because of scanty eggs, hence concentration technique is preferable.

(b) Concentration of ova in faeces by formal ether concentration method is preferable (Fig. 15.28).

C. Serological tests

Parasitic-specific IgG and IgE anti-paragonimus antibodies in patient's serum detected by ELISA using adult excretory-secretory antigens is very sensitive. Dot ELISA has also been used to detect parasitic antigen in human sera.

D. Eosinophilia

Eosinophilia is almost a constant finding.

SCHISTOSOMA HAEMATOBIUM

Species

Schistosoma species with their differential characteristics are shown in Table 15.10.

Diagnosis

A. Direct evidences

(a) **Microscopy** : Definitive diagnosis is made by detection of eggs.

1. Examination of centrifuged deposit of urine shows eggs with characteristic terminal spine. Occasionally hatched miracidia of *S. haematobium* may be found. Eggs may be also found in seminal fluid. They may also be found in faeces.

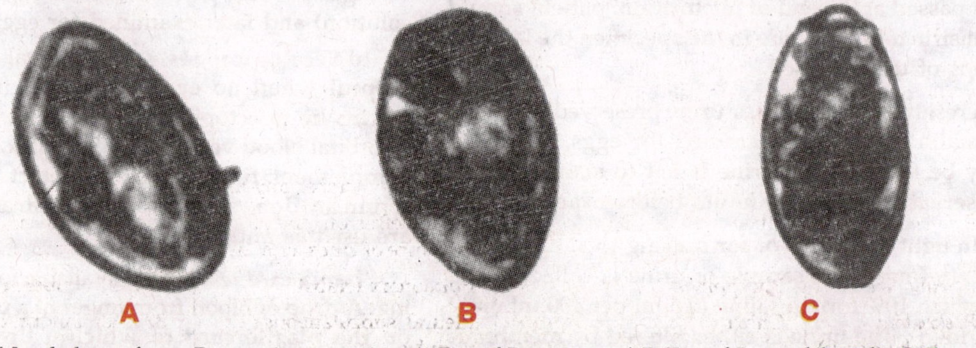

Fig. 15.28 : Morphology of eggs Paragonimus species : A. Egg of *P. westermani*; B. Egg of *P. uterobilateralis*; C. Egg of *P. africanus*

Table 15.10 : Differential features of Schistosomes of man

Feature	*S. haematobium*	*S. mansoni*	*S. japonicum*	*S. mekongi*	*S. intercalatum*
Morphology *Adult* Location in body (vein)	Veins surrounding bladder (vesical plexus)	Inferior mesenteric vein	Superior mesenteric vein	Mesenteric vein	Mesenteric vein
Length (mm) : Male	10-15 × 0.75	6-12 × 1.0	10-20 × 0.5	6-15 × 0.5	11-14 × 0.3-0.4
Female	16-20 × 0.25	10-20 × 0.25	20-30 × 0.3		10-14 × 0.15-0.2
Eggs Size (mm)	140-170 × 40-70	115–175 × 45-70	70-100 × 50-65	30-55 × 50-65	140-180 × 30-50
Shape	Elongate, terminal spined	Elongate, lateral spined	Round with small knob	Look like that of *S. japonicum*, lateral spine difficult to see	Elongate, terminal spined
Reaction to ZN staining	Negative	Positive	Positive	Positive	Positive
Distribution	Africa, Middle East, India, Portugal	Africa, Madagaskar, West Indies, Surinam, Brazil, Venezuela	China, Indonesia, Japan, Philippines	Mekong River Basin	Central and Western Africa
Reservoir hosts	Humans	Human, non-human primates	Dogs, cats, cattle, water buffalo, pigs	Human, dogs, rodents	Humans
Intermediate snail host (genus)	*Bulinus*	*Biomphalaria*	*Oncomelania*	*Lithoglyphopsis*	*Bulinus*
Diagnostic specimen for test	Urine, stool, (some cases), bladder biopsy, serology	Stool, rectal biopsy, serology	Stool, rectal biopsy, serology	Stool, rectal biopsy, serology	Stool, rectal biopsy, serology

In moderate to heavy infections, the urine is usually reddish in colour and cloudy due to presence of blood.

Since eggs are more abundant in the blood and pus passed at the end of micturition, patient should be instructed to include in the specimen the last few drops of urine passed.

Freshly passed urine or urine preserved with 10% formalin should be examined for eggs. Miracidia may be found if the urine is left to stand without preservative for a few hours before examination.

In light infections or for making total egg count, twenty-four hours sample of urine is collected and to which 10% formal saline (0.5 ml per 100 ml urine is added). The urine is either filtered by membrane filter or centrifuged and the deposit is used for microscopy (Fig. 15.29).

2. *Biopsy* : Eggs may also be found in the wall of the rectum as well as in the bladder wall. Detection of eggs in rectal or bladder mucosal biopsy may be done when infection is light. The biopsied tissue may be digested with potash solution (4% NaOH/KOH solution) and later examined for eggs.

(b) **Serological tests** : Serological tests may be helpful when no eggs are found (in case adult worms lie in ectopic sites, e.g. CNS, spinal vessels or orbital blood vessels). ELISA, latex agglutination, complement fixation test to detect antibodies in serum are done at some places. Animal schistosomes are used as antigen.

Plasma card test is now available for mass screening. A drop of blood from finger of a patient is taken on the plastic card to which a drop of antigen solution (prepared from adult worm or cercariae) containing charcoal powder is added. The slide is

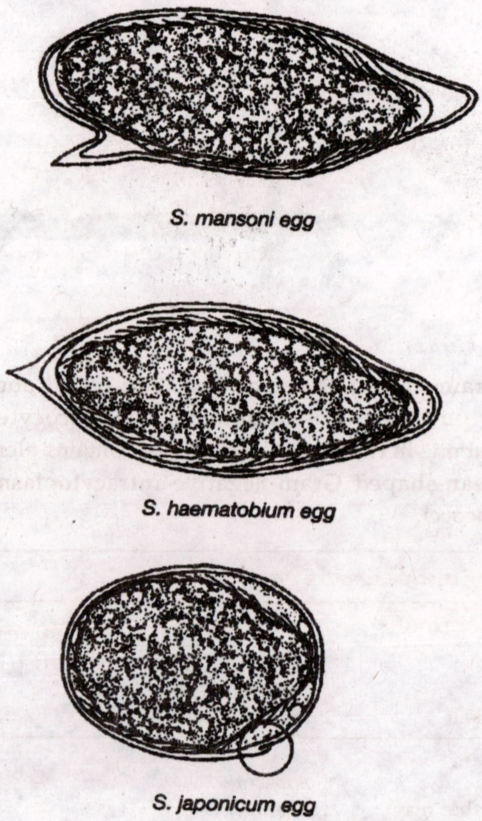

Fig. 15.29 : Diagrammatic representation of eggs of schistosomes. *S. mansoni* (top), *S. haematobium* (middle), *S. japonicum* (bottom). Eggs of *S.japonicum* are much smaller than the other two, also to note its small lateral spine marked by circle.

rotated for 2 minutes. Positive test shows precipitation.

B. Indirect evidences

1. *Haematuria and proteinuria,* caused by eggs penetrating the wall of the bladder, is a characteristic feature of *S. haematobium* infection. The use of **reagent strips** for detecting haematuria and proteinuria in areas of endemic infection has proven as useful screening test.

2. *Blood exam* : Eosinophilia is a common finding (Fig. 15.30).

SCHISTOSOMA JAPONICUM

Laboratory Diagnosis

Laboratory confirmation of *S. japonicum* infection is similar as in *S. mansoni.*

1. **Detection of eggs :**
   (a) Finding *S. japonicum* eggs in faeces.
   (b) Rectal biopsy is an important diagnostic test when eggs cannot be found in faeces.
2. **Serological tests :** ELISA, LA, CFT.
3. **Other findings :**
   (a) Mucus and blood are often present in stool.
   (b) Eosinophilia is present.

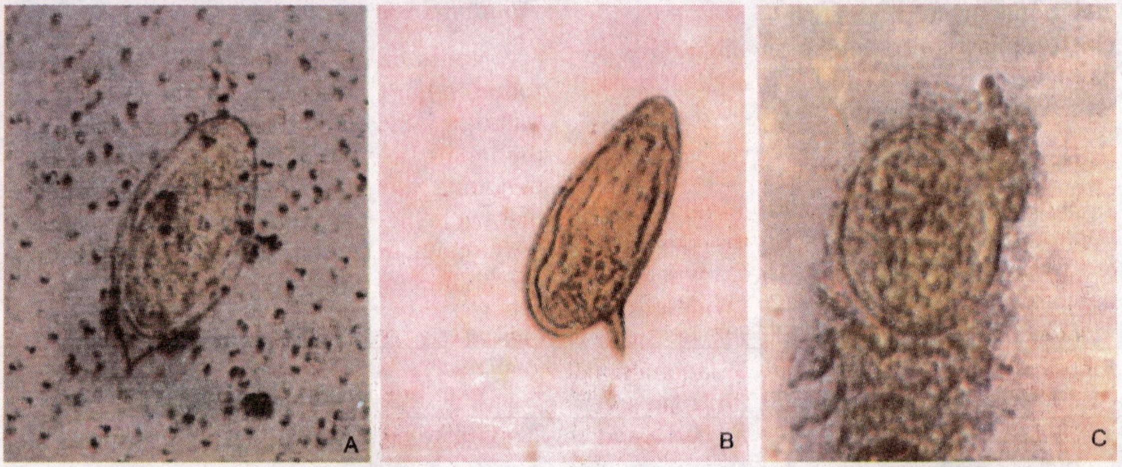

Fig. 15.30 : Microphotographs of eggs of schistosomes : *A.S. haematobium; B.S. mansoni; C.S. japonicum*

Laboratory Diagnosis of Sexually Transmitted Diseases (STDs)

16

URETHRITIS

Causative agents of urethritis are listed in Table 16.1.

Laboratory diagnosis

Specimen : Urethral, vaginal, cervical, and anal exudates are examined and cultured.

1. **Gonorrhoea** :

Gram-stained smear of discharge reveal abundant pus cells (polymorphonuclear leucocytes). About one in twenty of the pus cells, contains plenty of bean-shaped Gram-negative intracytoplasmic diplococci.

Table 16.1 : Urethritis : Characteristics of urethral discharge and diagnostic points

	Gonococcal urethritis	Non-gonococcal urethritis
1. ***Discharge***		
Quantity	Profuse	Scanty
Quality	Thick, purulent	Mucopurulent/serous
2. ***Symptoms***		
Type	Acute	Subacute
Urethral	Self limiting but may pass on to NGU	Chronic
3. ***Incubation period***	2-4 days	1-3 weeks
4. ***Microscopy***		
(a) *Gram-film*		
Intracellular Gram-negative diplococci	+	–
Pus cells (polymorphonuclear leucocytes) per oil-immersion field	> 5 (usually plenty)	> 5
(b) *Giemsa/ Macchiavello stains*		
Inclusion bodies :		
Intracytoplasmic	–	+ *(C. trachomatis)*
Intranuclear	–	+ *(HSV)*
Giant cells	–	+
(c) *Hanging drop* (cover slip preparation)	Not required	+ *(Motile T. vaginalis)*
(d) *Detection of specific antigen*		
Immunofluorescence/ ELISA (with monoclonal antibody)	+	+
5. ***Cultivation***		
Artificial media	Thayer-Martin medium	Tissue culture (McCoy cells)
6. ***Serology***		
CFT with patient's serum	+	+

(i) *Male patients* : A positive smear is virtually diagnostic of gonococci.

(ii) *Women* : It is sometimes difficult to interpret the smear finding in mixed normal flora in females. *Veillonella parvula* is also a Gram-negative diplo-coccus normally present in vaginal flora. Moreover, asymptomatic carriage is high in females, especially with endocervical lesion. Hence positive identification of the organism by culture or immuno-fluorescent study using genetic probes (e.g. DNA probe) is necessary to confirm the diagnosis.

2. **Trichomoniasis** : A direct wet film of freshly collected specimen shows motile trichomonad with polymorphonuclear leucocytes.

3. **Candidiasis** : Microscopical examination of vaginal secretions in 10% potassium hydroxide show yeast cells.

4. **Non-gonococcal urethritis**

(i) *Microscopy* : Smear stained by Giemsa stain shows intracytoplasmic inclusion bodies, suggestive of *C. trachomatis*. When diagnosis of *C. trachomatis* cannot be made by light microscopy, a definitive diagnosis is to be made by either culture or by antigen detection.

(ii) *Culture* : Specimen is inoculated into **McCoy** or **HeLa** cell tissue cultures. Tissue culture is not routinely available.

(iii) *Detection of antigen* : Smear made from exudate is examined by immunofluorescence test with a monoclonal antibody or by ELISA to detect LPS antigens (either soluble or in the elementary body cell wall) of *C. trachomatis*.

GENITAL ULCERS

Causes

1. Hard chancre (Syphilis) — by *T. pallidum*
2. Soft chancre (Chancroid) – by *H. ducreyi*
3. Herpes progenitalis – by *Herpes simplex* virus types 1 and 2, primarily type 2.
4. Donovanosis (granuloma inguinale) – by *Calymmatobacterium granulomatis.*
5. Lymphogranuloma venereum – by *C. trachomatis* types L1, L2, L3.

Laboratory diagnosis — See Table 16.2.

1. **Microscopy**

(i) **Dark-field microscopy** of specimen collected from a syphilitic primary chancre as well as secondary rash may reveal motile *Treponema pallidum.*

(ii) **Gram stain** of exudate from cases of chancroid may show Gram-negative ovoid bacilli. The bacteria *en mass* have configuration of "shoals of fish".

(iii) **Giemsa/Wright staining** of exudate of genital herpes often show multinucleated giant cells or intranuclear inclusions.

(iv) **Castaneda's method** : Chlamydiae though Gram-negative, but they stain well by **Castaneda's method** and **Giemsa** stain. The inclusions in cell culture are stained by both the stains well.

In donovanosis, Donovan bodies (round coccobacilli, 1 × 2 µm) may be found in smear from ulcer stained by Giemsa stain. The Donovan bodies lie within the cystic spaces in the cytoplasm of large

Table 16.2 : Laboratory diagnosis of genital ulcers

	Microscopy	Provisional diagnosis
Exudate		
Gram-film	Small Gram-negative bacilli occurring in strands	Chancroid (*H. ducreyi*)
Fontana's stain	Slender long (12-15 mm) spiral organisms	Syphilis (*T. pallidum*)
DGI	Motile spirochaetes	Syphilis
Scraping from ulcer		
Giemsa stain	Intracellular bodies (telephone handle appearance)	Donovanosis (*Calymmatobacterium granulomatis*)
	Intranuclear inclusion bodies, multinucleated giant cells	HSV types 1, 2

mononuclear cells. Capsule appears as a dense acidophilic zone around the bacterium, resembling a closed safety pin or **"telephone handle"**.

2. **Serological test**

(i) **Syphilis** : Syphilis is diagnosed in most patients on the basis of serological tests. Positive result is obtained from about two weeks after the appearance of primary sore. Two types of tests : **non-specific** (non-treponemal) and **specific** (treponemal) tests are used (Table 16.3) :

Table 16.3
Sensitivity of serological tests in syphilis (%)

Test	Primary	Secondary	Latent	Late
Non-treponemal				
VDRL	78	100	95	70
RPR	85	100	98	73
Treponemal				
FTA-ABS	84	100	100	96
MHA-TF	75	100	97	94

(a) *Non-specific tests* : Non-treponemal tests measure IgG and IgM antibodies (known as **reagin** antibodies) produced against lipids released from damaged cells during the early stage of the disease which are also present on cell surface of treponemes.

(b) *Specific or treponemal tests* : These are used to confirm positive VDRL or RPR tests. The most commonly used treponemal tests are FTA-ABS test and MHA-TP test. These tests can become positive before the non-treponemal tests in early syphilis, or remain positive when the non-treponemal tests revert to negative in some patients with late syphilis. Western blot test using whole cell *T. pallidum* as antigen has recently been used successfully to confirm non-treponemal tests.

VDRL and TPHA are more useful tests for diagnosis of syphilis in most laboratories. When these tests are done together, they provide an effective screen for early and late syphilis.

(ii) **Herpes genitalis** : Serological tests (e.g. CFT) with patient's HSV infection. The antibody titre is usually within 32, especially in genital herpes.

Treatment

1. **Syphilis** is best treated with large doses of penicillin. Long-acting benzathine penicillin is recommended in early syphilis, and penicillin G for congenital and late syphilis. Tetracycline and doxycyclines are alternative drugs.

2. **Herpes simplex** can be treated with acyclovir.

3. **Chancroid** is treated with sulfonamides or aminoglycosides.

VAGINAL DISCHARGE

Causes

Causes include *gonorrhoea,* infection due to *C. trachomatis,* bacterial vaginosis, *trichomonas vaginalis* and *Vulvovaginal candidiasis.*

The vaginal discharge may be due to more than one of the above mentioned microorganisms.

Laboratory diagnosis

1. *pH* — greater than 4.5.

2. *Amine test* — When vaginal fluid is mixed with a 10% solution of KOH, fishy odor is immediately liberated. The odor is due to volatile amines present in vaginal fluid.

3. *Saline microscopy* — Vaginal discharge contains *clue cells* (squamous epithelial cells coated with coccobacillary organisms). Leucocytes are virtually absent.

4. *Gram-film* — The normal vaginal flora of lactobacilli in vagina is largely replaced by *G. vaginalis* and other anaerobes.

QUESTIONS RELATED TO LABORATORY DIAGNOSIS OF SEXUALLY TRANSMITTED DISEASES

Q.1. *Name the complications of STD.*

Ans. 1. Infertility. 2. Ectopic pregnancy. 3. Premature birth/stillbirths/birth defects. 4. Heart diseases. 5. Degenerative nerve diseases. 6. Congenital and perinatal infections may lead to blindness, mental retardation and rarely to cancer.

Q.2. *What is NGU and the causative agents?*

Ans. See Table 16.1 of the text.

Q.3. *Name the aetiologic agents of genital ulcers.*

Ans. See Table 16.2 of the text.

4. *Name the tests employed in detection of STD.*

Ans. Ab Detection Tests : Detection of antibody is very important, particularly in those STDs in which culture is difficult or not possible. The tests included are :

For detection of Abs in Syphilis:

- VDRL
- *Treponema pallidum* immobilisation test
- Rapid plasma reagin test
- Fluorescent treponemal Ab absorption test

For detection of Abs in various bacterial and viral infections:

- *Treponema pallidum* haemagglutination test
- ELISA
- Western blot assay for HIV
- Radioimmunoassay
- Immunodiffusion test

For detection of Abs in various bacterial and viral infections:

- Reverse passive haemagglutination test
- Counter-current immunoelectrophoresis
- Agglutination test
- Complement fixation test

Miscellaneous Tests

- Limulus amoebocyte lysate assay test : for detection of endotoxin of Gram-negative bacteria.
- Nucleic acid hybridisation assay.
- DNA hybridisation assay.

SPACE FOR NOTES

Bacteriology of Water, Milk and Air

17

BACTERIOLOGY OF WATER

Introduction

Safe water should be free from microorganisms and chemical substances and drinking water in particular should not only be safe but also pleasant to drink, i.e. cool, clear, colourless and devoid of disagreeable taste or smell.

Faecal pollution of water supplies may lead to introduction of a variety of intestinal pathogens that comprise water-borne diseases (Table 17.1).

Bacteriological indicators

These are based on organisms indicative of water pollution by human/animal faeces, such as :

(i) *Escherichia coli* and coliform as a whole,

(ii) Faecal streptococci (*S. faecalis*) and

(iii) *Clostridium perfringens.*

While evaluating faecal pollution of water supplies, one has to keep in view the bacterial flora in water (Table 17.2) as natural water almost always contains a few harmless microorganisms.

Table 17.1 : Water-borne diseases

Group	Diseases
A. *Causes directly by infective agent*	
(a) Viral	Viral hepatitis (Hepatitis A, E), poliomyelitis, rotavirus diarrhoea in infants
(b) Bacterial	Cholera, typhoid, paratyphoid, *Esch. coli* diarrhoea, bacillary dysentery, *Yersinia enterocolitica, Campylobacter jejuni* and *E. coli* diarrhoea
(c) Protozoal	Amoebiasis, Giardiasis, *Balantidium coli* diarrhoea
(d) Helminthic	Roundworm, whipworm, threadworm, hydatid disease
B. *Diseases due to aquatic host*	
(a) Cyclope	Guineaworm, fish tapeworm
(b) Snail	Schistosomiasis

Table 17.2 : Bacterial flora in water

Source	Organisms
A. *Without faecal contamination*	
(1) Natural water bacteria (mainly derived from air by rains)	*Micrococcus, Pseudomonas, Serratia, Flavobacterium, Alcaligenes, Acinetobacter*
(2) Soil bacteria (washed into water)	*Bacillus subtilis, Bacillus megaterium, Klebsiella* spp.
B. *After faecal contamination*	
(1) Intestinal bacteria (through sewage)	*Esch. coli, Klebsiella* spp., *Streptococcus faecalis, Clostridium welchii*
(2) Sewage bacteria proper	*Proteus vulgaris, Clostridium sporogenes*, filamentous bacteria (e.g. *Nocardia* spp.)

1. **Coliforms** : The coliforms ferment lactose, e.g. *E. coli, Klebsiella* spp, *Enterobacter, Citrobacter* and *Edwardsiella* spp. *E. coli* is the typical example of faecal group and *Klebsiella aerogenes* is an example of non-faecal group of coliform.

2. **Faecal streptococci** (*Streptococcus faecalis*) are regularly found in faeces though their number is much less than *Escherichia coli*. Their presence in water is regarded as confirmatory evidence of recent faecal contamination of water in doubtful cases.

3. **Clostridium perfringens** also occurs in faeces regularly. They are also excreted in much smaller number than *Escherichia coli*. Presence of spores of the organism in water supplies indicate faecal pollution.

Bacteriological examination of water

1. Presumptive coliform test

(a) **Multiple-tube method** : By this test the most probable number (MPN) of coliform organisms are detected in 100 ml water.

Media : Double-strength and single strength modified MacConkey's fluid medium containing bromocresol purple sterilised in bottles/tubes containing Durham's tube (for indication of gas production).

Procedure : Measured amounts of sample of water are added by sterile graduated pipettes as follows :

(i) 50 ml water to 50 ml double strength medium.

(ii) 10 ml water to 10 ml double strength medium.

(iii) Five 1 ml quantities each to 5 ml single strength medium.

(iv) 0.1 ml quantities of water to each 5 ml single strength medium.

The tubes/bottles are incubated at 37°C for 48 hours. An estimate of coliform count is made from the tubes showing acid and gas production by the help of a statistical table (Tables 17.4 and 17.5). The reaction may occasionally be due to combination of organisms or due to other organisms. Organism is identified by biochemical test (Table 17.3).

(b) **Membrane-filter (MF) method** : A measured volume of water is filtered through a membrane specially made of cellulose ester. Bacteria are retained on the surface of membrane. The membrane is inoculated (face upwards) in suitable medium and incubated for 15-20 hours and the number of colonies are counted directly.

Table 17.3
Differential features of typical and atypical coliform bacilli

Gas at 44°C	Indole production at 44°C	Organism
+	+	Typical coliform bacilli
+	–	Irregular type of coliform bacilli
–	+	Other coliform bacilli
–	–	Other organisms (e.g. *C. welchii, S. faecalis*)

2. Detection of faecal streptococci and *Cl. welchii* :

Their presence in water provides useful confirmatory evidence of the faecal pollution of water in doubtful cases. These are identified by subculture in solid media.

Colony count : One ml test sample of water is placed in Petri dish (10 cm diameter) and then 10 ml melted yeast agar (45°–50°C) is poured on the water, mixed thoroughly and allowed to solidify. One more plate is prepared. One plate is incubated at 22°C and other at 37°C for about 18-24 hours.

Table 17.4
Probability Tables (according to McCrady)

Quantity of water	50 ml	10 ml	1 ml	
No. of samples of each quantity tested	1	5	5	
Number giving positive reaction (acid and gas)				Probable number of coliform bacilli in 100 ml of water
	0	0	0	0
	0	0	1	1
	0	0	2	2
	0	1	0	1
	0	1	1	2
	0	1	2	3
	0	2	0	2
	0	2	1	3
	0	2	2	4
	0	3	0	3
	0	3	1	5
Contd.	0	4	0	5

Table 17.4
Probability Tables (according to McCrady)
(continued from previous page)

Quantity of water	50 ml	10 ml	1 ml	
No. of samples of each quantity tested	1	5	5	
Number giving positive reaction (acid and gas)				Probable number of coliform bacilli in 100 ml of water
	1	0	0	1
	1	0	1	3
	1	0	2	4
	1	0	3	6
	1	1	0	3
	1	1	1	5
	1	1	2	7
	1	1	3	9
	1	2	0	5
	1	2	1	7
	1	2	2	10
	1	2	3	12
	1	3	0	8
	1	3	1	11
	1	3	2	14
	1	3	3	18
	1	3	4	20
	1	4	0	13
	1	4	1	17
	1	4	2	20
	1	4	3	30
	1	4	4	35
	1	4	5	40
	1	5	0	25
	1	5	1	35
	1	5	2	50
	1	5	3	90
	1	5	4	160
	1	5	5	180+

Table 17.5
Probability Tables (according to McCrady)

Quantity of water	10 ml	1 ml	0.1 ml	
No. of samples of each quantity tested	5	5	5	
Number giving positive reaction (acid and gas)				Probable number of coliform bacilli in 100 ml of water
	0	0	0	0
	0	0	1	2
	0	0	2	4
	0	1	0	2
	0	1	1	4
	0	1	2	6
	0	2	0	4
	0	2	1	6
	0	3	0	6
	1	0	0	2
	1	0	1	4
	1	0	2	6
	1	0	3	8
	1	1	0	4
	1	1	1	6
	1	1	2	8
	1	2	0	6
	1	2	1	8
	1	2	2	10
	1	3	0	8
	1	3	1	10
	1	4	0	11
	2	0	0	5
	2	0	1	7
	2	0	2	9
	2	0	3	12
	2	1	0	7
	2	1	1	9
	2	1	2	12
	2	2	0	9
	2	2	1	12
	2	2	2	14
	2	3	0	12
	2	3	1	14
	2	4	0	15
	3	0	0	8
Contd.	3	0	1	11

Table 17.5 *(continued)*
Probability Tables (according to McCrady)

Quantity of water	10 ml	1 ml	0.1 ml	
No. of samples of each quantity tested	5	5	5	
	Number giving positive reaction (acid and gas)			Probable number of coliform bacilli in 100 ml of water
	3	0	2	13
	3	1	0	11
	3	1	1	14
	3	1	2	17
	3	1	3	20
	3	2	0	14
	3	2	1	17
	3	2	3	20
	3	3	0	17
	3	3	1	20
	3	4	0	20
	3	4	1	25
	3	5	0	25
	4	0	0	13
	4	0	1	17
	4	0	2	20
	4	0	3	25
	4	1	0	17
	4	1	1	20
	4	1	2	25
	4	2	0	20
	4	2	1	25
	4	2	2	30
	4	3	0	25
	4	3	1	35
	4	3	2	40
	4	4	0	35
	4	4	1	40
	4	4	2	45
	4	5	0	40
	4	5	1	50
	4	5	2	55
	5	0	0	25
Contd.	5	0	1	30

Table 17.5 *(continued)*
Probability Tables (according to McCrady)

Quantity of water	10 ml	1 ml	0.1 ml	
No. of samples of each quantity tested	5	5	5	
	Number giving positive reaction (acid and gas)			Probable number of coliform bacilli in 100 ml of water
	5	0	2	45
	5	0	3	60
	5	0	4	75
	5	1	0	35
	5	1	1	45
	5	1	2	65
	5	1	3	85
	5	1	4	115
	5	2	0	50
	5	2	1	70
	5	2	2	95
	5	2	3	120
	5	2	4	150
	5	2	5	175
	5	3	0	80
	5	3	1	110
	5	3	2	140
	5	3	3	175
	5	3	4	200
	5	3	5	250
	5	4	0	130
	5	4	1	170
	5	4	2	225
	5	4	3	275
	5	4	4	350
	5	4	5	425
	5	5	0	250
	5	5	1	350
	5	5	2	550
	5	5	3	900
	5	5	4	1600
	5	5	5	1800+

***Interpretation of total count*:**

(i) *Growth at 22°C* indicates the amount of decomposing organic matter present in water.

(ii) *Growth at 37°C* is more important index of contamination of water sample.

3. Biological examination of water : Sometimes water may contain microscopic organisms, such as algae, fungi, yeast, protozoa, minute worms, etc. which are collectively known as 'plankton'. These plankton organisms are index of pollution and produce objectionable taste in water.

4. Interpretation of results : On the basis of repeated tests of water, a standard has been suggested by pioneer workers in the field into class 1, class 2, class 3 and class 4 types of water based on presumptive coliform count per 100 ml sample (Table 17.6) :

Table 17.6
Classification of drinking water according to bacteriological tests

	Presumptive coliform count per 100 ml	*E.coli* count per 100 ml
Class 1 Excellent	0	0
Class 2 Satisfactory	1-3	0
Class 3 Suspicious	4-10	0
Class 4 Unsatisfactory	More than 10	0, 1 or more

Bacteriological examination of sewage and sewage effluents

1. Concentration of the organisms in the sample yields better result. Sample may be concentrated by membrane filter technique. Pathogenic bacteria retained on the surface of membrane are transferred into a suitable differential medium and incubated.

2. Dilution method : As the number of pathogenic bacteria present may be scanty, larger volume of multiple samples may have to be examined for isolating the organisms. A volume of 10 ml of enrichment and selective media (selenite broth for *Salmonella* spp, alkaline peptone water for *Vibrio cholerae*) is mixed with nine times its volume of water and incubated for 24 hours and then subcultured in suitable media.

Isolated organisms are identified by biochemical test and serotyping.

BACTERIOLOGY OF MILK

Introduction

A. Presence of bacteria in milk

Milk always contain some bacteria derived from various sources :

(i) *Milk ducts of udder* : Even when best possible precautions are taken, some bacteria are derived from the udders (Table 17.7). Their number is highest in the fore-milk and lowest in milk obtained by strippings. Aseptically drawn raw milk may contain 10 bacteria to several thousand per ml.

(ii) *Milking equipment* : Unsterile milking equipment is a major contributor of bacteria of milk.

(iii) *The milker* : Milkers' hands also contribute to bacteria in milk which can be avoided by proper cleaning of hands before milking the animal.

(iv) *Unclean udders and dust in milking shed* : These are also sources of bacteria in milk.

(v) *Water* : Water used for cleaning the udders and for adulteration also partly contribute to bacteria in milk.

(vi) *Diseased animals* : Pathogenic organism causing infection in animals (e.g. mastitis, brucellosis, tuberculosis) may be excreted in milk.

(vii) *Carriers* : Carriers of infectious diseases (e.g. typhoid, paratyphoid, dysentery, food poisoning

Table 17.7 : Types of bacteria likely to be found in milk of healthy cows

Group	Organisms	Sources
Acid-forming	Lactic streptococci (e.g. *Str. lactis*), *Str. faecalis*, *Lactobacilli*, *Staphylococci*	Utensils, udders
Alkali-forming	*Alcaligenes* spp., *Achromobacter*	Environment
Gas-forming	Coliform bacilli, *Cl. welchii*, *Cl. butyricum*	Water, hands of milker
Proteolytic	*B. subtilis*, *B. cereus*, *Proteus vulgaris*	Environment

bacilli, coagulase positive staphylococci, or haemolytic streptococci) who milk the animal sometimes act as sources of pathogenic bacteria of milk.

B. Types of bacteria in milk

The various types of bacteria that may be encountered in milk are given in Table 17.7. Milk, even under best precautions, contains some bacteria. Fresh milk is bactericidal as well as bacteriostatic but this activity disappears a few hours after the milk has been withdrawn.

C. Types of bacteria in human milk

(a) *Prior to infant feeding* : *S. epidermidis* (100% samples), *S. mitis* (69%), *Gaffkya tetragena* (19%) and *S. aureus* (13%). Other organisms are found in about 10% samples.

(b) *After breast-feeding* : Same organisms as mentioned above are seen but most bacteria are derived from maternal skin and infant's mouth.

D. Milk-borne diseases (Table 17.8)

Milk is a good medium for bacteria and also a good vehicle for many organisms and may result from infection of animals, contaminated milk and infections of man.

Pasteurisation of milk

Pasteurisation of milk — heating to 72°C/161°F for 15 seconds followed by rapid cooling to 10°C/50°F—eliminates the risk of most infections (90%) including the more heat-resistant tubercle bacillus and Q fever organisms, but it does not destroy thermophilic bacteria and bacterial spores.

E. Biological standards of milk

Standards of milk as laid down under Milk Regulations Act of 1965 and 1972 in England and Wales is as follows :

(i) *Untreated milk* : Raw milk under most favourable conditions, may contain at least 500 bacteria per ml.

(ii) *Pasteurised milk* should not contain coliform in 0.1 ml milk and on submission to phosphatase test must give a reading not exceeding 10 μg of ρ-nitrophenol per ml of milk.

(iii) Sterilised milk must satisfy the turbidity test.

(iv) Ultraheated milk must contain less than 10 bacteria per 0.01 ml (i.e. 1,000 bacteria per ml).

Milk analysis

Sample is collected aseptically.

Sampling

(i) If the milk is contained in retain bottles, one unopened bottle is to be sent to laboratory.

(ii) When the milk is in a large container, sample is collected by a sterile dipper from the depth of milk by a sterile 4 oz screw-capped bottle.

A. Bacteriological tests

1. *Viable count* : This plate count method of test is done by serial dilutions of milk sample (1 : 10, 1 : 100, 1 : 1,000 in sterile Ringer's solution) incorporating in yeast extract milk agar in 10 cm Petri dish and then incubated at 30°-31°C for 72 hours. Number of colonies multiplied by dilution factor gives the colony count in the fixed amount of milk.

2. *Coliform test* : Varying dilutions of milk are inoculated into 3 tubes of MacConkey's fluid medium with Durham's tube and incubated at 37°C for 48 hours. Then production of acid and gas is noted. Contamination of milk by coliform bacilli usually occurs from dirty utensils, dust and dairy workers.

B. Chemical test

This test includes *methylene blue test*, phosphatase and turbidity tests.

Table 17.8 : Milk-borne diseases

Source	Diseases
Infections primarily of animals	Tuberculosis, brucellosis, streptococcal infections, enterotoxigenic staphylococci, salmonellosis, Q fever, cow pox, foot and mouth diseases, anthrax, leptospirosis, milker's nodes, *Campylobacter fetus*, *Y. enterocolitica*
Contaminated milk by ticks, rats	Tick-borne encephalitis, *Streptobacillus moniliformis* (rat-borne)
Infections primarily of man	Typhoid and paratyphoid fevers, cholera, shigellosis, enteropathogenic *E. coli*, staphylococcal food poisoning, streptococcal infections, tuberculosis, hepatitis

1. **Methylene blue test** : This simple test is an economical substitute of viable count. Viable bacteria reduce the dye in milk when kept in a cool dark place. Solution of methylene blue used gives a final concentration of 1/300,000. The milk is decolourised after reduction of methylene blue and the rate of reduction is related to the degree of bacterial contamination. Raw or untreated milk is considered satisfactory if it fails to decolourise methylene blue in 30 minutes under standard condition.

Resazurin test is also a dye reduction test similar to methylene blue test. Unlike methylene blue test, reduction of resazurin by bacteria passes through a series of colour changes : blue, lilac, mauve, pink to the final colourless state of complete reduction.

The *"Ten Minute Resazurin Test'* is usually done in creameries, in which change of colour of milk containing the dye is noted after 10 minutes and compared with a set of colour standards in a Lovibond comparator.

2. **Phosphatase test** : This is statutory test for pasteurised milk in England.

The test is done by adding 1 ml of milk to be tested to 5 ml buffer-substrate solution (buffer + disodium phenyl phosphate) in a test tube. The mixture is incubated in water bath at 37°C for 2 hours. A yellow coloured solution of ρ-nitrophenol is produced if the milk contains phosphatase. The colour is compared with a standard solution by a comparator or colorimeter. In a properly pasteurised milk, the concentration of ρ-nitrophenol is less than 10 µg per ml of milk.

C. Turbidity test

This test for sterilised milk distinguishes between pasteurised and sterilised milk. When milk is heated to at least 100°C for 5 minutes, the soluble proteins in milk get denatured and that cannot be precipitated by ammonium sulphate.

D. Detection of specific pathogens

(a) *Tubercle bacilli* : The milk is thoroughly mixed and 50 ml amounts are centrifuged in each of two tubes at 300 rpm for 30 minutes. Part of the deposit is used for AFB-film and part is used for inoculation into guinea pigs.

(b) *Brucella* : Isolation of *Br. abortus* is attempted by inoculating cream on serum dextrose agar. The cream and centrifuged deposit of milk may also be injected intramuscularly into guinea pigs.

The animals are killed after six weeks, serum is examined by *Br. abortus* suspension and spleen is used for culture of brucellae.

Brucellosis in animals can be detected by demonstrating antibodies against brucellae in milk by *milk ring test* and *whey agglutination test*.

BACTERIOLOGY OF AIR

The immediate environment of man comprises of air on which depends all forms of life. Since a man respires about 500 cft of air in a day, the content of air is important particularly so when the air contains pathogenic organisms.

I. Sources of air pollution

(i) *Human sources* : Man is an important source of spreading bacteria in the environment in droplet during coughing and sneezing. The air-borne bacteria may be derived by evaporation of droplets or by aerosols. The bacterial content in air increases with increased density of human and animal population. Pathogenic organisms do not multiply in air and are seldom carried from more than short distance. Infections that spread by droplet include tuberculosis, Q fever, psittacosis and coccidio-idomycosis, etc.

(ii) *Environmental sources* : Soil and vegetations contain non-pathogenic organisms such as Achromobacter, Sarcina, Micrococci, sometimes coliform bacilli, spores and fragments of moulds.

II. Pollution in different types of air

Bacterial content in air depends on location whether it is outdoor or indoor.

(i) *Outdoor air* : The bacterial content depends on type of soil and vegetation, humidity of air and density of population. The air above ocean is almost bacteria-free. However, outdoor air contains much less bacteria than indoor air and the organisms present are non-pathogenic, e.g. *Achromobacter, Sarcina, Micrococcus, Bacillus subtilis*, spores and fragments of moulds. The upper air contains much less bacteria. Pathogenic bacteria usually do not survive in outdoor air.

(ii) *Indoor air* : Indoor air also contains droplets of organisms disseminated by man and animals. Hospital air may contain droplet nuclei or skin scales carrying infective organisms.

III. Bacteriological examination

Bacteriological examination is necessary for

operation theatres, store house of food, pharmacy and hospital wards. There are two methods :

(i) *Sediment method* : Petri dish (9-10 cm diam) containing nutrient agar and blood agar are exposed to air for half to one hour and the plates are then incubated at 37°C for 24 hours. Colonies are then counted.

(ii) *Slit sampler method* : The number of bacteria in a measured volume of air is determined by this method. A known volume of air is directed onto a plate of culture medium through a slit of 0.25 mm wide. The plate is rotated mechanically so as to allow the organisms to spread out evenly in the medium. One cubic foot of air is made to pass through these slits. In the same way, 10 cubic feet is tested. The culture media are incubated and colonies counted which gives the number of bacteria present in the air.

IV. Interpretation

(i) Most bacteria found in the air are harmless saprophytes or commensals, and even in the wards of hospital and other closed rooms occupied by the patients and carriers. Approximately 1% of the air borne organisms in the wards or closed rooms are pathogenic. *Staphylococcus aureus* is the predominant air-borne organism, about 0.1 to 10 organisms are present in one cu. ft. air. *Streptococcus pyogenes* may be found in larger numbers in the air (10/cu. ft. air) in rooms occupied by patients with scarlet fever and streptococcal tonsillitis.

(ii) It is not definitely known what should be the minimum size of dose of organism that may cause infection following inhalation. This depends upon the type of pathogenic organisms and the host immune response. It has been found in guinea pig that as little as 0.00008 tubercle bacilli per cu. ft. air is sufficient to cause infection. Thus, a man may be infected even when he inhales only a single pathogen in 500 or so cu. ft. air that he respires during 24 hours.

(iii) The following limits of air pollution may be acceptable :

(a) Factories, offices, homes, etc. — 50 per cu. ft.

(b) Operation theatre — 10 per cu. ft.

(c) Dressing room, operation theatre for neurosurgery — 1 per cu. ft.

QUESTIONS RELATED TO BACTERIOLOGY OF WATER, MILK AND AIR

1. *How do you find viable bacterial count in milk?*

Ans. (i) It is detected by plate counts with serial dilutions of the milk samples. (ii) Dilute raw milk with sterile Ringer saline as 1:10, 1 : 100 and 1 : 1,000. Then 1 ml of appropriate dilution is mixed with 10 ml of medium and poured in plates. (iii) Incubate plates at 30°-31°C for 72 hours. (iv) Number of colonies are counted and multiplied by dilution factor and number of viable bacteria per millilitre of milk is determined. (v) Normally raw milk contains 500 to several million bacteria per millilitre.

2. *What is the indication of methylene blue test ?*

Ans. (i) It is an indirect technique for detection of microorganisms in milk.

(ii) An economical substitute for viable count.

(iii) **Technique** : 1 ml. of methylene blue is mixed with 10 ml of milk in a test tube and incubated in dark at 37°C.

(iv) **Finding** : (a) When bacteria are present, the milk is decolourised due to reduction of methylene blue by bacteria making the milk colourless — test is positive. (b) No change in colour — test is negative.

(v) **Remarks** : Milk is considered satisfactory if it fails to decolourise methylene blue in 30 minutes.

3. *Name the tests of detection of tubercle bacilli in milk.*

Ans. (a) Milk is centrifuged at 3,000 rpm for 30 minutes and sediment is inoculated into two guinea pigs and two L-J media.

(b) L-J media observed for growth and guinea pigs are observed for a period of 3 months for tuberculosis.

(c) Confirmation is done by using biochemical tests.

4. *What are the tests for detection of brucella bacilli in milk?*

Ans. By isolation of brucellae is attempted by :

(a) Inoculate cream from milk sample on serum glucose agar.

(b) Inject centrifuged deposit of the milk sample intramuscularly in guinea pigs.

Findings : The guinea pig can be sacrificed after 6 weeks and the spleen used for culture of brucella and serum used for demonstration of Abs by milk ring test.

The milk ring test is the highly sensitive test for brucella Abs in the milk of infected cows. The test is used for diagnosis of brucellosis in animals. The positive milk ring test is confirmed by Whey's agglutination test.

Note : In case of suspected food poisoning, the sediment of centrifuged milk is examined for :

- *Staph. aureus*
- *Salmonella* sp.
- *Campylobacter* sp.
- *Y. enterocolitica*

5. *Name methods for bacteriological examination of air.*

Ans. (a) Measuring the rate at which bacteria carrying particles settle down, e.g. settle plate method.

(b) Counting the number of bacteria carrying particles contained in a given volume of the air, e.g. slit sampler method.

SPACE FOR NOTES

Laboratory Animals : Care, Management, Particulars and Common Diseases

18

CARE AND MANAGEMENT OF ANIMALS

Laboratory animals in most countries are protected by the Law "Cruelty to Animals Act". One is to obtain licence from the Home Department for using them on experimental purposes.

The health and well-being of the animals depend on the care, human attitude of the animal-keepers (staff) of the animal house. To keep animals healthy, the staff has to look after cleanliness of the animal rooms and cages, provide proper food and water, to move to a cooler or warmer place and to provide air.

The general principles are outlined :

1. Fluid

They are to be provided with plentiful supply of fresh clean drinking water from a bottle (250 ml capacity) attached to the outside of the cage. The water is led in a 6-9 mm glass tubing through a rubber bung to an accessible position inside the cage; the outlet tubing is about 3 mm.

2. Diet

A balanced diet containing carbohydrate, fat, protein, vitamins and trace elements is to be given regularly. It is commercially in the form of cubes or pellets. Small quantities of green stuff are also to be supplied.

3. Cleanliness

Cleanliness of room and cages is essential unless they are kept in considerable risk of epidemic diseases. Animals, when breeding, should not have their cages changed too often. Clean cages should be used. Cages may be boiled in soapy water; alternatively, to be kept immersed in a solution of disinfectant such as 3% lysol. Lysol, however, should not be used in cleaning the cages of rabbit because its smell distresses the animals.

4. Litter

A layer of absorbent material (e.g. soft wood saw-dusts, sugarcane piths) should be spread to a depth of 1/2 to 1 inch (1.25–2.5 cm) on the bottom of the cages.

5. Cages

Each species of animal require its own type of cage. It should be large enough for movement and some exercise of the animal.

6. Labelling

Every case should be provided with a holder or socket for a small card of 6-9 cm for record of the experiment (date, identifying marks of animal, nature of experiment and specimen).

7. Ventilation

Animal room should be air-conditioned; or at least ten changes of air in each hour are needed.

8. Humidity

Humidity of animal house ranges between 45% for rabbits to 65% for mice.

9. Marking animals

White or light coloured animals are marked by staining the fur with a strong dye (e.g. carbol fuchsin, eosin). Rabbits may be marked in ears with a needle dipped in India ink. Rats and mice are punctured in ear and fowls are marked by numbered metal tags on legs clipped through the loose skin of the wing.

10. Detection of disease in animals

A routine tour of inspection of the animals should be made at least once a day with attention to the general condition of animals, amounts of food and water consumed and the nature of faeces. To see nose movements of the animals and to see any animal remaining quiet and still. Such animals may be separated and investigated for the cause of disease.

11. Recording animals' temperature

Clinical thermometer is liberally smeared with sterile petroleum jelly and the blunt-ended rectal thermometer is introduced into the rectum or vagina to a depth of about 3 to 3.5 cm.

12. Prevention of disease

(i) **Newly arrived animals** to be kept in a special quarantine room and kept under observation for 10-14 days. Animals falling sick during the period should be kept in quarantine and necropsis must be done for finding out the cause of the illness.

(ii) **Animal infected experimentally** with bacteria or viruses should be kept in separate isolation rooms to prevent spread of infection to other animals.

13. Insect pest

Bed bugs, fleas, lice, mites, ticks, flies, mosquitoes and cockroaches may all infest the animal house. These can be controlled by 0.5% insecticidal sprays or 10% DDT.

PARTICULARS OF SOME COMMON ANIMALS

Table 18.1 shows important datas on some of the animals.

RABBIT (Fig. 18.1)

Handling :

Animals should be handled with care. The rabbit is picked up from cage with the ears by one hand in a firm grip and another hand is placed under the hind-quarters to support the weight and then lifted gently. After removing from cage, the animal is placed in a non-slippery place as it otherwise feels insecure and becomes frightened.

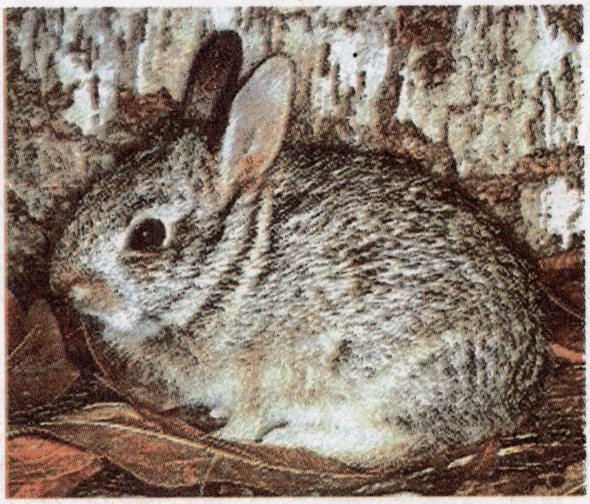

Fig. 18.1 : Rabbit

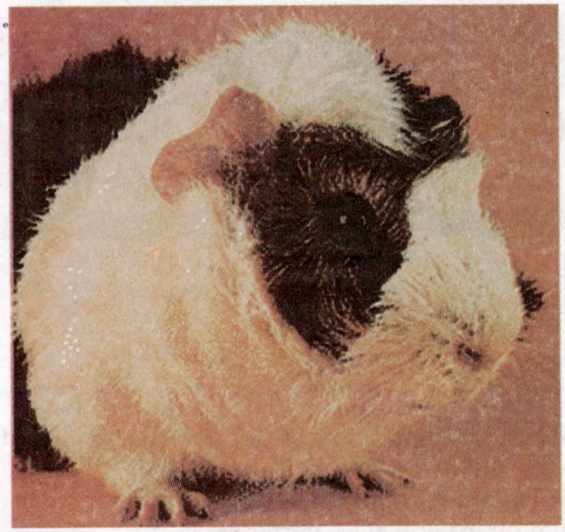

Fig. 18.2 : Guinea pig

Breeding :

When the doe (female) is on heat, vulva and vagina become red, swollen and moist. The doe is placed in the cage of buck (male).

GUINEA PIG (Fig. 18.2)

Handling :

One hand is placed across the back of the animal with the thumb behind the shoulders and the other fingers well forward on the opposite side. The animal is lifted gently supporting its weight with other hand placing the palm uppermost under the hind quarters.

ARMADILLO (Fig. 18.3)

When nine-banded armadillo is inoculated with lepra bacilli, generalised infection develops with

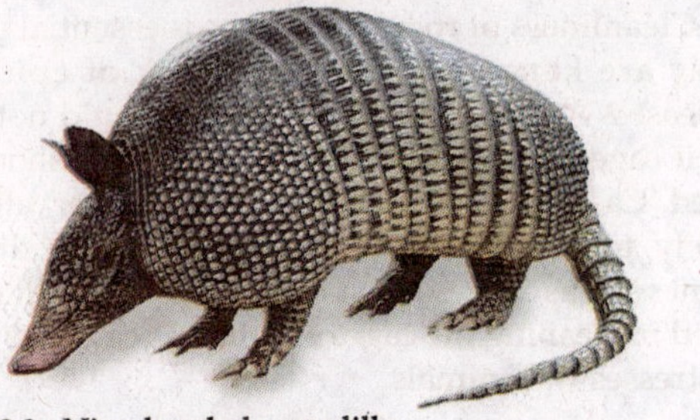

Fig. 18.3 : Nine-banded armadillo

Table 18.1 : Shows important datas of Laboratory Animals

Features	Rabbit	Guinea-pigs	Mice	Rats	Hamsters	Fowl
Rectal temperature (No temperature below 40°C is considered as pathological)	38.7° – 39°C	37.6° – 38.9°C	37.4°C	37.5°C	36.7° – 38°C	41° – 60°C
Oestrous cycle	—	—	4-5 days	4-5 days	4-5 days	—
Normal respiration rate	55	80	—	210	—	12
Pulse rate per minute	135	150	120	—	—	140
Gestation period	28-31 days	59-72 days	19-21 days	21-23 days	16-17 days	—
Weaning age	6-8 weeks	14-21 days	19-21 days	23-28 days	3-4 weeks	—
Mating age	6-9 months	12-20 weeks	6-8 weeks	70-84 days	7-9 weeks	—
Litters	4 yearly average litters – 4	3 yearly, average litters – 3	8-12 yearly, average litters 7-8	7-9 yearly average litters – 7	3-4 yearly average litters – 5	—
Room temperature	15.5°–18.5°C	18.5°–21°C	20°–21°C	18.5°–21°C	20°–22°C	—
Humidity	40 –45%	45%	50 –60%	45–55%	40–50%	—
Weight (*adult*)	0.9–6.7 kg	120 g	25–28 g	—	—	—
CAGES : Galvanised iron	2' × 2' × 1 1/2' (for one)	4' × 6' × 1' 8" (high) (for 25)	6" × 12" × 6" (deep) (for 6)*	Same as guinea pigs	17" × 7" × 9" (for one)	24" tall and 20" × 20"
Diet (*daily*)	Pellets or daily 30 g mixture of 1 part oats plus 3 parts of bran	Pellet diet	Pellet diet	Dry pellet	Pellet diet	Pellet diet
Diet supplemented by	Green vegetables plus hay Plenty	Cabbage 60g plus hay Plenty	— Plenty	— Plenty	Fresh green foods. Milk added to bran/oats Plenty	Green food Plenty

* Cages made of thick polypropyline (plastic) are now commercially available for mice which are commonly used

Key : foot = ' inch = "

extensive multiplication of the bacilli and the lesions produced resemble lepromatous leprosy. Natural infection by a mycobacterium resembling lepra bacillus has been observed in some wild caught armadillos in Texas and Mexico. The wild armadillo, therefore, should be screened for mycobacterial infection and kept in quarantine for 3 months before inoculation. **European hedgedog** bred in captivity is suitable for propagation.

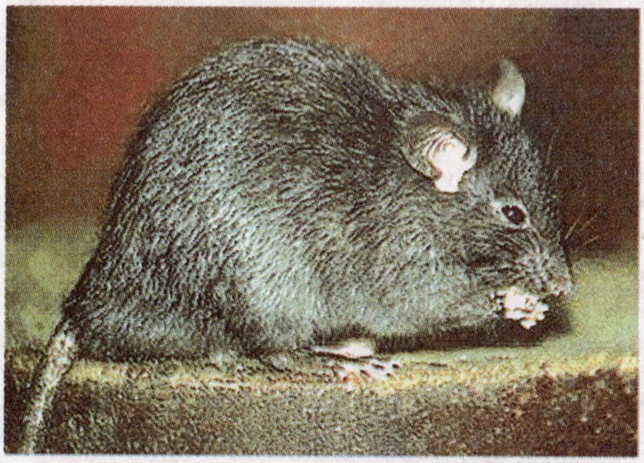

Fig. 18.4 : Rat

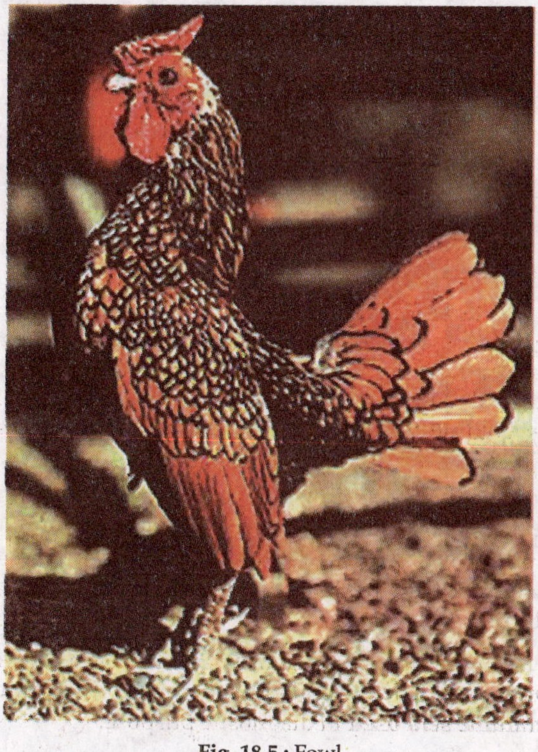

Fig. 18.5 : Fowl

MICE

Handling

Take the help of an assistant who holds the tail of the animal with the left hand and gently raises the hind limbs from floor of the cage. The mouse placed in such position cannot turn round and bite. By the help of right finger and thumb a fold of skin close to the head is held.

RAT (Fig. 18.4)

Rat is handled in the same way as guinea pig by experienced operator.

COMMON DISEASES OF LABORATORY ANIMALS

Diarrhoea due to *Salmonella typhimurium* is a common natural disease of rabbits, guinea pigs and mice. Coccidiosis (Protozoan disease) and pseudotuberculosis (caused by *Yersinia pseudotuberculosis)* are also common natural disease of animals. Explosive epizootics have been observed with *S. typhimurium* infection in which practically the whole of a colony of animals have been destroyed.

The natural diseases of the laboratory animals are given :

Rabbits : Coccidiosis (diarrhoea), pseudotuberculosis (caseous lymph nodes) and *Taenia pisiformis* (numerous cysts in omentum).

Guinea pigs : Protozoan diseases (coccidiosis toxoplasmosis), pseudotuberculosis, *S. typhimurium,* abscess in lymph node *(Streptococcus* group C), haemorrhagic septicaemia *(P. multocida)* and viral pneumonia and paralysis.

Mice : Mouse typhoid (caused by *S. typhimurium, S. enteritidis)* may be responsible for severe epizootics. Other diseases include : Ectromelia (mouse pox, caused by a pox virus related to the vaccinia virus), *Streptobacillus moniliformis,* infection, viral infections and *Taenia taeniae-formis* infection (large cysts in liver).

Hamsters : Streptococcal and staphylococcal infections, distemper (virus) and foot rot (caused by mites).

Fowls (Fig. 18.5) : Salmonellae of various types (e.g. *S. typhimurium* causing diarrhoea), *S. pullorum* (outbreak of typhoid), coccidiosis, avian leucosis (involving lymph node and bone marrow), parasitic infections due to lice and mite, virus diseases (infectious laryngotracheitis, fowl pest due to Newcastle virus).

MATERIALS INOCULATED

1. **Urine, CSF, blood and serous fluids**

These specimens are inoculated with a medium-bore needle but in case of tenacious material, like pus and sputum, is injected through a wide-bore needle.

2. **Culture materials**

Liquid cultures are inoculated through a medium-bore needle. Growths on solid media are first scraped off and suspended in broth or saline, alternatively, the diluting fluid may be poured on the culture which is then emulsified with a wire loop.

3. **Tissues**

Small fragments of tissues such as brain, spleen, liver and kidney are first homogenised by crushing these materials with a suitable diluent in a tissue grinder. When tissue is well-ground, more saline is added and allowed to stand for a short time. After the tissue has settled to the bottom of the mortar, the supernatant fluid is drawn into a syringe. When intravenous injection is to be given, care must be taken that no large particles are injected. The suspension must be centrifuged at a low speed and the supernatant fluid is used for intravenous administration.

EXPERIMENTAL PROCEDURE INOCULATION OF MATERIAL

1. **Scarification**

Procedure : At first the animal is clipped and its flank is shaved to remove the hair. Alternatively, depilating powder (mixture) may be used to remove hair. Skin is cleansed with alcohol and allowed to evaporate. Several parallel scratches are made by a sharp sterile scalpel, just enough to draw blood. The specimen is then rubbed into the scarified area with the side of the scalpel.

Use : This technique is mainly employed for the propagation of Vaccinia virus in rabbit.

2. **Subcutaneous inoculation**

Procedure : Subcutaneous inoculation is made in the loose tissue about the flank or into the abdominal wall. Hair is clipped. The skin is sterilised with iodine and alcohol and then pinched up, and the needle is inserted. Amounts up to 5 ml can be introduced. A 2 ml or 5 ml syringe is conveniently used.

Use : This method is the same for rabbit and guinea pig and obviates superficial ulceration when tuberculous specimen is injected. In fowls, subcutaneous inoculation is done in pectoral or thigh regions.

3. **Intracutaneous inoculation**

Procedure : Hair is removed from the flanks of the animal either by plucking or shaving or by depilating powder. A 1 ml all-glass tuberculin syringe, fitted with short needle No. 25 or 26 gauge is used. After pinching up the skin of the animal between the thumb and forefinger, the point of the needle is inserted at the top of the fold so that the level of the needle is towards the surface of the skin. The needle passes into the dermis only, as near as the surface. Usually, a volume of 0.2 ml is injected. When several tests are to be done, injections are to be given about one inch apart and not too near the middle line of the abdomen. No more than ten injections should be made in one animal.

Use : This method is mainly used in testing cultures of the diphtheria bacillus for toxigenicity. Usually white guinea pigs (300-400 g) are used.

4. **Intraperitoneal inoculation**

Procedure : Animal is held by assistant as above and the material is inoculated in the peritoneum in the midline in the lower half of the abdomen. Not more than 5 ml can be inoculated intraperitoneally.

Use : It is done mostly in guinea pig and sometimes mice are also intraperitoneally inoculated.

5. **Intravenous inoculation**

By this method, specimen is directly introduced into the circulation.

Procedure : Intravenous inoculation is done in rabbit, guinea pig, mouse and rat as follows :

(a) ***Rabbit*** : For this, the marginal vein of the ear is most convenient. The hair over the ear is removed by dry shaving with a sharp razor. Vein may be distended by rubbing with a piece of cotton wool or by holding the ear on an electric bulb (heat dilates blood vessels).

The rabbit is held by an assistant or placed in a special box so that only its head protrudes. The operator faces the animal and holds the ear horizontally by left hand and injects the material into the vein by a sterile syringe.

Uses : Rabbits are mainly used for diagnostic purposes. They are also used for production of immune sera used in diagnostic purpose.

(b) ***Mouse and rat*** : Intravenous injection may be

given into a vein at the root of the tail by a fine needle. The tail vein is dilated by placing in water at about 45°C. A maximum volume of 0.5 ml can thus be inoculated.

(c) ***Fowl*** : Fowl is placed on its side and feathers over an area in the elbow are plucked and a large brachial vein is seen on the bone beneath the skin. Intravenous administration of specimen or culture is made carefully with fine needle.

6. **Intracerebral inoculation**

(a) ***Rabbit*** : The animal is anaesthetised with ether, hair over the head is shaved. After disinfection of skin of head, a short incision is made by a scalpel through the scalp at a point 2 mm lateral to the sagittal suture and 1.5 mm anterior to the lambdoidal suture. The skull is perforated with a trephine or mechanical drill. A 0.45 ml of material is introduced into the occipital lobe of brain by a needle (cut down to 5/18 inch).

Rabbits may also be inoculated in frontal lobe of brain, at a point 2 mm lateral to the median plane joining the two external canthi of the eyes.

(b) ***Mouse and rat*** : The area of skull is disinfected as above. A 0.03 ml of fluid is injected directly by a one ml syringe at a site midway between the outer canthus of the eye and the point of attachment of the pinna of the ear about 3 mm from the midline. About 1/8 to 1/6 inch point of needle is introduced through skull.

7. **Intratesticular**

Rabbit : Testes lie in abdomen. The animal lies on the back and the testes are made to descend on scrotum by steady pressure on the belly. After fixing the testes by an assistant, skin is disinfected and then 0.2 to 0.4 ml of inoculum is directly introduced into the centre of a testis by a hypodermic needle.

8. **Ophthalmic**

Rabbit : Only one eye is inoculated by dropping a drop of material through a Pasteur pipette. Before installation of the material, one eye may be scarified by anaesthesia.

9. **Intranasal inoculation**

(a) ***Mouse*** : It should preferably be kept in an inoculating chamber specially designed for the purpose so that the operator is not at a risk of inhaling the infective material. Failing this, the operator should use a mask. The animal is anaesthetised with ether and as soon as its breathing has become deep, a volume of 0.1 ml is introduced into the anterior nares one side only by an automatic pipette.

(b) ***Ferrets and fowls*** : Under light ether anaesthesia, as soon as the regular respiration is established, 0.5 to 1.5 ml material is dropped from a Pasteur pipette into the nares.

Use : For studies of *Distemper* virus in ferret and NewCastle virus and other virus infections in fowls.

Inoculation of infant mice

Suckling mice of 48 hours old or less are employed for the isolation of herpes simplex, enteric and other arboviruses. The litters should be handled with great care and cleanliness to avoid biting from their mothers.

The following dose of injections can be used :

(i) 0.03 ml subcutaneously
(ii) 0.05 ml intraperitoneally
(iii) 0.03 ml intracerebrally.

Sometimes two routes — intraperitoneal and intracerebral — inoculations are done together in the same animal.

EXPERIMENTAL PROCEDURE

Collection of material

1. **Ear Vein**

About 20-30 ml blood may be collected from the ear vein of a large rabbit. The ear is shaved and sterilised with sterile gauze soaked in 70% alcohol. Before operation, heated (by Bunsen burner) petroleum jelly is kept ready in a container. When the jelly becomes cool but still fluid, the jelly is painted over the vein — both on margin and underside of the ear. The ear is held forward and the vein is made prominent by means of a small spring clip at the base of the ear. The vein is incised with a small sharp sterile scalpel. The blood is allowed to drop into a sterile flask containing glass beads.

The ear vein can be dilated by holding on an electric bulb under it or by rubbing with a piece of cotton soaked xylol.

Use : This technique is mainly used in rabbit and sometimes in guinea pig (for collection up to 0.5 ml blood).

2. **Cardiac puncture**

Larger volumes of blood can be collected by cardiac puncture :

(a) ***Guinea pig*** : After lightly anaesthetising with

ether, the animal laid on its back with its front limbs drawn forwards. An area over the fourth and fifth left intercostal spaces is plucked and the skin painted with tincture of iodine. The location of the apex beat of the heart is defined by digital palpation and thereafter, a needle (No. 20 gauge mounted on a syringe) is inserted at this point between the ribs. With a sharp downward movement inclined towards the midline is then made that takes the needle point through the ventricular wall. As much as 15 ml of blood from the heart of guinea pig may be obtained from a 350-400 g animal, though smaller amounts are advisable if the guinea pig is to survive. For the success of this operation very sharp needles are essential.

(b) **Rabbit** : The animal is anaesthetised and then fastened to a board with the body axis quite straight and the fur clipped over the left side of the chest; the area is shaved and then sterilised with alcohol and ether. A 100 ml bulb pipette (*vide* Fig. 18.6) that has been cut down at both ends to 9 in in length, one end being slightly tapered and the other end stoppered with cotton-wool. It is wrapped in kraft paper and sterilised in the hot-air oven. A wide-bore transfusion needle is fitted into a short length (1 $^1/_2$ in) of thick rubber tubing and sterilised by boiling. When the animal is anaesthetised, the rubber tubing is attached to the tapered end of the pipette and to the other end is fitted a mouthpiece such as that used in pipetting. After inserting the needle into the left side of the chest, suction applied. The needle should lie in the right ventricle of the heart, and blood rapidly flows into the pipette. Volume of 50 ml of blood per kg of body-weight can be obtained. Thereafter, the blood is transferred to a sterile 500 ml flask or bottle containing glass beads for defibrination.

(c) **Fowls** :

Method (1) : The fowl is anaesthetised and placed on its right side. The needle is inserted over the heart of the bird between the second and third ribs at a point close to the edge of the breast muscle which can be felt. At a depth of 1$^1/_2$ inch (3.75 cm) the needle enters the ventricle. This technique carries a risk of lung puncture and required experience before it can be used with confidence. *Method* (2) is perhaps easier. The bird is placed on its back, ventral side uppermost, and stretch its neck over the edge of the table. Pluck the base of the neck and the skin is cleaned with alcohol as before. A 20 ml syringe with a No. 17 or 18 gauge needle 2 in long is inserted horizontally just deep to the sternum; it should be tilted very slightly downwards and will enter the heart at a depth of 1$^1/_2$ inch (3.75 cm).

NECROPSY

Postmortem examination should be done routinely for all experimental animals, whatever may be the cause of death. When a virulent pathogen such as the bacillus of plague or of anthrax has been injected into animals, special care must be taken to avoid dissemination of infection, with danger to the operator and other workers.

The procedure in conducting a necropsy and also the method used when dealing with highly infectious organisms should be mentioned.

Since the principal application of necropsy is to recover organisms previously injected into the animal, hence, the *postmortem* examination must be conducted with strict aseptic precautions.

Materials required : A suitable animal board or table, on the top of which the carcase can be fixed in the supine position should be used.

Instruments : Instruments include three scalpels; scissors, ordinary size, four pairs; mouse-toothed forceps, four pairs; small bone forceps, if the skull is to be opened; a searing iron—a 4-oz soldering bolt is suitable for the purpose; sterile glasswares like capillary pipettes; Petri dishes, test tubes and tubes, bottles or plates of media.

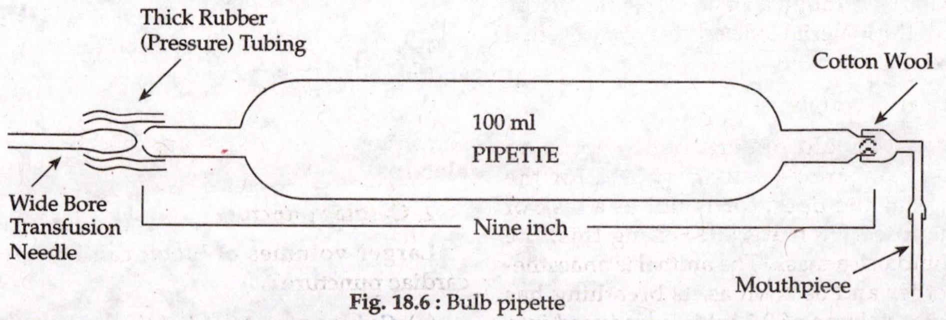

Fig. 18.6 : Bulb pipette

Knives are properly sterilised in strong lysol (about 20%) and then placed in a weaker solution (2%). Metal instruments are sterilised by boiling in a sterilising bath, e.g. an enamelled "fish-kettle". The tray of sterile instruments is lifted out of the steriliser and laid on a spread towel which has previously been soaked in 1 : 1,000 solution of mercuric chloride.

Where cultures are to be made, first to immerse the animal completely in weak lysol solution (3%) for a few moments. This technique not only destroys most of the surface organisms, but prevents the dust in the fur from getting into the air and thereby contaminating other materials. Animal is then fixed to the board and towels moistened with antiseptic solution are placed over the head and lower extremities of the animal.

Instruments are removed from the steriliser. A long median incision is now made through the skin of the abdomen and chest and then the skin is widely dissected, exposing the abdominal and chest muscles. The peritoneal cavity is opened with second set of instruments and the abdominal wall is reflected to each side. The spleen is removed with fresh instruments and placed in a sterile Petri dish. Other organs like the liver, kidneys and renals may be similarly removed. The ensiform cartilage is now tightly gripped with the help of a pair of strong forceps, and by means of a sterile pair of strong scissors a cut is made on either side of the chest through the costal cartilages. Sternum is raised and pulled towards the head. The heart is now exposed. A sterile capillary pipette, furnished with a teat, or a sterile syringe is passed through the heart wall. Blood can thus be withdrawn and inoculated into various media. When the necropsy has been properly performed, it is not necessary to scar the surface of the heart. The lungs are then removed with fresh instruments by cutting each organ free at the hilum. Care must be taken not to open into the oesophagus if the lungs are to be used for cultivation.

After the removal of the organs these are placed in separate Petri dishes.

Naked-eye appearances of the organs are studied. For culture the spleen gives the best results, but the other solid viscera may also similarly be used. The organ is cut open with sterile instruments and a small portion which is taken up with a stiff wire and smeared on the surface of solid media. The liquid media are inoculated with a small fragment of the tissue.

While conducting postmortem examinations, one should be familiar with various animal diseases, such as worm infestation, coccidiosis, pseudotuberculosis, etc. which may be noticed, and the worker should have clear idea of their appearances.

When the animal is inoculated with highly pathogenic organisms the worker should always wear rubber gloves. After soaking the carcase in antiseptic solution as before it is nailed to a rough piece of board of the appropriate size. This board is then placed in a large enamelled iron tray. Necropsy should be performed carefully in the usual way. Carcase is finally covered with 10% lysol, that flows over the board and into the tray. The entire contents of the tray-board and carcase are then destroyed in an incinerator or furnace. Rubber gloves, instruments and tray are thoroughly sterilised. The wearing of a large overall made of waterproof material is strongly recommended in all PM examination and, in addition, the use of some form of glasses or goggles to protect the eyes is to be done.

SPACE FOR NOTES

Medium for Cultivation and Preservation of Bacteria and Fungi

19

INTRODUCTION

Microorganisms need nutrients, ambient temperature, gaseous environment and proper pH for their survival and growth. Except the obligate intracellular bacteria, rest can be grown in artificial media, supplying the essential nutrients (C,H,OH_2O, minerals, vitamins, growth factors, etc.) and maintaining optimum pH. For identification of bacteria and fungi their biochemical properties (e.g. carbohydrate, protein and amino acid, lipid and fatty acids utilisation pattern as well as elaboration of different enzymes, toxin, metabolic products, and ability to grow on special nutrient source and composition, etc.) are studied, which require formulation of special types of medium. In addition, indicator, transport, preservation medium are required in the laboratory for the special purposes. A list of commonly utilised medium in the laboratory is given :

I. Simple medium

(a) Peptone water

(b) Nutrient broth

(c) Nutrient agar.

II. Enriched medium

(a) Blood agar

(b) Dorset egg

(c) Loeffler serum slope

(d) Chocolate agar

(e) Lowenstein-Jensen medium.

III. Selective medium

(a) Bile salt agar (BSA)

(b) Desoxycholate citrate agar (DCA).

IV. Selective and indication medium

(a) MacConkey's agar

(b) SS agar

(c) TCBS agar

(d) Sabouraud's dextrose agar with chloramphenicol and cycloheximide.

V. Transport medium

(a) Cary-Blair medium

(b) Stuart's transport medium

(c) Amies's modification of Stuart transport medium.

VI. Biochemical test media

(a) OF test medium

(b) Carbohydrate fermentation media

(c) Amino acid decarboxylase media

(d) Gelatin liquefaction test medium

(e) Tween 80 hydrolysis medium

(f) MR-VP test medium

(g) Urease test medium

(h) Simmon's citrate medium

(i) Potassium nitrate broth.

VII. Antibiotic sensitivity test medium

(a) Mueller-Hinton agar.

PEPTONE WATER

Composition :

Peptone	...	1 gm
Sodium chloride	...	0.5 gm
Distilled water	...	1,000 ml

Mix – heat to melt – adjust pH to 7.4 – pour in 75 mm × 12 mm test tubes in 2.5 ml quantities – plug with non-absorbent cotton — sterilise by autoclaving at 15 lb pressure for 15 minutes.

NUTRIENT BROTH

(a) Preparation of Beef Heat Infusion :

Remove all fat and membranes from finely minced 1kg of beef heart. Add to it 2 litres of distilled water and keep at 4°C for 24 hours. Next day, boil it for 30 minutes. Adjust the volume to 2 litres. Then filter through absorbent cotton, to get clear light yellow extract.

(b) Preparation of complete medium :

Composition:

Beef heat infusion	...	2000 ml
Peptone	...	20 gm i.e. 1%
NaCl	...	10 gm i.e. 0.5%

Dissolve — adjust pH to 7.6 with 4% NaOH solution — Autoclave at 15 lb pressure for 15 minutes.

Next day, dispense the clear fluid in flasks and steam for 30 minutes. Then filter through Whatman filter paper No. 1, adjust the pH to 7.6 and distribute in tubes (75 mm × 12 mm) in 2-3 ml quantities. Sterilise at 15 lb pressure for 15 minutes.

[**Note** : (1) Instead of beef heart, lean meat may be used.

(2) Commercial beef extract/lab lemco is available to replace the infusion. This is used in 1 gm% quantity].

NUTRIENT AGAR (See Fig. 19.1)

Composition : Nutrient broth ... 1,000 ml
Agar Agar ... 2.5 gm

Heat to melt. Adjust pH to 7.5. Dispense in tubes for making slants. To make plates, the material is kept in flasks. Tubes and flasks containing melted medium is plugged and autoclaved at 121°C for 15 min. Content of the flask is used to make plates and tubes and kept in slanting position to make small but a large slant-surface.

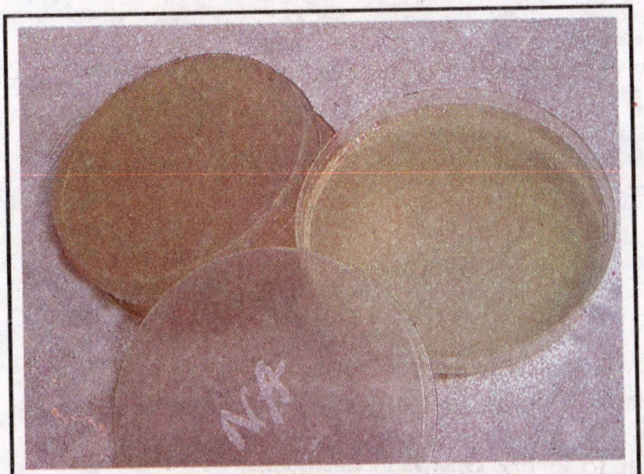

Fig. 19.1 : Nutrient Agar medium

BLOOD AGAR (Fig. 19.2)

Composition : Sterile defibrinated sheep blood ... 5 ml
Nutrient agar (Melted and temp. brought to 55°C) ... 100 ml

(i) Pour 8 ml of nutrient agar in a sterile Petri dish to form a base.

(ii) Add 5 ml sterile defibrinated sheep blood to the remaining melted nutrient agar — mix and pour over the Petri dishes containing the base medium already poured.

[**Note** : (1) Human blood is unsuitable.

(2) Alternative to sheep blood, horse blood may be used.

(3) Blood agar may be prepared without agar base.

(4) Bilayer medium, as mentioned above, is most suitable for demonstration of haemolysis.

(5) After addition of blood to base medium, control heating at 80°C in water bath will lyse the RBC to make it chocolate agar medium.]

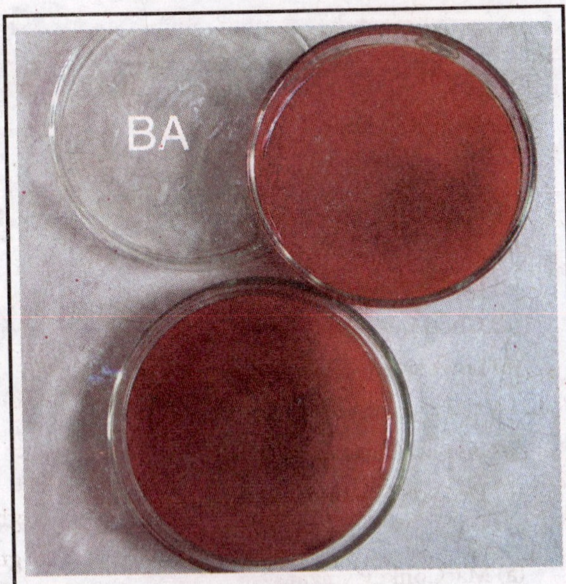

Fig. 19.2 : Blood agar medium

MACCONKEY'S AGAR

Composition :

Part I :

Sodium taurocholate or bile salt	...	5 gm or 0.5%
Peptone	...	20 gm or 2%
Sodium chloride	....	5 gm or 0.5%
Agar agar	...	25 gm or 2.5%
Distilled water	...	1,000 ml

Mix — melt by heating – adjust pH to 7.6 – sterilise by autoclaving at 15 lbs pressure for 15 minutes.

Part II :

Neutral red (indicator) solution	...	10 cc i.e. 1% v/v
Lactose	...	10 gm i.e. 1%

Add these ingredients to sterile Part I component in melted condition. Mix well, steam it at 100°C for 1/2 hour. Pour plates.

[**Note** : Preparation of neutral red solution : Required water is sterilised by autoclaving. To it 2% neutral red powder in 50% ethanol is added and incubated at 37°C for 7 days.]

BILE SALT AGAR (BSA)

Composition :

Sodium taurocholate	...	5 gm i.e. 0.5%
Peptone	...	10 gm i.e. 0.1%
Lab-Lemco	...	5 gm i.e. 0.5%
Sodium chloride	...	5 gm i.e. 0.5%
Agar agar	...	20-25 gm i.e. 2-2.5%
Distilled water	...	1,000 ml

Melt the ingredients by heating. Adjust pH at 8-8.2. Sterilise by autoclaving at 15 lb pressure for 15 minutes. Pour plates.

DEOXYCHOLATE CITRATE AGAR (DCA)

Composition :

Proteose peptone, No. 3	...	10 gm
Lactose	...	10 gm
Sodium citrate	...	20 gm
Ferric ammonium citrate	...	2 gm
Sodium deoxycholate	...	5 gm
Agar agar	...	20-25 gm
Neutral red (1% solution in 50% ethanol)	...	1 ml
Lab-lemco	...	5 gm
Distilled water	...	1,000 ml

Dissolve meat extract in 50 ml distilled water by heating. Make the reaction just alkaline to phenolphthalein by adding 4% NaOH. Boil it at 100°C and filter through Whatman filter paper No.1. Adjust pH to 7.4. Add proteose peptone, sodium citrate, ferric ammonium citrate and agar agar. Melt – recheck pH. Then add neutral red, lactose. Steam at 100°C for 1 hour. Add deoxycholate – dissolve and pour plates.

SALMONELLA-SHIGELLA AGAR (SS AGAR) (Fig. 19.3)

Usual constituents:

Beef extract	...	0.5 gm
Peptone	...	0.5 gm
Bile salt	...	0.85 gm
Lactose	...	1 gm
Sodium citrate	...	0.85 gm
Sodium thiosulphate	...	0.85 gm
Ferric citrate	...	0.1 gm
Brilliant green	...	0.33 mg
Neutral red	...	1 ml
Agar agar	...	2-2.5 gm
Distilled water	...	100 ml

The ingredients, except lactose, is dissolved by heating. pH is adjusted to 7.6. 1 ml of 1% neutral

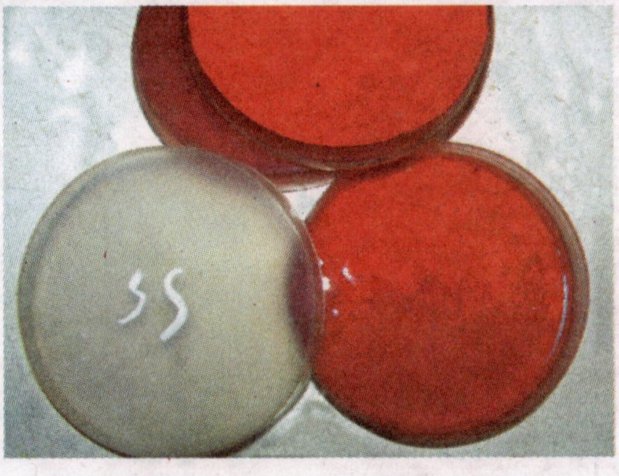

Fig. 19.3 : Salmonella-Shigella Agar (SS Agar)

red solution with lactose is added. Boil for 1 minute with frequent agitation. It is cooled to 45°C-50°C and plates are poured.

Often the medium prepared from ingredients (a complex mixture) does not work properly. It is recommended to procure commercially available dried powder of the medium. In our experience, 'Difco' brand works well.

THIOSULPHATE CITRATE BILE SUCROSE (TCBS) AGAR (Fig. 19.4)

Usual constituents :

Na citrate	...	1 gm
Yeast extract	...	0.5 gm
Peptone	...	1 gm
Sodium thiosulphate ($Na_2S_2O_35H_2O$)	...	1 gm
NaCl	...	1 gm
Ferric citrate	...	0.1 gm
Ox bile	...	0.8 gm
Sucrose	...	2 gm
Bromothymol blue	...	0.004 gm
Thymol blue	...	0.004 gm
Agar agar	...	2–2.5 gm
Distilled water	...	100 ml
pH	...	8.6

Dissolve the ingredients. Adjust pH to 8.6. Boil for 1 min. Bring down the temperature to 45°-50°C and pour plates.

The complex nature of the ingredients make the preparation of the sodium difficult. It is recommended to use the dried powder of commercially available medium. In our experience, 'Difco' brand works well.

LÖWENSTEIN-JENSEN MEDIUM

Composition : Part A – Mineral salt solution

Potassium dihydrogen phosphate (KH_2PO_4)	...	AR 0.4% or 2.6 gm
Magnesium sulphate ($MgSO_4$)	...	AR 0.04% or 0.24 gm
Magnesium citrate $Mg_3(C_6H_5O_7)_2$	...	AR 0.1% or 0.6 gm
Asparagine	...	0.6% or 3.6 gm
Glycerol	...	AR 2% or 12 ml
Distilled water	...	600 ml

Dissolve the ingredients by heating. Autoclave at 121°C for 20 minutes to sterilise. Sterilised solution may be stored in suitable amounts at 4°C.

Composition : Part B – Egg fluid

Malachite green solution	...	20 ml
Egg solution	...	1,000 ml

Clean fresh hen's eggs and disinfect the surface by keeping immersed in 70% alcoholic solution for half an hour. The eggs must be less than 4 days old and 20-22 eggs are needed to make 1 litre egg fluid. Handling aseptically, crack eggs using a sterile knife and collect the content in a sterile beaker. Beat the eggs with a sterile glass-rod.

Malachite green solution : Make 2% solution of Malachite green in distilled water. Incubate for 2 hours.

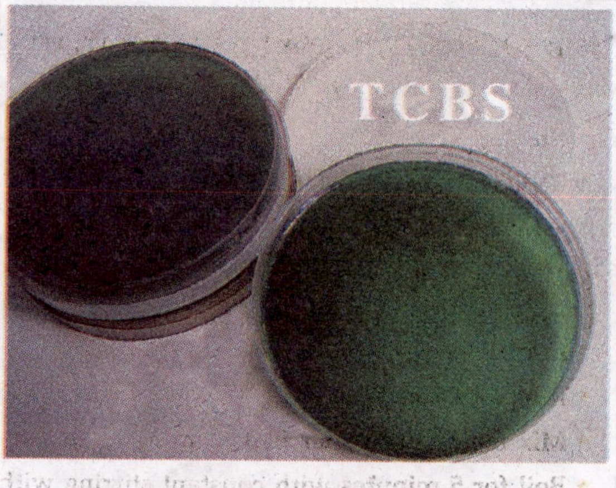

Fig. 19.4 : T.C.B.S. Agar

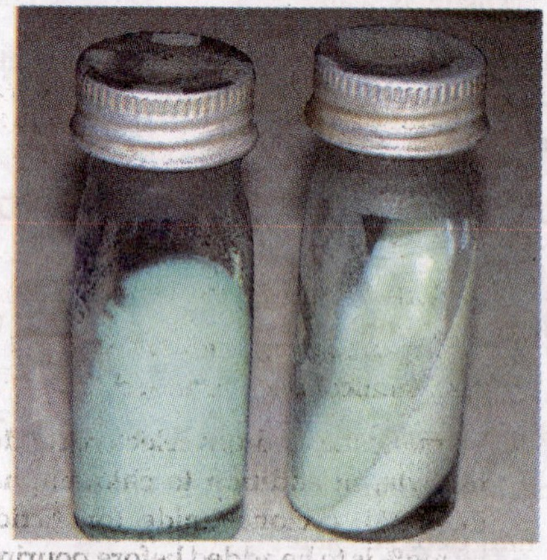

Fig. 19.5 : Löwenstein-Jensen Medium

Preparation of complete medium :

Mineral salt solution	...	600 ml
Malachite green solution	...	20 ml
Egg fluid	...	1,000 ml

Distribute in 5 ml arounds in sterile McCartney bottles, screw the cap tightly.

Sterilisation : Lay the bottles on their slides and inspissate at 80°-85°C for 50 minutes. Inspissate at 80°C for 2 hours on 1st day, 1 hour on 2nd day and 1 hour on 3rd day.

MUELLER-HINTON AGAR

Composition :

Beef extract/Lab-Lemco	...	20 gm
Casein hydrolylate	...	17.5 gm
Starch (soluble)	...	1.5 gm
Agar agar	...	2 gm
Distilled water	...	1,000 ml
pH	...	7.4 ± 0.2

Ingredients are dissolved by heating. pH is adjusted, followed by autoclavity at 121°C for 20 minutes. Pour plates of 4 mm thick.

SABOURAUD DEXTROSE AGAR

Composition :

Dextrose	...	4 gm
Neopeptone	...	10 gm
Agar agar	...	2 gm
Distilled water	...	1 L
pH	...	5.6

Mix and dissolve the ingredients by heating. Adjust the pH with N/10 HCl. Pour in 5-7 ml quantities in 15 × 125 mm clean glass tubes. Plug it with non-absorbent cotton. Sterilise by autoclaving at 121°C for 10 minutes. Cool the tubes in slanting position.

[**Note**: 1. Prolonged heating may char dextrose.

2. To inhibit bacterial growth 5 mg % chloramphenicol may be added.

3. To make the medium selective for dermatophyte, in addition to chloramphenicol (5 mg%), cycloheximide (or Actidione) 50 mg% is to be added before pouring and autoclaving].

LAKED BLOOD TELLURITE AGAR

Part I : Basal medium

Composition :

Lab-lemco	...	1% or 10 gm
NaCl	...	0.5% or 5 gm
Agar agar	...	2-2.5% or 20-25 gm
Peptone	...	1% or 10 gm
Distilled water	...	1 L
pH	...	7.8

Dissolve ingredients by heating. Adjust pH to 7.8. Sterilise by autoclaving at 121°C for 20 minutes.

Part II: Preparation of laked blood

Prepare sterile (by autoclaving) Sodium Citrate solution (10 gm in 10 ml DN) in screw-cap bottle. This is used to collect 250 ml of sheep blood. To this add 1.25 ml formalin and 30 ml ether. Shake gently. Colour of the solution will turn inky black. Store this laked blood in refrigerator. It keeps well for several months.

Part III: Tellurite solution

Potassium tellurite	...	0.7 gm
Sterile DW	...	20 ml

Store in tightly closed screw-capped bottle. Keep in dark.

Final medium : To each 200 ml of molten (basal medium, brought to 50°C, add 10 ml of laked blood and 2 ml Tellurite solution. Keep in water bath at 75°C to 80°C for 15 minutes. Pour plates.

ROBERTSON'S COOKED MEAT AGAR (Fig. 19.6)

Ingredients :

A. Dried minced meat.

B. Beef infusion broth.

Preparation of meat :

- Take 500 gm of lean meat, free from fat and fascia.
- Mince in a mincer.
- Mix meat with water in 1 : 2 ratio.
- Boil for 5 minutes with constant stirring with glass rod.

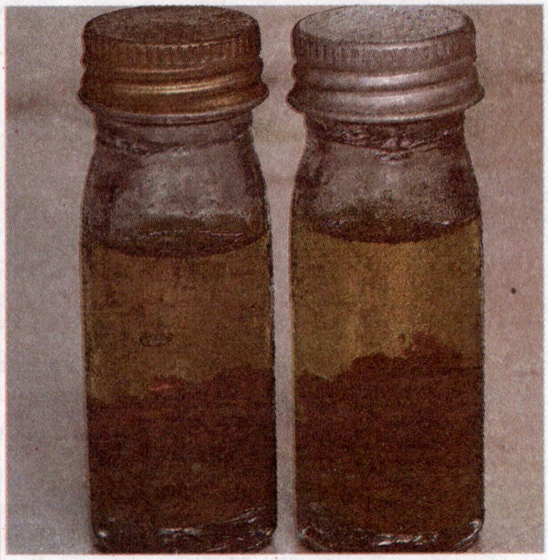

Fig. 19.6 : Robertson's cooked meat medium

- Change water twice in this manner to remove fat.
- Drain-off any excess hot water.
- Add N/20 NaOH enough to cover the chopped meat and boil for 20 minutes.
- Leave it at 4°C in refrigerator overnight.
- Decant off N/20 NaOH solution. Wash in cold tap water 2-3 times to remove traces of NaOH solution.
- Spread out the treated minced meat particles on filter paper. Place the whole thing in a hot air oven at 45°C. Make it dry.

Preparation of complete medium :

- Distribute the dry meat in screw-capped bottles (McCartney) to a height of 3 cm. Then add nutrient broth (pH 7.4-7.6) in meat filled bottles to get a height of about 1 cm above the meat surface. Caps to be replaced tightly.
- Sterilise by autoclaving at 121°C for 20 minutes.

CARY-BLAIR TRANSPORT MEDIUM

Composition :

Sodium chloride (NaCl)	...	5 gm
Disodium phosphate	...	1.1 gm
Sodium thioglycolate	...	1.5 gm
Agar agar	...	5 gm
Distilled water	...	991 ml

Prepare the medium in chemically clean glassware, rinsed with Sorensen's buffer 0.067 M buffer (pH 8.1). Heat to dissolve the ingredients. Cool to 50°C and add 9 ml of freshly prepared calcium chloride ($CaCl_2$). Adjust pH to 8.4. Dispense in 7 ml quantities into previously rinsed and sterilised 9 ml screw-capped bottles. Steam the bottles for 15 minutes. Cool and tighten the caps.

SUGAR FERMENTATION TEST MEDIUM

Composition for 100 ml medium :

(A) Base :	Distilled water	...	100 cc
	Peptone	...	1 gm
	Sodium chloride	...	0.5 gm
	pH	...	7.6
(B) Andrade indicator :			
	Acid fuchsin	...	0.5 gm
	Distilled water	...	100 cc
	(N) NaOH solution	...	17 cc

Incubate the mixture for 7 days.

(C)	Required Sugar (Glucose/Sucrose/Lactose/ Mannitol/Maltose, etc.)	...	1 gm

Method :

Dissolve the ingredients of base medium by boiling. Adjust pH at 7.6. Add IV (i.e. 1 cc) Andrade indicator and 1% (i.e. 1 gm) of the required sugar. Dissolve. Pour in 100 mm × 12 mm test tubes in 2 ml quantities. In each glucose tubes, additionally add one Durham's tube in inverted position. Sterilisation by steaming at 100°C for 3 successive days.

SIMMON'S CITRATE AGAR (Fig. 19.7)

Composition :

Sodium chloride	...	5 gm
Magnesium sulphate ($MgSO_4$)	...	0.2 gm
Ammonium dihydrogen phosphate ($NH_4H_2PO_4$)	...	1 gm
Potassium dihydrogen phosphate (K_2HPO_4)	...	1 gm
Sodium citrate, ($Na_3C_6H_5O_72H_2O$)	...	5 gm

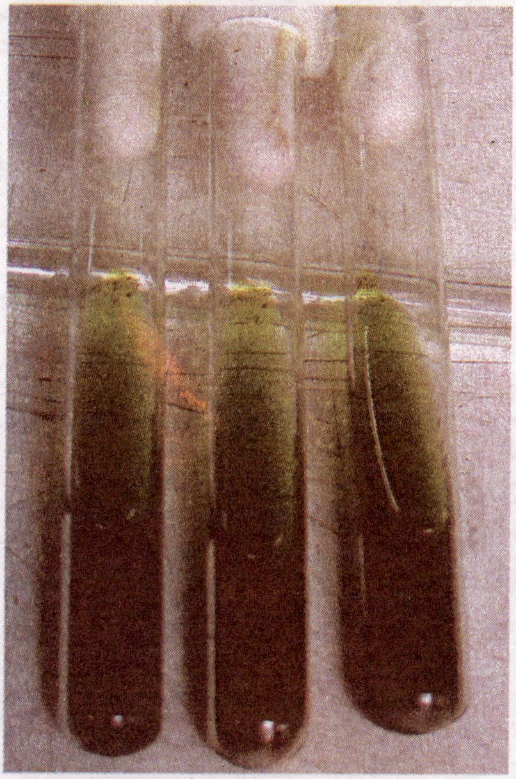

Fig. 19.7 : Simon's Citrate Agar

Agar agar	...	20 gm
Bromothymol blue (1/500 aqueous solution)	...	40 ml
Distilled water	...	1,000 ml

Mix and dissolve the ingredient (except bromothymol blue) by heating. Adjust pH to 6.9. Add bromothymol blue. Pour in 3-4 ml quantities in 100 mm × 12 mm test tubes. Autoclave. Keep the tubes in slanting position to form slopes.

CHRISTENSEN'S UREA AGAR

Composition :

Agar base:

Peptone	...	1 gm
Sodium chloride (NaCl)	...	5 gm
Disodium hydrogen phosphate (K_2HPO_4)	...	2 gm
Phenol red (Aqueous solution 1 : 500)	...	6 ml
Agar	...	20 gm
Distilled water	...	1 litre

Dissolve the ingredients. Adjust pH to 6.8. Then add phenol red.

SPACE FOR NOTES

SPACE FOR NOTES

Antimicrobial Susceptibility Test(s)

20

INTRODUCTION

One of the prime duty of clinical microbiology laboratory is to undertake antimicrobial susceptibility test(s) if an isolated bacteria is found to be pathogenic and whose antimicrobial susceptibility pattern cannot be predicted empirically. Aim of these tests is to determine the phenotypic property of resistance or sensitivity profile of the isolate to help clinician to prescribe suitable antimicrobial agent(s). In addition to this routine practice this is done for research purposes, e.g. surveillance of antimicrobial agent susceptibility of bacteria causing diarrhoeal disease (*V. cholerae*, E.T.E.C.*, diarrhoeagenic serovars of *Salmonella* etc.)

Categories of antimicrobial susceptibility

(a) **Sensitive** — Ordinary recommended dose achieve a systemic concentration which is > M.I.C.** of the antimicrobial agent tested against the isolate.

(b) **Intermediate sensitive** — Isolate is amenable to treatment with a larger dose of the antimicrobial agent, so that concentration at the site of infection is above the breakpoint value to tackle with high M.I.C. value of the isolate.

(c) **Resistance** — M.I.C. value of the isolate is so high that the required concentration is unachievable at the site of infection.

Methods:

A. Tube dilution method

B. Agar dilution method

C. Disc diffusion method :

(a) Kirby Bauer Method

(b) Stoke's Method

* E.T.E.C. = Enterotoxigenic E. coli.

** M.I.C. = Minimum inhibitory concentration.

(A) Tube dilution method :

Principle: Ability (i.e. resistance) or inability (i.e. sensitive) of the test bacterium to grow in tubes containing broth medium with serial dilution of a given antibiotic, is noted to determine M.I.C. value. If M.I.C. > breakpoint value, the test organism is considered resistant.

Method

1. Medium — A number of tubes with nutrient broth are taken. Serial dilutions of antibiotic to be tested are to be prepared in broth. The concentrations are determined according to breakpoint*** value of the antibiotic. For an initial test some tubes are adjusted above the breakpoint value and others below. One tube is kept aside as control without antibiotic.

2. Inoculum — One loopful of overnight broth culture of the isolate to be tested.

3. Incubation — 37°C for overnight period is the usual method. If 'time killing curve'‡ is desired, serial subculture is to be done at hourly or $^1/_2$ hourly interval.

4. Reading — (a) Growth in control tube validates the result. (b) Tubes where there is growth or no growth are noted. (c) The highest concentration where growth occurs and lowest concentration where no growth occurs are noted. Concentration in between these two values is the M.I.C. value of this antimicrobial agent for the isolate tested.

*** Breakpoint = Breakpoint value is the concentration of an antibiotic/antimicrobial agent achievable in blood by usual route of administration with the maximum possible dose, without producing a toxic effect.

‡ Time-killing curve = Graphic showing rate of decrease of viable bacterial number by the effect of a bactericidal antimicrobial agent.

5. Interpretation :

Resistance — MIC value > Breakpoint value

Sensitive — MIC value < Breakpoint value

Advantages :

1. An accurate method for MIC determination.

2. Mutants if grown in between tubes showing no growth could be easily recognised.

3. Compounds of high molecular weight and poorly diffusible in agar plates could be tested.

4. Whether the agent is bacteriostatic or bactericidal, could be determined by subculture from tubes showing no growth.

Disadvantages :

1. A cumbersome and laborious test method.

2. Mutants grown in tube adjacent to the tube showing growth of the bacteria under test could not be recognised. This may lead to false interpretation of MIC value.

3. Unsuitable method for clinical microbiology laboratory, where large number of organisms are to be tested.

4. Fastidious organism could not be tested.

(B) Agar dilution method

Principle : Ability (i.e. resistance) or inability (i.e. sensitive) to grow, in Müller Hinton Agar plates containing different concentrations of a given antibiotic, is noted.

Method :

1. Medium — M.H.A. plates are to be poured with different concentrations of antibiotic to be tested. Like tube dilution method, concentrations of antibiotics are adjusted at above and below the breakpoint value. One plate is incorporated without antibiotic as control.

2. Inoculum — With loop of internal diameter 1 mm, from young broth culture adjusted to 0.5 Macfarland standard, inoculums are lifted and spot inoculation is done.

3. Incubation — 37°C for overnight period.

4. Reading :

- Growth on the plate without antibiotic validates the result.
- Spots showing no growth or growth of upto 3 colonies, indicates susceptibility at that concentration.
- Spots showing growth of more than 3 colonies indicates resistance at that concentration.

5. Interpretation :

Resistance — M.I.C. value > Breakpoint value

Sensitive — M.I.C. value < Breakpoint value

Advantages :

1. A number of isolates could be tested in a single test.

2. M.I.C. value could be determined.

3. Any mutant or contaminants developed in inoculum, could be recognised immediately.

Disadvantages : (1) Only one antimicrobial agent could be tested in a single set of test.

(C) Disc diffusion method

(a) Kirby Bauer Method

Principle : Production of inhibitory zone of a recommended size as recommended in Kirby Bauer Chart in a lawn culture of an isolate around an antimicrobial agent impregnated filter paper disc indicates sensitivity.

Medium : Nature of the medium affects the result of susceptibility test. A totally defined medium which support reproducible result is yet to be formulated with satisfaction. Factors related to the media affecting the result :

- Quality of agar — affects diffusibility of antimicrobials.
- Quality of protein hydrolysate — Varies from batch to batch affecting the result.
- Final pH of the stored medium — affects the action of antimicrobial.
- Cationic (Mg^{++} and Ca^{++}) concentration — affects the result.
- Presence of thymidine and thymine at higher concentration antagonises the action of antimicrobials (sulfonamides) which are inhibitors of folate metabolism.
- Hydration, unless optimum, might influence the diffusibility of antimicrobials.

Considering the above facts, it has been recommended by CLSI, the international agency for quality control of antimicrobial susceptibility test, to use 'Mueller-Hinton Agar' in Kirby–Bauer method for non-fastidious bacteria.

Media recommended for non fastidius bacteria—

(a) *N. gonorrhoeae* — G.C. Agar (Difco) supplemented with 10% (final concentration) saponin lysed horse/sheep blood.

(b) *Fastidious anaerobes* — Wilkin–Chalgren Agar (Oxoid) supplemented with 5% (final concentration) saponin lysed horse/sheep blood.

(c) *Other fastidious bacteria* — Isosensitest agar (oxoid) supplemented with 5% saponin lysed horse /sheep blood and 10 mg/L nicotinamide adenine dinucleotide (NAD).

Inoculum : Inoculum is to be prepared from pure culture. Its concentration affects the result. A heavy inoculum may cause reduction of zone size and indistinctness of margin of the zone. Optimum inoculum should produce, evenly distributed semi-confluent colony after overnight incubtion.

Preparation of inoculum — Bacteria is picked up by a loop touching the tip of similar looking 5 colonies. A suspension is to be made in peptone water. The opacity is adjusted to Macfarland opacity tube 0.5. This will produce a concentration of 1.5×10^8/ml bacteria. Macfarland 0.5 capacity tube is prepared by mixing 0.5 ml concentrated H_2SO_4 with 99.5 ml of saturated solution of $BaCl_2$.

Choice of disc

Choice of disc depends on the following considerations :

- Identity of the organism isolated
- Prevalent resistance patterns and antibiotic prescription policy of the hospital.
- Site of infection
- Method used

Organisms isolated — Antimicrobials to which the organism is intrinsically resistant are excluded from the test, e.g. Vancomycin in gram –ive isolates. Similarly, the same consideration may be applied for the antimicrobials, specifically developed for a particular bacteria but not others, e.g. ceftazidime for use against P. aeruginosa but not against staphylococcus.

Prevalent resistance patterns — Routine testing is not warranted for an antimicrobial, against which resistance is quite prevalent across the isolates. If gram –ive rods commonly shows resistance to cephalexin, it could be omitted from test battery. On similar ground more potent agents need not be tested.

Site of infection :

- Nitrofurantoin to be applied for urinary isolated, as it is not effective elsewhere.
- Urinary isolates need high potency discs.

Method used — Cefotaxime could be tested by tube dilution only, so should be omitted in disc diffusion method.

Method

- Preparation of Muller Hinton Agar plate — 4 mm thick solidified medium in 90 mm diameter petri plates. It is properly dried before use. Medium older than 7 days, even if properly preserved should not be used. Medium should not contain too much water or be too dry.
- Inoculum size — young culture in liquid medium containing 1.5×10^8 bacteria, matching Macforland opacity tube 0.5 standard.
- Inoculation on plate — A sterile swab soaked in the inoculum is streaked evenly on all parts of agar surface. Inoculum is allowed to dry before application of disc.
- Application disc — using flammed forceps, discs are lightly pressed on to the surface of the agar plates. A 90 mm diameter plate accommodates 5 discs at periphery and one at centre. It is desirable discs should be placed 20 mm apart.
- Preincubation — Next plates are kept for $^1/_2$ hour in refrigerator at 8-10°C for prediffusion of antibiotic in medium.
- Incubation — Incubation is done at 35°–37°C for 18-24 hours in humidified air.

Interpretation — Zone of inhibition is measured using caliper or template. Noted size is compared with Kirby-Bauer interpretative chart. Result is expressed as sensitive, intermediate sensitive or resistant as the interpretative chart dictates.

Quality assurance — The result of Kirby Bauer method of disc diffusion test may be influenced by the following factors leading to variations of inhibitory zone size.

(i) Medium — Composition, hydration status, thickness of the medium influence the zone size.

(ii) Disc — Thickness and size of the disc affects its absorptive powder, consequently the concentration of antibiotic too.

(iii) Inoculum size — More the size of the inoculum, less is the size of inhibitory zone and vice versa.

(iv) Incubation period and preincubation — If preincubation time is shortened, zone size is reduced. Over incubation reduces the zone size too and development of mutant.

To overcome these factors, the following measures are undertaken in clinical microbiology laboratory :

(i) Medium — Muller Hinton medium of 4 mm thickness and preferably used within 7 days of preparation.

(ii) Disc — 6 mm diameter discs are to be used punched out from Whattmann No.1 thickness filter paper disc for preparation of antibiotic impregnation. Concentrations of disc is determined according to CLSI guideline.

(iii) Inoculum size — An young culture in liquid medium matching turbidity standard of Macfarland 0.5 (equivalent to 1.5×10^8 bacteria/ml) is to be used for preparation for a semiconfluent lawn.

(iv) Preincubation and incubation — $^1/_2$ hr. preincubation followed by overnight incubation is the guideline.

(v) Check for the newly procured or prepared medium and discs —

Using reference strains, disc and medium is checked regularly for the recommended zone range according to CLSI guideline. If the experiment fails, the medium or disc batch is to be discarded.

(vi) External quality control — in collboration with reference centre of repute.

(b) STOKE'S METHOD

Stoke's method of disc diffusion test for antimicrobial sensitivity test overcomes many of the questions raised regarding quality assurance, accuracy and reproductibility of result in Kirby Bauer's Method. In Stoke's Method, inbuilt control measures are incorporated for quality assurance. Here in the same plate both control (E. coli NCTC 10418 for rapid growing gram –ive isolates, S. aureus NCTC 6571 for gram +ive non-fastidious cocci) and test strains are inculated as shown in the Fig. 20.1.

Method

- Inoculum preparation — The same method as is described in Kirby Bauer's Method is followed both for test and control strain.
- Inoculation — Inoculation done with swab on M.H. Agar plate to get semiconfluent colony as shown in Fig. 20.1. A narrow zone of uninoculated area should be kept to keep apart the control and test bacteria.
- Placement of disc — Antibiotic inpregnated discs of recommended concentration are placed over the uninoculated line in such a way, so that disc margins just covers a short area of both inoculated zones. In 90 mm diameter plate, it is recommended that 4 discs could be placed.

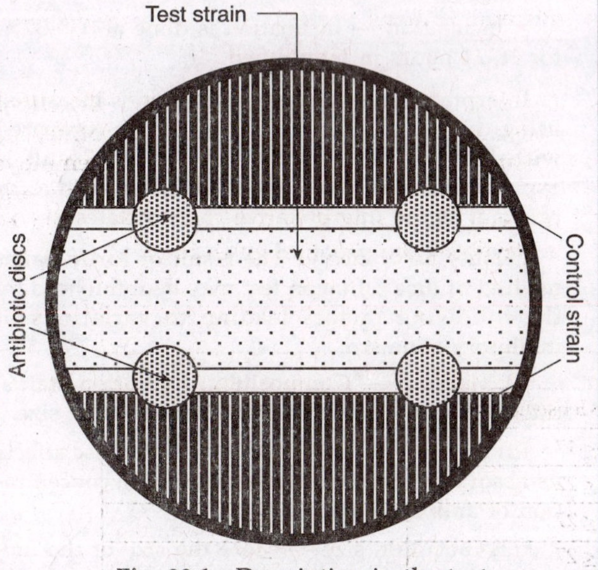

Fig. 20.1 : Description in the text

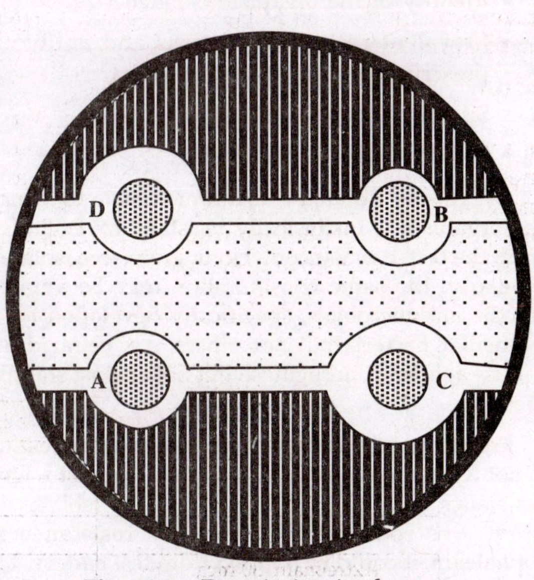

Fig. 20.2 : Description in the text

• Incubation — Preincubation at 10°C in refrigerator for $^1/_2$ hour is to be followed by incubation at 35°–37° for overnight period.

• Interpretation of result (Fig. 20.2) :

Sensitive : (1) Inhibitory zone of test is equal to that of control (A).

(2) Inhibitory zone is of test is greater than control (B).

(3) Inhibitory zone diameter of test is lesser than than control but not more than 3 mm (C).

Resistent : Inhibitory zone diameter of test is lesser than control by more than 3 mm (D).

Advantage : Both tests and control bacteria are tested on same medium, using same disc and environment. As the control bacteria is sensitive to all the discs, a comparison of inhibitory zone diameter of test yields a quality assured report.

Disadvantage : Only 4 antibiotics could be tested in a single plate. If 3 discs are applied on the line, the inhibitory zone diameter might overlap.

Some areas of difficulties in disc diffusion test :

(i) Test to detect Methicillin sensitivity — requires special medium (Columbia agar containing 5% v/v horse/sheep blood with NaCl 2%), 5 μg methicillin disc (freshly prepared) and incubation at 30°C. As methicillin is not stable for a long time, alternatively Oxacillin (2 μg) disc may be used. Recent reports shows Cefoxitin (30 μg) disc may be used as a surrogate marker on M.H. Agar media to detect methicillin resistance.

(ii) Tests to detect 'Extended Spectrum β-Lactamase (ESBL)' producing bacteria — ESBLs, found in a wide range of Gram-negative rods, are plasmid mediated enzymes capable of hydrolyzing and inactivating a wide variety of β-lactams, including 3rd generation cephalosporins, penicillins and aztreonam, but sensitive to cephamycin (cefoxitin). These enzymes are the result of mutations of TEM-1 and TEM-2 and SHV-1. Widespread use of 3rd generation cephalosporins and aztreonam is believed to be the major cause of mutation in these enzymes that has led to the emergence of ESBLs. These enzymes mediate resistance to β-lactam antibiotics containing an oxyimino-group such as oxyimino-cephalosporins (e.g. ceftazidime, ceftriaxone, cefotaxime) as well as oxyimino-monobactam (aztreonam) but have no detectable activity against cephamycins and carbapenems. Because of greatly extended substrate range, these enzymes were called extended spectrum β-lactamases. Generally, they are inhibited by β-lactamase-inhibitors such as clavulanate and tazobactam.

ESBL is very frequently detected in *K. pneumoniae, K. oxytoca* and *E. coli* and infrequently in *Enterobacter spp, Salmonella spp, Morganella morganii, Proteus mirabilis, Serratia marcescens, Pseudomonas aeruginosa, Acinetobacter spp, Burkholderia cepacia and Alcaligenes fecalis.*

Classical ESBLs have evolved from the widespread plasmid-encoded enzymes families TEM (> 130 type), SHV (> 50 type), cefotaxime (CTX-M) and oxacillin (OXA). New ones are being found every week.

Treatment failure rate is high and may exceed 90% when cephalosporins were used for serious infections caused by ESBL producing organisms, particularly when the MICs for used cephalosporins are elevated (e.g., 4 or 8 μg/ml) but are still within susceptible range.

Methods of detection

Different ESBL types express variable levels of resistance to third generation cephalosporine. So, routine clinical microbiology laboratory employs ESBL detection methods which are sensitive enough to recognize the level of resistance that would be achieved by the situation given in *vivo*.

Table 20.1

Antibiotic and disk content	Zone dimeter	
	E. coli/Klebsiella spp.	Proteus mirabilis
Cefpodoxime, 10 mcg	≤ 17	≤ 22
Ceftazidime, 30 mcg	≤ 22	≤ 22
Cefotaxime, 30 mcg	≤ 27	≤ 27
Aztreonam, 30 mcg	≤ 27	–
Ceftriaxone, 30 mcg	≤ 25	–

(A) Screening test : Initial screening, by disc diffusion test using cefpodoxime, cefotaxime, ceftriaxone, ceftazidime or aztreonam to note reduced susceptibility, if any, is done. Next, phenotypic confirmatory test is recommended. As proposed by the CLSI, M100-S-16 document suggests the use of more than one of the five indicaor cephalosporins will improve the sensitivity of detection. But, if it is necessary to rely on a single screening substance, ceftazidime or cefpodoxime is suggested as the best choice.

The breakpoint zone diameter used in this study for ESBL, producers, as per CLSI guidelines (2007) is shown below in the table 20.1.

Note that the above criteria is different from Kirby-Buer interpretative inhibition zone criteria as depicted below (see table 20.2).

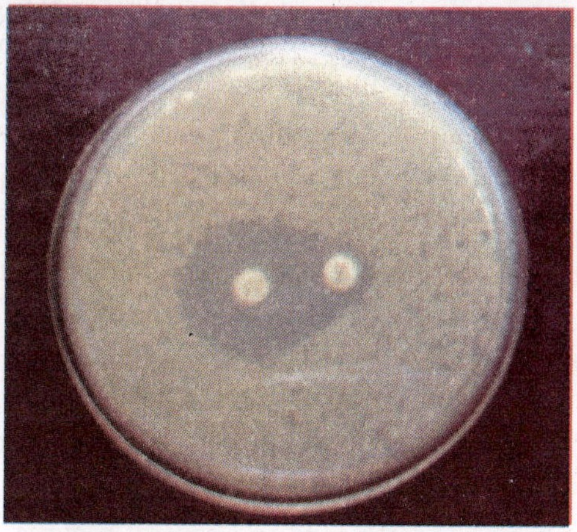

Fig. 20.3 : Positive Double disc synergy test [Amoxyclav (L) with ceftazidime (R)]

Table 20.2

Antibiotic	Disk content	Zone diameter (mm)		
		Sensitive (S)	Intermediate (I)	Resistant (R)
Cefoxitin (CN)	30 µg	≥ 18	15-17	≤ 14
Cefotaxime (Ce)	30 µg	≥ 23	15-22	≤ 14
Ceftriaxone (Ci)	30 µg	≥ 21	14-20	≤ 13
Ceftazidine (Ca)	30 µg	≥ 18	15-17	≤ 14
Cefipime (Cpm)	30 µg	≥ 18	15-17	≤ 14
Cefpodoxime (Cep)	10 µg	≥ 21	17-20	≤ 17

(B) Phenotypic test

(a) **Double Disc Synergy (DDS)**

The Jarlier double disc approximation of double disk synergy (DDS) was the first detection test described in 1980's. DDS is a disc diffusion test in which 30 mg antibiotic discs of ceftazidine, ceftriaxone, cefotaxime and aztreonam are placed on the plate, 30 mm (center to center) from the amoxicillin/clavulanate (20 µg/10 µg) disc. A clear extension of the edge of the antibiotic's inhibition zone towards the disk containing clavulanate is interpreted as synergy, indicating the presence of an ESBL (Fig. 20.3 & Fig. 20.4). The use of cefpodoxime as the expanded spectrum cephalosporin of choice has been suggested as evaluation of DDS has shown sensitivities and specificities ranged from 79% to 97% and 94% to 100% respectively in two reports. False negative results have been observed with isolates harboring SHV-2,

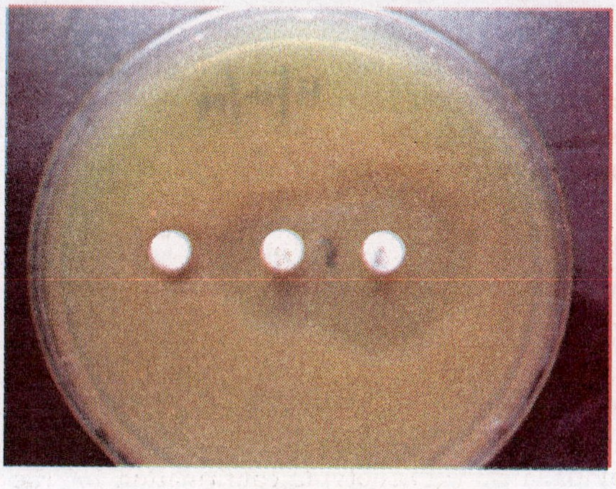

Fig. 20.4 : Positive Double disk synergy test. [Amoxyclav(M) with ceftazidime (L) and cefotaxime (R)]

SHV-3 and TEM-12. In isolates which are suspicious for harboring ESBLs but are negative using the standard distance of 30 mm between disks, the test may be repeated with closer (e.g., 20 mm) or more distant (e.g. 40 mm) disks. The test remains a reliable, convenient and inexpensive method of screening for ESBLs. However, the interpretation of the test is quite subjective. Sensitivity may be reduced when ESBL activity is very low leading to wide inhibition zones around the cephalosporin and aztreonam.

The disc on the left is cefotaxime (30 μg); the disc in the centre is coamoxyclav (20+10 μg); the disc on the right is ceftazidime (30 mg). Note the expansion of the zones around the cefotaxime and ceftazidime discs adjacent to the co-amoxyclav. The organism is *E. coli* with a TEM-24 enzyme.

Principle

It is based on the resistance that ESBLs confer to oxyimino-beta-lactams (cefotaxime, ceftriaxone and ceftazidime) and the ability of a beta lactam inhibitor, usually clavulanic acid, to block this resistance.

Materials required

(1) Disks of ceftazidime (30 μg); cefotaxime (30 μg); ceftriaxone (30 μg).

(2) Disk of amoxycillin/clavulanic acid (20 μg/ 10 μg).

Procedure : A 0.5 McFarland turbidity matched of test isolate was swabbed on Mueller-Hinton agar plate and 30 mg antibiotic disks of ceftazidime or ceftriaxone or cefotaxime were placed on the plate, 30 mm (center to center) from the amoxicillin/clavulanate (20 μg/10 μg) disk. The plate was incubated at 35°C for 18-24 hours.

Inference : A clear extension of the edge of ceftazidime or ceftriaxone or cefotaxime inhibition zone towards the disk containing clavulanate is interpreted as synergy, indicating the presence of an ESBL.

(b) **Combined disk method (Fig. 20.5)**

Cepha-losporin/clavulanate combination disks are used. The CLSI recommened use of cefotaxime (30 μg) or ceftazidime (30 μg) disks with or without clavulanate for phenotypic confirmation for the presence of ESBLs in *Klebsiella* and *E.coli*. The CLSI recommends that the disk test performed with semi confluent growth on Mueller-Hinton agar. A difference of ≥ 5 mm between the zone diameters of either of the cephalosporin disks and their respective cephalosporin/clavulanate disk is considered to be phenotypic confirmation of ESBL production. The use of both antibiotic disks is advisable since the use of ceftazidime alone has resulted in the inability to detect CTX-M-producing organisms.

Principle

It is an inhibitor potentiated disk diffusion method where the combination of cephalosporin and clavulanic acid shows an increase inhibitory zone diameter by ≥ 5 mm or 50% than that of cephalosporin alone.

Materials required

(a) Disk of ceftazidime, Ca (30 μg).

(b) Disk of ceftazidime + clavulanic, Cac (30 μg/ 10 μg).

Procedure : A disk of ceftazidime (30 μg) alone and a disk of ceftazidime + clavulanic acid (30 μg/ 10 μg) were used for this test. Both the disks were placed independently, 30 mm apart, on a lawn culture of 0.5 McFarland opacicity of the test isolate on Mueller Hinton Agar (MHA) plate and incubated for 18-24 hours at 35°C.

Inference : An increase of ≥ 5 mm or 50% in zone inhibition diameter around the ceftazidime/clavulanic acid in comparison to ceftazidime alone confirmed ESBL production.

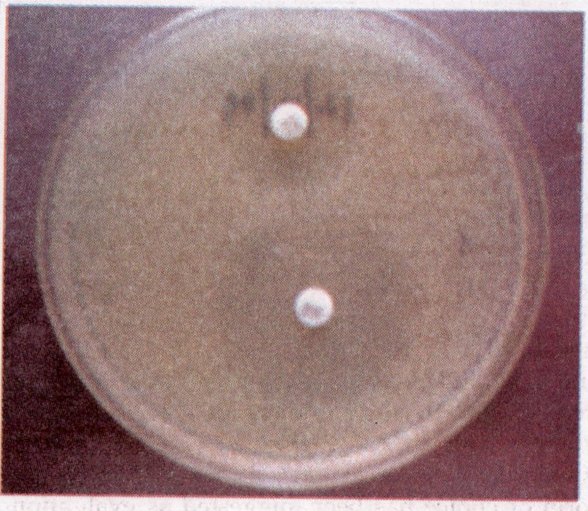

Fig. 20.5 : Positive Combined disk test [Ceftazidime (30 mcg) at above and Ceftazidime (30 mcg)/clavulanic acid (10 mcg) at lower part]

(c) **MIC reduction test**

Phenotypic confirmatory testing can also be performed by broth microdilution assays using ceftazidime (0.25 to 128 mg/ml), ceftazidime plus clavulanic acid (0.25/4, 128/4), cefotaxime (0.25 mg to 64 mg/ml) and cefotaxime plus clavulanic acid (0.25/4 to 64/4). The use of both antibiotics is recommended. The test is done using standard methods. Phenotypic confirmation is considered as > 3-two-fold-serial-dilution decrease in MIC of either cephalosporin in the presence of clavulanic acid to its MIC when used alone.

Materials required :

(a) Antimicrobial powder (ceftriaxone, ceftriaxone-tazobactam, ceftazidime and ceftazidimetazobactam).

(b) Sterile distilled water.

(c) Nutrient agar test tubes (each of 15 ml).

(d) Micro-pipettes (50 µl, 100 µl, 500 µl, 1000 µl).

Procedure :

- Stock solution preparation of ceftazidime
  - weight 54.4 mg of ceftazidime and dissolve in 2 ml of sterile D.W.
  - to achieve a concentration of 27200 µg/1000 µl.
- Working solution preparation and pouring of plates :

Tube No.	7	6	5	4	3	2	1
Stock solution	10 µl	10 µl	10 µl of 6	10 µl of 5	10 µl of 4	10 µl of 3	10 µl of 2
D.W.	Nil	10 µl	10 µl	10 µl	10 µl	10 µl	10 µl
	Add 10 µl of each dilution to 15 ml of molen 15 ml MHA brought to 55°C, and pour plates						
Final conc. (µg/ml)	128	64	32	16	8	4	2

Make 2 sets of such plates. In the second set before pouring plate add Clavulanic acid to each tube achieve a final concentration of 4 µg/ml.

Thus in 1st set conc. of Ceftazidime range from 2-128 µg/ml; in the 2nd set the conc. of ceftazidime/clavulanic acid range from 2/4 to 128/4 µg/ml.

After the plates were set, they were further dried in an incubator at 35C for 20-30 minutes. The plates were divided by a market pen on the lids for the desired number of isolates. In a 90 mm plate, a total of 25 isolates could be inoculated.

The test strains were spot inoculated with a wire loop calibrated to deliver 0.001 ml and the final inoculum on the agar surface should be approximately 10 colony forming unit per spot. A control nutrient agar plate without antibiotics was inoculated with the test strains. The test and the control plates were incubated at 35 C for 18-24 hours.

Inference : The antibiotic concentration of the plate showing ≥ 99% inhibition is taken as the MIC for the organism. Hazy growth and one or two colonies were ignored and considered as mutants. Growth of more than three colonies were taken as resistant. A minimum of ≥ 3 fold reduction in MIC of these strains when tested in combination of ceftriaxone-tazobactam or ceftazidime-tazobactam as compared to MIC for ceftriaxone or ceftazidime alone, confirmed that the strains were ESBL producer.

(d) **Etest ESBL strip (Fig. 20.6)**

The Etest ESBL strip is a two-sided strip in which clavulanate is added to one side of a dual oxyimino-beta lactam gradient looking for a reduction in the MIC of cephalosporins of more than three fold in the presence of clavulanate. The availability of cefotaxime as well as ceftazidime strips improves the

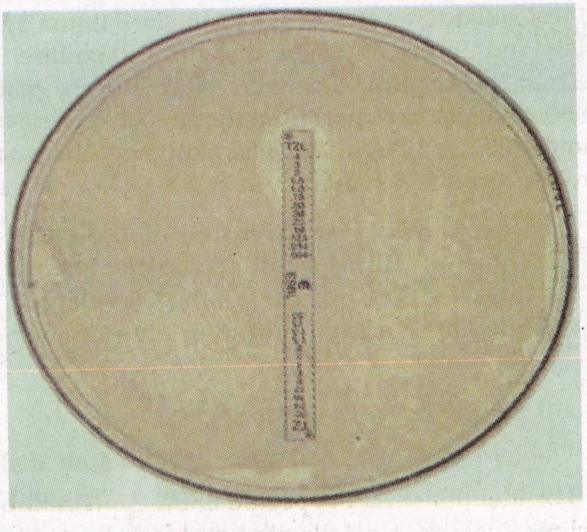

Fig. 20.6 : ESBL strips of ceftazidime TZ (0.5-32 µg/ml) and TZL ceftazidime (0.064-4 µg/ml) plus 4 µg/ml clavulanic acid are used to confirm representative isolates positive for ESBL production by disc diffusion tests.

ability to detect ESBL types which preferentially hydrolyze cefotaxime such as CTX-M-types enzymes. This method is useful for both screening and phenotypic confirmation of ESBL production. Sometime due to weak enzyme production, indeterminate results may be obtained. The reported sensitivity as a phenotypic confirmatory test for ESBL is 87 to 100% and specificity is 95 to 100%. The test is limited by its indeterminate results, difficulties in recognizing subtle zone deformities and cost.

(e) **The automated ESBL microbial susceptibility test system**

The automated antimicrobial susceptibility test systems (Vitek, MicroScan and BD phoenix) also produce ESBL test.

- The **Vitek ESBL test** utilizes cefotaxime and ceftazidime alone and in combination. A predetermined reduction in the growth of the cefotaxime or ceftazidime wells containing clavulanate, compared with the level of growth in the well with cephalosporin alone indicates a positive test. Sensitivity and specificity of the method exceed 90%. False-negative results have been observed in *Klebsiella pneumoniae* isolates producing both an ESBL and AmpC-type beta lactamase. *Klebsiella oxytoca* strains hyperproducing the K1 β-lactamase will usually be recorded as positive on the Vitek ESBL test.

- The **Micro Scan** panels which contain combinations of ceftazidime or cefotaxime plus β-lactamase inhibitors have appeared highly reliable.

- The **Phoenix ESBL test** uses growth response to cefpodoxime, ceftazidime, ceftriaxone and cefotaxime with or without clavulanate to detect the production of ESBLs. The results are usually available within six hours. The Phoenix ESBL method detects ESBL production in greater than 90% of strains genotypically confirmed to produce ESBL. The method correctly detects ESBL production by *Klebsiella, E. coli, Enterobacter, Proteus* and *Citrobacter spp.*

Molecular Methods

For identification of specific ESBL expressed by a clinical isolate, the following molecular detection methods can be applied :

(a) **Iso-electric focusing** — gives a presumptive identification since many of them possess identical isoelectric points.

(b) **Specific DNA probes** — Labour intensive. Applicable for TEM and SHV enzymes.

(c) **PCR with oligonucleotide primers oligotyping** — For PCR with oligonucleotide primers, several molecular methods that will aid in the detection and differentiation of ESBLs without sequencing have been suggested. However, PCR will not discriminate among different variants of TEM or SHV. These probes are less sensitive for the detection of mutations which are responsible for the extended substrate range. In some cases these mutations lead to the appearance or disappearance of restriction sites.

(d) **PCR followed by restriction fragment length polymorphism analysis (RFLP)** : Amplification of the relevant part of the gene by PCR followed by restriction enzyme analysis can thus indicate the presence or absence of specific TEM or SHV derived ESBLs.

(e) **PCR-single-strand conformation polymorphism (PCR-SSCP)** has also been applied to the study of ESBLs with satisfactory results. This method has been used to detect a single base mutation at specific location within the beta-lactamase gene. The combination of PCR-SSCP with PCR-restriction fragment length polymorphism (PCR-RFLP) allows the identification of newer SHV variants.

(f) **Ligase chain reaction** : The ligase chain reaction (LCR) is used for the identification of SHV genes. LCR allows the discrimination of DNA sequences that differ by a single base pair.

These techniques are available only in research centres and are beyond the scope of routine clinical microbiology laboratories.

Regarding the reporting of ESBL producing isolates, the microbiology laboratory report should state that the strain produced ESBL and should be considered resistant to all penicillins, cephalosporins and aztreonam.

(iii) Tests to detect 'AmpC-β-lactamase' producing bacteria :

(a) **AmpC Disk Test (Figs. 20.7A&B)** :

AmpC class β-lactamase is a cephalosporinase, substrate range of which includes third generation of cephalosporins (as E.S.B.L) including cephamycin and poorly inhibited by clavulanic acid. AmpC-β-lactamase are encoaded by genes located both in

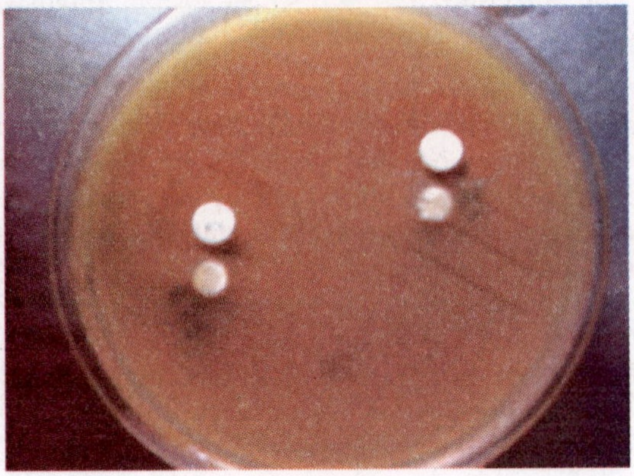

Fig. 20.7A : Positive AmpC disc test showing flattening

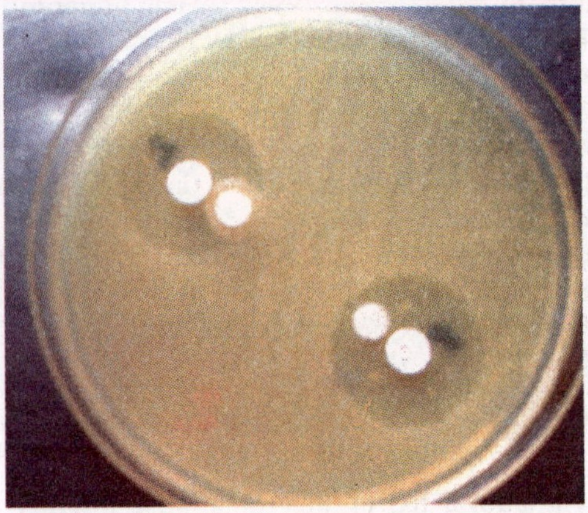

Fig. 20.7B : Negative AmpC disc test

plasmid and chromosome. It is demonstrated in *K. pneumoniae, E. coli, Salmonella spp. Proteus mirabilis, Citrobacter freundii, Enterobacter spp, Acinetobacter spp* and *Pseudomonas spp.*

Principle : A known sensitive strain shows blunting or indentation of flattening of the inhibitory zone around the Cefoxitin (30 mg) disc in response to placement of a sterile blank filter paper (6 mm in diameter, Whatman filter paper No.2) inoculated with several colonies of AmpC-β-lactamase.

Materials required :

(a) E.coli ATCC 25922

(b) Cefoxitin disk (30 μg)

(c) Peptone water

(d) Muller Hinton Agar plate

(e) Micro-pipette

(f) Sterile blank filter paper disc (6 mm in diameter, Whatman filter paper No.2)

Procedure : A lawn culture of *E. coli* ATCC 25922 was prepared on MHA plate. Sterile disks (6 mm) were moistened with sterile saline (20 μl) and inoculated with several colonies of test organism. The inoculated disc was then placed beside a cefoxitin disk (almost touching) on the inoculated plate. The plates were incubated overnight at 35°C.

Inference : A positive test appeared as a flattening or indentation of the cefoxitin inhibition zone in the vicinity of the test disc. A negative test had an undistorted zone.

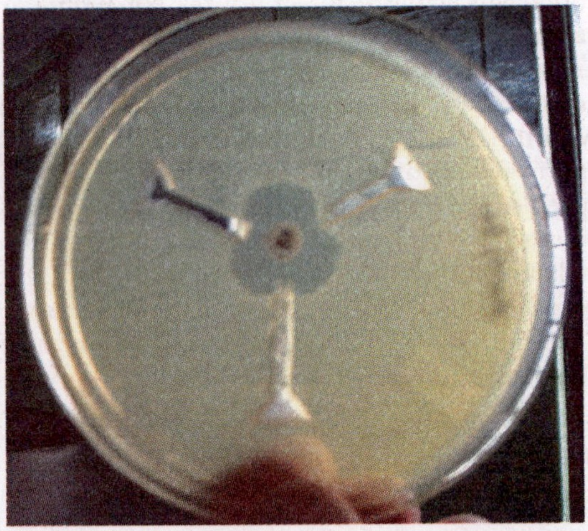

Fig. 20.8 : Positive modified three dimensional test showing distortion in two isolates

(b) **Modified three dimensional test (Fig. 20.8)**

Principle : A known sensitive strain shows blunting or indentation or flattening of the inhibitory zone around the Cefoxitin (30 mg) disc in response to addition of culture filtrate of AmpC β-lactamase producing strains.

Materials required :

(a) E. coli ATCC 25922

(b) Cefoxitin disk, (30 μg)

(c) Peptone water

(d) Mueller Hinton Agar plate

(e) Micro-pipette (50 μl)

(f) No. 15 surgical scapel blade with handle

Procedure : The suspected isolate of AmpC β-lactamase producer from MHA plate was suspended in peptone water and incubated overnight at 35°C. The growth in the peptone water was then centrifuged at 3000 rpm for 15-20 minutes and the supernatant was used as a crude enzyme extract for the test. Lawn culture of *E. coli* ATCC 25922 was prepared on MHA plates and cefoxitin (30 μg) disk were placed on the plates. Linear slits (3 cm) were cut using sterile surgical blade, 3 mm away from cefoxitin disk. At the other end of the slit a small circular well was made and the enzyme extract was loaded. A total of 30 μl of extract was loaded in the well at a 10 μl increment. The plates were kept upright for 5 to 10 minutes until the liquid dried and were incubated at 35°C for 18-24 hours.

Inference : Enhanced growth of the surface organism at the point where the slit inserted the zone of inhibition of cefoxitin was considered a positive three-dimensional test and was interpreted as evidence for the presence of AmpC β-lactamases. Three different results were recorded. Isolates showing clear distortion of the zone of inhibition were considered as AmpC producers. Isolates showing minimal distortion were taken as intermediate strains and isolates with no distortion as negative strains.

Detection of ESBL in presence of AmpC β-lactamases

For the detection of the co-existence phenotype of both ESBL and AmpC, a double disk synergy test (DDST) using a cefepime disk (30 μg) separated by a distant of 20 mm (center to center) from a amoxycillin/clavulanate disk (20 μg/10 μg) was performed.

After incubating at 35°C for 18-24 hours, an increase in zone of inhibition of cefepime towards the disk of amoxycillin-clavulanate was considered positive for ESBL production.

(iv) Tests to detect 'Metallo-β-lactamase'

Metallo-beta-lactamase pose a perplexing problem. These enzymes are capable of hydrolyzing β-lactams from all chemical classes except the monolactams and the beta-lactamases inhibitors as clavulanic acid or tazobactam are ineffective against it. The IMP-1 metalloenzyme was initially confined to Japanese isolates and was thought to be a major threat when it appeared on a transposable element in 1991. Now it is being reported all over the world including our country.

Metallo-beta-lactamases have been found in a limited number of species, such as *Bacteroides fragilis*, *Klebsiella pneumonia*, *Pseudomonas aeruginosa* and other members of gram-negative nonfermenters that frequently cause nosocomial outbreaks, and selection pressure for this enzyme is increasing.

Method (IMP-EDTA combination disk diffusion) (Figs. 209 and 20.10)

The inoculum was prepared emulsifying 5-6 colonies of the suspected isolate in Mueller Hinton broth and turbidity adjusted to 0.5 McFarland opacity standard. Two 10 μg Imipenem discs w ere

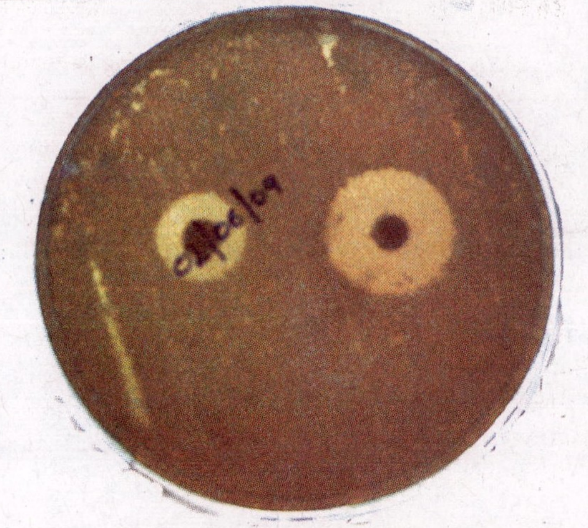

Fig. 20.9 : IMP and IMP–EDTA combination disk diffusion method

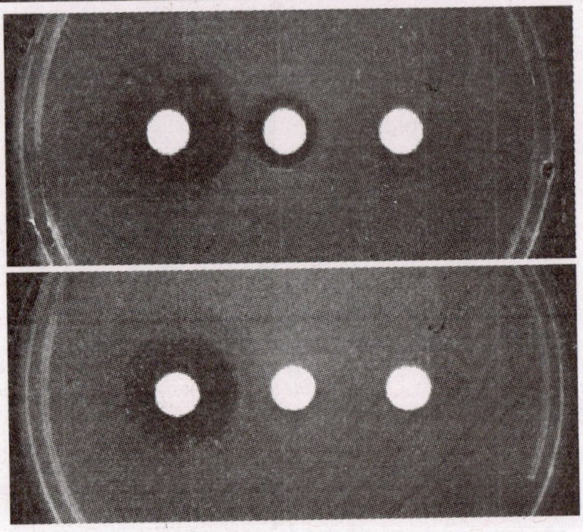

Fig. 20.10 : IMP [1], IMP–EDTA[2] and EDTA[3] combination disc diffusion method.
1 = Middle 2 = Left 3 = Right

placed on the Mueller Hinton (MH) media inoculated with test organism. To one of the Imipenem discs, 10-25 mm apart a blank filter study disc was placed to which 5 μL 0.5 M EDTA solution was added. The combinations used in DDST was I (10 μg) + EDTA (5 μL of 0.5 M. solution).

Interpretation : After 24 hours of incubation at 35°C, the zone of inhibition around Imipenem and Imipenem + EDTA discs were compared. If the zone of inhibition of Imipenem + EDTA discs compared to Imipenem alone is greater than 7 mm, then the test organism can be considered as MBL producing.

The zone of inhibition around Imipenem disc if expands towards EDTA disc, compared to the other Imipenem disc, placed on the far side, could also be interpreted as a positive result.

SPACE FOR NOTES

Appendices

APPENDIX I

Zone size Interpretative Chart
(according to CLSI-2007)
Based on Results obtained using Mueller Hinton Agar

APPENDIX II

A model set of question paper for
MBBS Examination (Microbiology)

APPENDIX III

A model set of question paper for
MD Microbiology Practical and Oral Examination

ZONE SIZE INTERPRETATIVE CHART (according to CLSI–2007)

(Based on Results obtained using Mueller Hinton Agar)

Antimicrobial Agent	Concentration	Resistant	Intermediate	Sensitive	Quality Control Limits					
		mm or less	mm	mm or more	*E. coli* ATCC 25922	*S. aureus* ATCC 25923	*Ps. aeruginosa* ATCC 27853	*H. influenzae* ATCC 49247	*S. pneumoniae* ATCC 49619	*N. gonorrhoeae* ATCC 49226
Amikacin	30 mcg	14	15-16	17	19-26	20-26	18-26	–	–	–
Amoxycillin/Clavulanic acid	20/10 mcg (30 mcg)									
Haemophilus spp.										
Staphylococci		19	–	20	–	28-36	–	15-23	–	–
Ampicillin	10 mcg									
Staphylococci		28	–	29	–	27-35	–	–	–	–
Haemophilus spp.		18	19-21	72	–	–	–	13-21	–	–
S. pneumoniae		–	–	–	–	–	–	–	30-36	–
Streptococcus other than *S. pneumoniae*		18	19-25	26	–	–	–	–	–	–
Ampicillin/Sulbactam	10/10 mcg									
Staphylococci		11	12-14	15	19-24	29-37	–	–	–	–
Haemophilus spp.		19	–	20	–	–	–	14-22	–	–
Azithromycin	15 mcg	13	14-17	13	--	21-26	--	--	19-25	--
Haemophilus spp.		--	--	12	--	--	--	13-21	--	--
Aziocillin	75 mcg	17	--	18	--	--	24-30	--	--	--
Aztreonam	30 mcg									
Ps. aeruginosa		15	16-21	22	28-36	--	23-29	--	--	--
Haemophilus spp.		--	--	26	--	--	--	30-38	--	--
Bacitracin	10 units	8	9-12	13	--	12-22	--	--	--	--
Carbenicillin	100 mcg									
Ps. aeruginosa		13	14-16	17	--	--	18-24	--	--	--
Cefaclor	30 mcg	14	15-17	18	23-27	27-31	--	--	--	--
Streptococci		--	--	--	--	--	--	--	24-32	--

ZONE SIZE INTERPRETATIVE CHART (according to CLSI–2007)
(Based on Results obtained using Mueller Hinton Agar) contd.....

Antimicrobial Agent	Concentration	Resistant	Intermediate	Sensitive	Quality Control Limits					
		mm or less	mm	mm or more	*E. coli* ATCC 25922	*S. aureus* ATCC 25923	*Ps. aeruginosa* ATCC 27853	*H. influenzae* ATCC 49247	*S. pneumoniae* ATCC 49619	*N. gonorrhoeae* ATCC 49226
Cefamandole	30 mcg	14	15-17	18	26-32	26-34	–	–	–	–
Cefazolin	30 mcg	14	15-17	18	21-27	29-35	–	–	–	–
Cefdinir	5 mcg									
Staphylococci		16	17-19	20	24-28	25-32	–	–	–	–
N. gonorrhoeae		–	–	–	–	–	–	–	–	40-49
S. pneumoniae		–	–	–	–	–	–	–	26-31	–
Cefepime	30 mcg									
Ps. aeruginosa & *Staphylococci*		14	15-17	18	31-37	23-29	24-30	–	–	–
Haemophilus spp.		–	–	26	–	–	–	25-31	–	–
N. gonorrhoeae		–	–	31	–	–	–	–	–	37-46
Streptococcus other than *S. pneumoniae*		21	22-23	24	–	–	–	–	–	–
S. pneumoniae		–	–	–	–	–	–	–	28-35	–
Cefixime	5 mcg									
Gram-negative enteric organisms,		15	16-18	19	23-27	–	–	–	–	–
Haemophilus spp.		–	–	21	–	–	–	25-33	–	–
N. gonorrhoeae		–	–	31	–	–	–	–	–	37-45
S. pneumoniae		–	–	–	–	–	–	–	16-23	–
Cefmetazole	30 mcg									
Gram-negative enteric organisms, *Staphylococci*		12	13-15	16	26-32	22-28	–	16-21	–	–
N. gonorrhoeae		27	28-32	33	–	–	–	–	–	31-36
Cefoperazone	75 mcg	15	16-20	21	28-34	24-33	23-29	–	–	–
Cefpodoxime	10 mcg									
Gram-negative enteric organisms, *Staphylococci*		17	18-20	21	23-28	19-25	–	–	–	–
Haemophilus spp.		–	–	21	–	–	–	25-31	–	–
N. gonorrhoeae		–	–	29	–	–	–	–	–	35-43
S. pneumoniae		–	–	–	–	–	–	–	28-34	–

ZONE SIZE INTERPRETATIVE CHART (according to CLSI–2007)

(Based on Results obtained using Mueller Hinton Agar) contd....

Antimicrobial Agent	Concentration	Resistant	Intermediate	Sensitive	Quality Control Limits					
		mm or less	mm	mm or more	*E. coli* ATCC 25922	*S. aureus* ATCC 25923	*Ps. aeruginosa* ATCC 27853	*H. influenzae* ATCC 49247	*S. pneumoniae* ATCC 49619	*N. gonorrhoeae* ATCC 49226
Cefprozil	30 mcg									
Gram-negative enteric organisms, *Staphylococci*		14	15-17	18	21-27	27-33	–	–	–	–
S. pneumoniae		–	–	–	–	–	–	–	25-32	–
Ceftazidime	30 mcg	14	15-17	18	25-32	16-20	22-29	–	–	–
Haemophilus spp.		–	–	26	–	–	–	27-35	–	–
N. gonorrhoeae		–	–	31	–	–	–	–	–	35-43
Ceftizoxime	30 mcg	14	15-19	20	30-36	27-35	12-17	–	28-34	–
N. gonorrhoeae		–	–	38	–	–	–	–	–	42-51
Haemophilus spp.		–	–	26	–	–	–	29-39	–	–
Ceftriaxone	30 mcg	13	14-20	21	29-35	22-28	17-23	–	–	–
Haemophilus spp.		–	–	26	–	–	–	31-39	–	–
S. pneumoniae		–	–	–	–	–	–	–	30-35	–
Streptococcus other than *S. pneumoniae*		24	25-26	27	–	–	–	–	–	–
N. gonorrhoeae		–	–	35	–	–	–	–	–	39-51
Cefuroxime Sodium (Parenteral)	30 mcg	14	15-17	18	20-26	27-35	–	–	–	–
N. gonorrhoeae		25	26-30	31	–	–	–	–	–	33-41
Haemophilus spp.		16	17-19	20	–	–	–	–	–	–
Cephalothin	30 mcg	14	15-17	18	15-21	29-37	–	–	26-32	–
Cephotaxime	30 mcg	14	15-22	23	29-35	25-31	18-22	–	–	–
Haemophilus spp.		–	–	26	–	–	–	31-39	–	–
S. pneumoniae		–	–	–	–	–	–	–	30-35	–
Streptococcus other than *S. pneumoniae*		25	26-27	28	–	–	–	–	–	–
N. gonorrhoeae		–	–	31	–	–	–	–	–	38-48

ZONE SIZE INTERPRETATIVE CHART (according to CLSI–2007)

(Based on Results obtained using Mueller Hinton Agar) contd....

Antimicrobial Agent	Concentration	Resistant	Intermediate	Sensitive	Quality Control Limits					
		mm or less	mm	mm or more	*E. coli* ATCC 25922	*S. aureus* ATCC 25923	*Ps. aeruginosa* ATCC 27853	*H. influenzae* ATCC 49247	*S. pneumoniae* ATCC 49619	*N. gonorrhoeae* ATCC 49226
Cephoxitin	30 mcg	14	15-17	18	23-29	23-29	–	–	–	–
N. gonorrhoeae		23	24-27	28	–	–	–	–	–	33-41
Chloramphenicol	30 mcg	12	13-17	18	21-27	19-26	–	–	–	–
Haemophilus spp.		25	26-28	29	–	–	–	31-40	–	–
S. pneumoniae		20	–	21	–	–	–	–	23-27	–
Streptococcus other than *S. pneumoniae*		17	18-20	21	–	–	–	–	–	–
Cinoxacin	100 mcg	14	15-18	19	26-32	–	–	–	–	–
Ciprofloxacin	5 mcg	15	16-20	21	30-40	22-30	25-33	–	–	–
Haemophilus spp.		–	–	21	–	–	–	34-42	–	–
N. gonorrhoeae		27	28-40	41	–	–	–	–	–	48-58
Clarithromycin	15 mcg									
Streptococci		16	17-20	21	–	–	–	–	25-31	–
Staphylococci		13	14-17	18	–	26-32	–	–	–	–
Haemophilus spp.		10	11-12	13	–	–	–	11-17	–	–
Clindamycin	2 mcg									
Staphylococci		14	15-20	21	–	24-30	–	–	–	–
Streptococci		15	16-18	19	–	–	–	–	19-25	–
Colistin	10 mcg	10	–	11	11-17	–	11-17	–	–	–
Co-trimoxazole (Trimethoprim/ Sulphamethoxazole)	1.25/ 23.75 mcg	10	11-15	16	23-29	24-32	–	24-32	–	–
S. pneumoniae		15	16-18	19	–	–	–	–	20-28	–
Doxycycline Hydrochloride	30 mcg	12	13-15	16	18-24	23-29	–	–	–	–
Enoxacin	10 mcg									
Gram-negative enteric organisms, *Staphylococci*		14	15-17	18	28-36	22-28	22-28	–	–	–
N. gonorrhoeae		31	32-35	36	–	–	–	–	–	43-51

ZONE SIZE INTERPRETATIVE CHART (according to CLSI–2007)

(Based on Results obtained using Mueller Hinton Agar) contd....

Antimicrobial Agent	Concentration	Resistant	Intermediate	Sensitive	Quality Control Limits					
		mm or less	mm	mm or more	*E. coli* ATCC 25922	*S. aureus* ATCC 25923	*Ps. aeruginosa* ATCC 27853	*H. influenzae* ATCC 49247	*S. pneumoniae* ATCC 49619	*N. gonorrhoeae* ATCC 49226
Erythromycin	15 mcg									
Staphylococci		13	14-22	23	–	22-30	–	–	–	–
Streptococci		15	16-20	21	–	–	–	–	25-30	–
Fosfomycin	200 mcg									
Gram-negative enteric organisms		12	13-15	16	22-30	–	–	–	–	–
Staphylococci		–	–	–	–	25-33	–	–	–	–
Gentamicin	10 mcg	12	13-14	15	19-25	19-27	16-21	–	–	–
Gatifloxacin	5 mcg	–	–	–	30-37	27-33	20-28	33-41	24-31	45-56
Gram-negative enteric organisms,		14	15-17	18						
Staphylococci		19	20-22	23						
Haemophilus spp.		–	–	18						
Streptococci		17	18-20	21						
N. gonorrhoeae		33	34-37	38						
Imipenem	10 mcg	13	14-15	16	26-32	–	20-28	–	–	–
Haemophilus spp.		–	–	16	–	–	–	21-29	–	–
Kanamycin	30 mcg	13	14-17	18	17-25	19-26	–	–	–	–
Levofloxacin	5 mcg									
Staphylococci		15	16-18	19						
Gram-negative enteric organisms and *Streptococci*		13	14-16	17	29-37	25-30	19-26	–	–	–
Haemophilus spp.		–	–	17	–	–	–	32-40	20-25	–
Linezolid	30 mcg				–	25-32	–	–	25-34	–
Staphylococci		–	–	21						
Streptococci		–	–	21						
Lomefloxacin	10 mcg	18	19-21	22	27-33	23-29	22-28	–	–	–
N. gonorrhoeae		26	27-37	38	–	–	–	–	–	45-54
Haemophilus spp.		–	–	22	–	–	–	33-41	–	–

ZONE SIZE INTERPRETATIVE CHART (according to CLSI–2007)

(Based on Results obtained using Mueller Hinton Agar) contd....

Antimicrobial Agent	Concentration	Resistant	Intermediate	Sensitive	Quality Control Limits					
		mm or less	mm	mm or more	*E. coli* ATCC 25922	*S. aureus* ATCC 25923	*Ps. aeruginosa* ATCC 27853	*H. influenzae* ATCC 49247	*S. pneumoniae* ATCC 49619	*N. gonorrhoeae* ATCC 49226
Meropenem	10 mcg									
Gram-negative enteric organisms, *Staphylococci* and *Ps. aeruginosa*		13	14-15	16	28-34	29-37	27-33	–	–	–
Haemophilus spp.		–	–	20	–	–	–	20-28	–	–
S. pneumoniae		–	–	–	–	–	–	–	28-35	–
Methicillin	5 mcg	9	10-13	14	–	17-22	–	–	–	–
Mezlocillin	75 mcg	17	18-20	21	23-29	–	19-25	–	–	–
Minocycline	30 mcg	14	15-18	19	19-25	25-30	–	–	–	–
Moxalactam	30 mcg	14	15-22	23	28-35	18-24	17-25	–	–	–
Moxifloxacin	5 mcg				28-35	28-35	17-25	31-39	25-31	–
Staphylococci		20	21-23	24						
Haemophilus spp.		–	–	18						
Streptococci		14	15-17	18						
Nafcillin	1 mcg									
Staphylococci		10	11-12	13	–	16-22	–	–	–	–
Nalidixic Acid	30 mcg	13	14-18	19	22-28	–	–	–	–	–
Neomycin	30 mcg	12	13-16	17	17-23	18-26	–	–	–	–
Netillin (Netilmicin Sulphate)	30 mcg	12	13-14	15	22-30	22-31	17-23	–	–	–
Nitrofurantoin	300 mcg	14	15-16	17	20-25	18-22	–	–	23-29	–
Norfloxacin	10 mcg	12	13-16	17	28-35	17-28	22-29	–	–	–
S. pneumoniae		–	–	–	–	–	–	–	15-21	–
Novobiocin	30 mcg	17	18-21	22	–	22-31	–	–	–	–

ZONE SIZE INTERPRETATIVE CHART (according to CLSI–2007)
(Based on Results obtained using Mueller Hinton Agar) contd....

Antimicrobial Agent	Concentration	Resistant	Intermediate	Sensitive	Quality Control Limits					
		mm or less	mm	mm or more	*E. coli* ATCC 25922	*S. aureus* ATCC 25923	*Ps. aeruginosa* ATCC 27853	*H. influenzae* ATCC 49247	*S. pneumoniae* ATCC 49619	*N. gonorrhoeae* ATCC 49226
Ofloxacin	5 mcg	12	13-15	16	29-33	24-28	17-21	–	–	–
Haemophilus spp.		–	–	16	–	–	–	31-40	–	–
Streptococci		12	13-15	16	–	–	–	–	16-21	–
N. gonorrhoeae		24	25-30	31	–	–	–	–	–	43-51
Staphylococci		14	15-17	18						
Oxacillin	1 mcg									
Staphylococci		10	11-12	13	–	18-24	–	–	–	–
coagulase negative *Staphylococci*		17	–	18	–	–	–	–	–	–
S. pneumoniae		–	–	–	–	–	–	–	≤ 12	–
Oxolinic acid	2 mcg	10	–	11	20-24	10-13	–	–	–	–
Penicillin G	10 units									
Staphylococci		28	–	29	–	26-37	–	–	–	–
S. pneumoniae		–	–	20	–	–	–	–	24-30	–
Streptococcus other than *S. pneumoniae*		19	20-27	28	–	–	–	–	–	–
N. gonorrhoeae		26	27-46	47	–	–	–	–	–	26-34
Piperacillin	100 mcg									
Ps. aeruginosa		17	–	18	–	–	25-33	–	–	–
Gram-negative enteric organisms		17	18-20	21	24-30	–	–	–	–	–
Piperacillin/Tazobactam	100/10 mcg									
Gram-negative enteric organisms		17	18-20	21	24-30	–	–	–	–	–
Staphylococci and *Ps. aeruginosa*		17	–	18	–	27-36	25-33	–	–	–
Haemophilus spp.		–	–	–	–	–	–	33-38	–	–
Polymyxin-B	300 units	11	–	12	13-19	–	14-18	–	–	–
Pristinamycin (Quinupristin/ Dalfopristin)	15 mcg	–	–	–	–		–	–	–	–
Staphylococci and *Streptococci*		15	16-18	19	–	21-28	–	–	19-24	–
Haemophilus spp.		–	–	–	–	–	–	15-21	–	–

ZONE SIZE INTERPRETATIVE CHART (according to CLSI–2007)
(Based on Results obtained using Mueller Hinton Agar) contd....

Antimicrobial Agent	Concentration	Resistant	Intermediate	Sensitive	Quality Control Limits					
		mm or less	mm	mm or more	*E. coli* ATCC 25922	*S. aureus* ATCC 25923	*Ps. aeruginosa* ATCC 27853	*H. influenzae* ATCC 49247	*S. pneumoniae* ATCC 49619	*N. gonorrhoeae* ATCC 49226
Rifampicin	5 mcg									
E. coli		–	–	–	8-10	–	–	–	–	–
Staphylococci and *Haemophilus spp.*		16	17-19	20	–	26-34	–	22-30	–	–
S. pneumoniae		16	17-18	19	–	–	–	–	25-30	–
Sparfloxacin	5 mcg	15	16-18	19	–	27-33	21-29	–	21-27	–
E. coli		–	–	–	30-38	–	–	–	–	–
N. gonorrhoeae		–	–	–	–	–	–	–	–	43-51
Haemophilus spp.		–	–	–	–	–	–	32-40	–	–
Spectinomycin	100 mcg	14	15-17	18	–	–	–	–	–	23-29
Streptomycin	10 mcg	11	12-14	15	12-20	–	–	–	–	–
Staphylococci		–	–	–	–	14-22	–	–	–	–
Sulphafurazole (Sulfisoxazole)	300 mcg	12	13-16	17	15-23	24-34	–	–	–	–
Teicoplanin	30 mcg	10	11-13	14	–	15-21	–	–	–	–
Tetracycline	30 mcg	14	15-18	19	18-25	24-30	–	–	–	–
Haemophilus spp.		25	26-28	29	–	–	–	14-22	–	–
Streptococci		18	19-22	23	–	–	–	–	27-31	–
N. gonorrhoeae		30	31-37	38	–	–	–	–	–	30-42
Ticarcillin	75 mcg									
Ps. aeruginose		14	–	15	–	–	21-27	–	–	–
Gram-negative enteric organisms		14	15-19	20	24-30	–	–	–	–	–
Ticarcillin/Clavulanic acid	75/10 mcg									
Gram-negative enteric organisms		14	15-19	20	24-30	–	–	–	–	–
Ps. aeruginosa		14	–	15	–	–	20-28	–	–	–
When testing *Staphylococci*		22	–	23	–	29-37	–	–	–	–
Tobramycin	10 mcg	12	13-14	15	18-26	19-29	19-25	–	–	–

ZONE SIZE INTERPRETATIVE CHART (according to CLSI–2007)
(Based on Results obtained using Mueller Hinton Agar) contd....

Antimicrobial Agent	Concen-tration	Resistant	Inter-mediate	Sensi-tive	Quality Control Limits					
		mm or less	mm	mm or more	*E. coli* ATCC 25922	*S. aureus* ATCC 25923	*Ps. aeru-ginosa* ATCC 27853	*H. influ-enzae* ATCC 49247	*S. pne-umoniae* ATCC 49619	*N. gono-rrhoeae* ATCC 49226
Trimethoprim	5 mcg	10	11-15	16	21-28	19-26	–	–	–	–
Vancomycin	30 mcg									
Staphylococci		–	–	15	–	17-21	–	–	–	–
Streptococci		–	–	17	–	–	–	–	20-27	–

Note : 1. For control of Gentamicin 120 mcg using *E. faecalis* ATCC 29212, standard inhibitory zone size range is 16-23 mm.

2. For control of Streptomycin 300 mcg using *E. faecalis* ATCC 29212, standard inhibitory zone size range is 14-20 mm.

APPENDIX II

A model set of question paper for MBBS Examination (Microbiology)

Use separate answer scripts for each group

Group A

1. A 15 year old boy presented with mild fever, malaise, loss of appetite and yellow discolouration of eyes. He has a recent history of injury, 2 months back, treated by injections and wound repair in a clinic. What are the possible diagnoses ?

   What is/are the aetiological agent/s? How will you establish the laboratory diagnosis?

   What prophylaxis could have been offered to prevent the condition? 1+1+5+3

Or

A man of 50 years complains of sudden onset fever with chills and rigor. The fever subsided with sweating after a few hours. On examination he revealed a mild hepatosplenomegaly. What is the clinical diagnosis? What are the possible aetiological agents? Which are the vectors transmitting the agent/s? Write, with diagram, the life cycle of the agent. Give an outline of the laboratory diagnosis of the condition. 1+1+1+4+3

Group B

2. Write short notes on (*any three*) : 3 × 4

   (a) Dengue haemorrhagic fever
   (b) Larva migrans
   (c) Eumycotic mycetoma
   (d) Extra-intestinal amoebiasis

Group C

3. Comment on (*any three*) : 3 × 4

   (a) In post-transfusion benign tertian malaria, there is no relapse.
   (b) Wood's lamp examination helps diagnosis of taenia capitis.
   (c) The trophozoites of *Plasmodium falciparum* are usually not found in peripheral blood smear.
   (d) Examination of discharging granules indicate aetiological diagnosis of mycetoma.

Group D

4. Differentiate between : 3 × 2

   (a) Definitive host and intermediate host.
   (b) Hyphae and pseudohyphae.
   (c) Antigenic shift and drift in influenza virus.

APPENDIX III

A model set of question paper for MD Microbiology Practical and Oral Examination

FIRST DAY at 10 a.m

Bacteriology

1. You are supplied with a pure growth of an organism in—(a) Nutrient Agar Slant. (b) Nutrient Broth. Please identify the organism as far as possible and do an antibiogram report.

2. (a) You are supplied with a stool sample of a patient suffering from diarrhoea.

   (b) You are supplied with a wound swab from a patient suffering from surgical wound infection/ Throat swab from a patient suffering from sore throat. Please identify the aetiologic agents as far as possible.

(1st Day) at 12 Noon

SHORT VIVA VOCE

Serology

3. (a) You are supplied with a serum from a patient suffering from PUO.

   (b) You are supplied with the serum of a patient having a primary chancre. Perform the required serological test.

   Discuss the interpretation of your results.

(1st Day) at 1.30 p.m. **SHORT VIVA VOCE**

(1st Day) at 2 p.m. **LUNCH BREAK**

(1st Day) at 2.30 p.m. **Animal Experiment and/Post-mortem**

4. (a) There is sudden death of a large number of animals in the animal room.

   Please do a post-mortem to find out the causative organism.

   Demonstrate the technique of mice handling and intraperitoneal injection with the given suspension of microorganism.

   Or

   (b) Demonstrate the technique of blood letting from the Marginal Ear Vein of rabbit. Demonstrate animal handling in case of rabbits. Discuss in details the usefulness of the above two procedures in diagnostic microbiology.

(1st Day) 3.30 p.m. to 4.30 p.m. : 1, 2 and 3 continued

SECOND DAY

(2nd Day) 10 a.m : 1, 2, 3 and 4 continued.

(2nd Day) at 11 a.m. **SHORT VIVA VOCE**

PARASITOLOGY

5. You are supplied with a stained smear from a patient suffering from fever and chills. Examine the smear carefully and identify the organism as far as possible.
6. You are supplied with stool from a patient suffering from malnutrition and diarrhoea. Examine the stool for any parasites that may be present giving labelled diagram of identifying features.
7. You are supplied with four slides. Identify the organism giving labelled diagrams in support of your diagnosis.

(2nd Day) at 1 p.m. **SHORT VIVA VOCE**

(2nd Day) at 2 p.m. **LUNCH BREAK**

(2nd Day) at 2.30 p.m. **VIROLOGY**

8. You have been provided with blister fluid from a patient suspected of having Herpes Simplex lesions. How will you proceed for isolation of the virus in embryonated egg.

(2nd Day) at 3 p.m. **SHORT VIVA VOCE**

(2nd Day) at 4 p.m. **MYCOLOGY**

9. Two cultures of fungi are provided. Please make needle mounts and identify them by reporting positive findings. (SHORT VIVA)

THIRD DAY

(3rd Day) 10 a.m : 1, 2, 3 and 4 continued and conclusion.

(3rd Day) 10.30 a.m : Short Viva Voce on overall practical work.

(3rd Day) 11.30 a.m : Viva Voce on thesis submitted by the candidates.

(3rd Day) 12 p.m **GRAND VIVA VOCE**

SPACE FOR NOTES

Index

I

J

K

L

M

R

S

T

U

V

W